D1352022

P R A C T I C A L

ANAESTHESIA

—— AND ——

ANALGESIA

—— FOR ——

DAY SURGERY

P R A C T I C A L

ANAESTHESIA
— AND —
ANALGESIA
— FOR —
DAY SURGERY

J.M. Millar
Consultant Anaesthetist
Nuffield Department of Anaesthetics
John Radcliffe Hospital, Oxford, UK

Honorary Senior Clinical Lecturer
University of Oxford, Oxford, UK

G.E. Rudkin
Senior Lecturer in Day Surgery
Department of Surgery
The Queen Elizabeth Hospital, Woodville, Australia

M. Hitchcock
Senior Registrar
Sir Humphry Davy Department of Anaesthesia
Bristol Royal Infirmary, Bristol, UK

*β*IOS
SCIENTIFIC
PUBLISHERS

BIOS Scientific Publishers Ltd
9 Newtec Place, Magdalen Road, Oxford OX4 1RE, UK
Tel. +44 (0)1865 726286. Fax +44 (0)1865 246823
World Wide Web home page: http://www.bios.co.uk

DISTRIBUTORS

Australia and New Zealand
    Blackwell Science Asia
    54 University Street
    Carlton, South Victoria 3053

India
    Viva Books Private Limited
    4325/3 Ansari Road, Daryaganj
    New Delhi 110002

Singapore and South East Asia
    APAC Publishers Services
    Block 12 Lorong Bakar Batu #05–09
    Kolam Ayer Industrial Estate
    Singapore 348745

USA and Canada
    BIOS Scientific Publishers
    PO Box 605, Herndon
    VA 20172-0605

Important Note from the Publisher
The information contained within this book was obtained by BIOS Scientific Publishers Ltd from sources believed by us to be reliable. However, while every effort has been made to ensure its accuracy, no responsibility for loss or injury whatsoever occasioned to any person acting or refraining from action as a result of information contained herein can be accepted by the authors, publishers or sponsors.

The reader should remember that medicine is a constantly evolving science and while the authors and publishers have ensured that all dosages, applications and practices are based on current indications, there may be specific practices which differ between communities. You should always follow the prescribing information provided by the manufacturers of specific products and the relevant authorities in the country in which you are practising.

Typeset by Creative Associates, Oxford, UK.
Printed by Biddles Ltd, Guildford, UK.

Contents

Contributors

Hitchcock, M. Senior Registrar, Sir Humphry Davy Department of Anaesthesia, Bristol Royal Infirmary, Bristol BS2 8HW, UK

Millar, J.M. Consultant Anaesthetist, Nuffield Department of Anaesthetics, Oxford Radcliffe Hospital Trust, John Radcliffe Hospital, Oxford OX3 9DU, UK

Morton, N.S. Consultant in Paediatric Anaesthesia and Intensive Care, Department of Anaesthesia, Royal Hospital for Sick Children, Glasgow G3 8SJ, UK

Ogg, T.W. Vice President: International Association for Ambulatory Surgery, 11 Worts Causeway, Cambridge CB1 4RJ, UK

Rudkin, G.E. Senior Lecturer in Day Surgery, Department of Surgery, The University of Adelaide, The Queen Elizabeth Hospital, Woodville Road, Woodville, SA 5011, Australia

Abbreviations

ASA	American Association of Anesthesiologists
BADS	British Association of Day Surgery
BMI	body mass index
BP	blood pressure
CCF	congestive cardiac failure
CNS	central nervous system
COAD	chronic obstructive airways disease
COSHH	Control of Substances Hazardous to Health
CT	computerized tomography
CVA	cerebrovascular accident
D&C	dilatation and curettage
DSU	day surgery unit
DVT	deep-vein thrombosis
ECG	electrocardiogram
EEG	electroencephalograph
EMLA®	eutectic mixture of local anaesthetics
ENT	ear, nose and throat
ERPC	evacuation of retained products of conception
ESWL	extracorporeal shock wave lithotripsy
FASA	Federated Ambulatory Surgery Association
FRC	functional residual capacity
GP	general practitioner
GTN	glycerol trinitrate
Hb	haemoglobin
HIV	human immunodeficiency virus
5HT	5-hydroxytryptamine
IAAS	International Association for Ambulatory Surgery
IDDM	insulin-dependent diabetes mellitus
ILMA	intubating laryngeal mask airway
IM	intramuscular(ly)
IPPV	intermittent positive pressure ventilation
IV	intravenous(ly)
IVRA	intravenous regional anaesthesia
LMA	laryngeal mask airway

LOS	lower oesophageal sphinter
LOSP	lower oesophageal sphincter pressure
MAC	monitored anaesthesia care
MI	myocardial infarct
MIS	minimally invasive surgery
MRI	magnetic resonance imaging
MW	molecular weight
NIDDM	non-insulin-dependent diabetes mellitus
NPO	*nil per os* (fasting)
NSAIDs	non-steroidal anti-inflammatory drugs
PACU	postanaesthesia care unit
PADSS	postanaesthesia discharge scoring system
PCA	patient-controlled analgesia
PCS	patient-controlled sedation
PEFR	peak expiratory flow rate
pLMA	prototype laryngeal mask airway
PO	*per os* (by mouth)
PONV	postoperative nausea and vomiting
PR	*per rectum*
prn	*pro re nata* (whenever necessary)
RSV	respiratory syncytial virus
s.c.	subcutaneous(ly)
SIDS	sudden infant death syndrome
SVR	systemic vascular resistance
TCI	target-controlled infusions
TENS	transcutaneous electric nerve stimulation
TIA	transient ischaemic attack
TIVA	total intravenous anaesthesia
TLC	total lung compliance
TOP	termination of pregnancy
V/Q	ventilation/perfusion ratio

Preface

The expansion of day surgery, and the invasiveness of the procedures now undertaken as day cases, are challenges to the anaesthetist. As 50% of elective surgery in the UK, and more in other countries, is already carried out on a day case basis, there will be few anaesthetists who do not anaesthetize day cases. Reduced numbers of in-patient beds mean that unplanned admissions after day surgery may disrupt the care of more than just that individual patient, and poor recovery after discharge may increase the work load on community health services. Good quality recovery is therefore imperative, not least for the patient.

Even experienced anaesthetists, faced with increasing amounts of day surgery, may find that their usual techniques are inappropriate. The aim of this book is to give the information needed for good day surgery anaesthetic practice – safe selection of patients, the best anaesthetic techniques and the most effective analgesia. The Day Surgery Unit is no place for amateurs or beginners, so we will not tell you how to give an anaesthetic, only how to choose the best one to ensure that patients go home safely and comfortably. We hope that anaesthetic trainees will find this useful.

We are practical day surgery anaesthetists; we have given you the evidence but we have also applied clinical common sense. We have tried to answer the questions that we get asked about day surgery anaesthesia. Although we recognize that cost is important, it is neither the only nor the most important consideration, and the true cost of a poor outcome in day surgery may be more complicated than just adding up the prices of the anaesthetic drugs used.

The role of the anaesthetist is crucial in good quality day surgery, and in its outcome for the patient and the hospital. We hope we can help you to do it better.

J.M. Millar
G.E. Rudkin
M. Hitchcock

CHAPTER 1

Introduction

T.W. Ogg

The world-wide expansion of day surgery over the past few years has been one of the success stories in health-care provision. For instance, in the UK during 1995–6 a total of 1.9 million day operations were recorded, and this figure represents a 3-fold increase over an 8-year period. There are three distinct reasons for this dramatic expansion. First, medical practice has changed and patients are now encouraged to become mobile shortly after surgery. Indeed, this action has resulted in a steady decrease in the length of in-patient stay. Secondly, there have been technological advances in both surgery and anaesthesia. Nowadays anaesthetists have access to drugs which produce rapid induction of anaesthesia and equally swift patient recovery with minimal postoperative sequelae. In addition, surgeons have developed minimally invasive surgical techniques which, with advances in laser surgery and fibre-optics, have all fuelled day surgery expansion. Thirdly, and perhaps most importantly, all countries are currently attempting to provide a first-class patient service while reducing their health-care costs.

> *A surgical day case is a patient who is admitted for investigation or operation on a planned non-resident basis and who none the less requires facilities for recovery. The whole procedure should not require an overnight stay in a hospital bed.*

The Royal College of Surgeons of England stated in 1992, 'Day surgery is now considered the best option for 50% of all patients undergoing elective surgical procedures though the proportion will vary between specialties'[1]. Many countries now share this aspiration as day surgery has been shown to provide safe, cost-effective treatment for a whole range of minor and intermediate surgical conditions. Furthermore, day surgery also offers a means whereby key objectives confronting health purchasers and providers can be tackled. For instance, the British Patients' Charter standards may be met, waiting list times for treatment can be reduced and 'value for money' health care may therefore be provided. The advantages of day surgery are listed in *Table 1.1*.

The National Heath Service Executive Task Force Report on Day Surgery (1993) indicated that all English hospitals ought to perform 50% of their non-emergency surgery on a day basis by the year 2000[2]. If other countries were to adopt such a proposal, then many surgeons, anaesthetists, nurses and managers would have to change their attitudes to day surgery.

In the present economic climate many countries are struggling to provide health-care and for many years the stimulus to increase day surgery has been a lack of financial resources, poor staffing levels and long surgical waiting lists. Throughout Europe many day surgery programmes are now being planned as managers begin to appreciate that resources for health provision are indeed limited.

Table 1.1. The advantages of day surgery

Acceptable to the majority of doctors, nurses, managers and patients
Psychological benefits, especially for children
Low incidence of postoperative morbidity
Reduced wound infection rates
Excellent nurse recruitment
High volume patient throughput
Reduced elective surgical waiting lists
Economic benefits, e.g. reduction of hotel costs and in-patient beds
Smaller hospitals required
Lends itself to audit

Much of the progress in Britain has been spearheaded by the British Association of Day Surgery (BADS), founded in 1989 with the objectives to expand day surgery, organize scientific meetings and to produce a journal applicable to this growth speciality. In 1995, 13 countries, including Australia, Belgium and Britain, combined to form an International Association for Ambulatory Surgery (IAAS).

What may the reader expect from this book?

There are several books on this subject, usually including lengthy discussion on the historical development and planning involved in the establishment of a viable day surgery unit. However, the authors of this book have decided to avoid these aspects and concentrate on a practical, common-sense approach to their subject. Their main aim is to target all anaesthetists practising day surgery, together with their trainees and medical students involved in this specialized care. In addition, since day surgery benefits from a multidisciplinary approach, all nurses, especially anaesthetic nurses, working with day surgery patients will find this book useful.

Many of the problems in day surgery (*Table 1.2*) can be influenced by the anaesthetist, both in his or her individual practice and as part of a multidisciplinary team. This book will look at how some of these problems can be reduced.

The authors of this book each have considerable experience in day surgery. Their individual chapters have been written to provide sensible advice for anaesthetists, trainees and nurses, without attempting to produce a basic anaesthetic textbook. The information is practical, concise, current and affordable.

Table 1.2. The potential problems of day surgery

High initial capital costs, e.g. equipment and facilities
Resistance from senior medical staff and managers
Patient selection must be consistently good
The ideal anaesthetic has not yet been introduced
Postoperative morbidity may limit the suitability of surgical procedures
Postdischarge problems may be significant
Community workload may increase, especially if geriatric day cases increase
Education, audit and research should be identified and funded

The future challenge?

The challenge of day surgery has brought a changing role for the modern anaesthetist. Many have become directors of day units and, in addition to their clinical duties, they have become budget holders and are encouraged to introduce programmes of quality assurance, research and education.

Previously many countries have failed to develop day surgery because of their medical staffs' preference for a more traditional approach to surgery. Other barriers have included a lack of information, inadequate facilities and poor management. However these arguments have now changed, prompting one prominent British surgeon[3] to write that 'Day Surgery is the surgery of today'. Once readers have read this book, I am sure they will agree with this statement and indeed acclaim that 'Day Surgery is the surgery of the future'.

As the next millennium approaches there can be few health-care professionals who doubt the wisdom of offering an efficient day surgery service. The rapid advances in surgery and anaesthesia have made this possible and the range of operations performed increases annually. The age of the large teaching hospital with its emphasis on in-patient teaching is past. The future is day surgery and transfer of the patients to the community. The aim of this book, written by acknowledged day case enthusiasts, is to convince readers to keep an open mind on the subject and to introduce change into their medical and nursing practices after due consideration of the expert advice offered. The end result has to be a first class service to patients.

References

1. **Commission on the Provision of Surgical Services** (1992) *Guidelines for Day Case Surgery.* Royal College of Surgeons of England, London.
2. **Report by the Day Surgery Task Force** (1993) *Day Surgery.* N.H.S. Management Executive, London.
3. **Bevan PG (NHS Management Executive, Value for Money Unit)** (1989) *The Management and Utilisation of Operating Departments.* HMSO, London. pp. 33–34.

CHAPTER 2

Selection and investigation of adult day cases

J.M. Millar

The selection of suitable patients for day surgery is the key to ensuring safe and effective treatment. Selection involves recognition and evaluation of risk and possible complications for both the surgical procedure and the individual patient so that an informed decision can be made as to suitability for day surgery. The place of investigations in day surgery is controversial and these should be looked at critically to decide whether they are necessary and cost effective. Assessment is the process by which potential patients' suitability is evaluated and investigations carried out according to clinical need.

The possible risks of poor selection for day surgery are described in *Table 2.1*. The major risks of day surgery are low. Warner and colleagues[1] found that only 33 patients out of 38 585 day cases died or had major morbidity: a risk of 0.0009% or 1:1366. Of the four patients who died, two were involved in car accidents where they were not the driver, and two suffered myocardial infarcts, all within the first week. Of the 31 cases of medically related morbidity and mortality, which included non-fatal myocardial infarct, pulmonary embolus, stroke and respiratory failure, only four occurred within 8 hours of surgery, 15 in the next 40 hours and the rest within the next 28 days. In a Canadian study[2] of nearly 7000 day cases, no deaths and few major events occurred.

Table 2.1. Aims of selection and investigation in day surgery – reduction of risk

Major risks – potential for serious harm
Life-threatening anaesthetic complications
Major surgical morbidity
Major postdischarge morbidity and mortality

Minor risks – little potential for serious harm
Cancellation on the day of surgery
Minor anaesthetic complications
Intraoperative surgical difficulty
Unanticipated overnight admission
Unacceptable levels of pain after discharge
Unpleasant postoperative morbidity

Social factors

Patients must have a responsible and physically able adult (over 16 years of age) carer both to collect them and to care for them overnight after their operation. This is mandatory and, if it cannot be arranged, the patient should be admitted overnight.

Overnight accommodation in a hospital hotel may be an option[3]. Teenage children under 16 and very elderly or disabled partners are unsuitable carers.

For humanitarian and safety reasons, the patient should normally live within 1 hour's travelling distance from the day surgery unit (DSU). Travel home by public transport is undesirable. However, the travelling time, distance and mode of transport are arbitrary. Although well-motivated patients were satisfied after day surgery when travelling time by car or train exceeded 1 hour, many felt that it had contributed to increased pain and nausea[4]. In a Norwegian study, patients were happy to travel 100–200 km by boat or ferry, provided that their treatment was good enough[5].

More difficult to assess are the patient's home circumstances. Decent sanitary arrangements, access to a telephone and few stairs to climb are essential. The patient's referring general practitioner (GP) should be able to help identify patients where this is a problem. Assessment nurses are also better at picking up these problems than doctors.

> *If the patients do not satisfy these conditions, they must be admitted overnight, no matter how fit they are or how minor the procedure. If this is explained to them in advance, they may be able to make suitable arrangements.*

Surgical procedures

Type of surgery
In general the surgery should have little risk of postoperative bleeding or other complications after discharge. The boundaries for this are not fixed – many procedures previously considered too risky to undertake are acceptable in some centres, where adenotonsillectomy[6,7], laparoscopic cholecystectomy[8,9], lumbar microdiscectomy[10] and laser transurethral prostatectomy[11] are carried out as day cases. Open abdominal, thoracic, intracranial and major vascular procedures are universally considered to be completely unsuitable.

Pain
Pain should be controllable with oral or rectal analgesics. In future more sophisticated drug delivery systems may make this criterion optional but, at present, day surgery implies that patients have no immediate medical or nursing care after discharge from the hospital, and that their pain is manageable at home.

Duration
The duration of the procedure is generally limited to less than 90–120 minutes. Procedures lasting longer than 2 hours have been associated with increased rates of complications in some studies[12,13] but not in others[14].

The invasiveness of the procedure is a more relevant factor than its duration. The surgical procedure is the main predictor of complications[12–16]. Lower abdominal surgery[13], urology[13], laparoscopy[17], dental procedures[14] and cataract extraction[15] are particularly associated with morbidity. Recovery times may be longer for more invasive operations; these should be carried out earlier in the day, and a higher rate of overnight admission can be expected.

The boundaries of what may be considered suitable day case procedures are continually being extended by improvements in anaesthesia, pain management and surgical techniques.

> *When introducing new procedures as day cases, have a trial run on patients who are treated in the same way but admitted overnight. If this goes well, start slowly with careful monitoring of the complications and patient follow-up. A higher overnight admission rate may be needed, especially initially. Curb surgical enthusiasm until you have got it right.*

Patients

Are anaesthetic complications predictable? In the Canadian study[2], intraoperative but not postoperative events were related to pre-existing respiratory problems such as asthma or chronic obstructive airways disease (COAD), hypertension and obesity, but no definition of these conditions was given. The Federated Ambulatory Surgery Association (FASA)[12] studied 87 492 day cases. Patients with symptomatic heart disease, chronic lung disease or hypertension had a significantly increased risk of complications. However, asthma, insulin-dependent diabetes (IDDM), smoking and age did not increase the risk. Stable ASA 3 (American Association of Anesthesiologists' physical classification; see *Table 2.2*) patients have not been shown to be more likely to be admitted after day case surgery[13], and an increased rate of complications in ASA 3 patients has been related to the surgical procedure[13,15]. For major and emergency surgery, the risk of complications has been shown to increase with worsening ASA status[18], but this would not seem to be true for day surgical procedures.

Table 2.2. The American Society of Anesthesiologists' physical status classification (ASA status)

ASA 1	A healthy patient
ASA 2	Mild systemic disease, no functional limitation
ASA 3	Severe systemic disease, some functional limitation
ASA 4	Severe systemic disease, incapacitating and a constant threat to life
ASA 5	Moribund patient not expected to survive for 24 hours with or without operation

> *The general statement that strict selection criteria are needed, and that only ASA 1 or 2 patients are suitable for day surgery, is unhelpful. Even ASA 1 and 2 patients may need preoperative assessment and investigation. Stable ASA 3 and even selected ASA 4 patients are increasingly being treated as day cases, but these patients need more careful assessment and must be anaesthetized and operated on by senior and experienced medical staff.*

Age
Physiological age is more important than chronological age. Once corrections have been made for the fitness of the patient and the surgical procedure, recovery or complications are not significantly increased by age alone[13–15]. The likelihood of cardiovascular, respiratory and other diseases does increase with age. Elderly patients may also have elderly carers and poor support systems at home. However, they may benefit from a return to familiar surroundings and minimal time in hospital which can be disorienting to the elderly.

The procedure and type of anaesthesia is important. Local anaesthesia is well tolerated with no or minimal sedation[19], but postoperative confusion may still occur[20]. Hypotension and hypoxaemia may contribute to this. Newer anaesthetic agents such as desflurane with rapid recovery and minimal metabolism may improve recovery in the elderly[21].

> *Arbitrary age limits for day surgery are illogical, but the older the patient, the more important the preoperative assessment of fitness and social conditions.*

Hypertension

The hazards of anaesthesia in untreated hypertensive patients are well recognized[22,23], and hypertensive patients have been shown to have more complications in day surgery[12]. Controlled hypertension in otherwise fit patients does not make the patient unsuitable for day surgery, but the level of 'controlled' blood pressure (BP) may be difficult to set[24]. It has been suggested that elective surgery should be cancelled if the diastolic arterial pressure exceeds 110 mmHg[25] or even 120 mmHg[26]. Mild hypertension should be treated but this may not influence perioperative morbidity[27].

Uncontrolled BP is the most common preventable cause of anaesthetic cancellation on the day of surgery. Usually this is because the BP has not been checked, or high BP has not been treated. A pre-admission BP is useful in deciding whether the patient has chronic hypertension or is merely nervous, and for planning appropriate treatment.

'White coat' hypertension is a recurring source of strife between anaesthetists, surgeons and GPs. Patients with white coat hypertension have been found to have similar abnormalities of left ventricular function compared with persistently hypertensive patients[28]. Also, preoperative hypertension on admission was found to be a predictor of silent preoperative[29] and intraoperative[30] myocardial ischaemia, which in turn may be risk factors for postoperative myocardial ischaemia[22,31]. A single admission BP of ≥170/100 mmHg was found to be as good a predictor of perioperative ischaemia as three or more diastolic readings of >100 mmHg[29]. However, other studies have not confirmed an increased cardiovascular risk associated with admission hypertension[32] or perioperative ischaemia[33], particularly in non-vascular surgical patients[34].

In the day surgery setting this confusing evidence needs to be interpreted according to the circumstances. An extremely anxious, but otherwise fit, middle-aged woman for removal of a potentially malignant breast lump who is found to be hypertensive on admission may not have the same risk as an obese elderly chronic smoker for hernia repair, who has attended his GP over the years with labile hypertension.

Treatment with beta-blockers provides better protection against myocardial ischaemia than diuretics alone[23]. However, treating hypertension immediately preoperatively with beta-blockers may cause intraoperative hypotension[35]. Reducing BP with sedation, a popular strategy, does not treat the underlying disease.

Hypertensive patients for general anaesthesia may require an electrocardiogram (ECG), and electrolytes may need to be checked for those on diuretics. These patients should also be instructed to take their antihypertensive drugs as usual on the day of admission, to help prevent hypertensive episodes.

> *Hypertension in day case patients should be taken seriously and treated before admission. If hypertension (diastolic BP ≥110 mmHg) on admission does not settle rapidly without treatment, patients for general anaesthesia should be treated before rebooking for surgery at a later date. Discussing the patient's management with the GP is helpful.*

Cardiac disease

Fleisher and Barash[36] reviewed the relationship of cardiovascular disease and surgery. High-risk procedures are vascular, intrathoracic or intra-abdominal surgery. Peripheral non-vascular procedures which are suitable for day surgery do not significantly increase the risk.

Patients with asymptomatic valvular disease and normal exercise tolerance are suitable for day surgery with antibiotic cover.

Risk factors associated with cardiac disease[36–38] have been summarized with reference to day surgery in *Figure 2.1*.

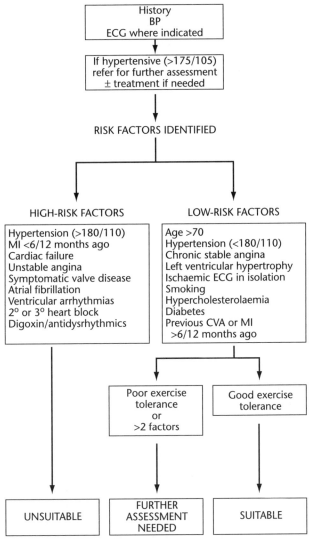

Figure 2.1. Cardiac evaluation of patients undergoing surgical procedures associated with low to moderate risk of perioperative ischaemia.
CVA, cerebrovascular accident; MI, myocardial infarct.

> *Pre-admission assessment is important to identify at-risk cardiac patients and plan their care.*

Asthma

Asthma is now one of the most common diseases encountered in day surgery, especially in younger patients. A well-controlled patient on inhalers with good exercise tolerance seldom causes problems. Those who have required steroids or hospitalization for their asthma in the past need further anaesthetic assessment. Peak expiratory flow rate (PEFR) and lung spirometry (FEV1/FVC) provide more useful information than a chest radiograph, but clinical anaesthetic assessment is even better.

Asthmatics with current upper respiratory tract infections should have their procedure postponed.

It is useful to know whether asthmatics have taken non-steroidal anti-inflammatory drugs (NSAIDs) without symptoms of bronchospasm in the past, as this suggests that they are in the 95% of asthmatics who can tolerate these drugs[39].

Chronic obstructive airways disease (COAD)

Patients with COAD without a productive cough and with normal exercise tolerance are suitable for day surgery. Patients with restricted pulmonary function will need further assessment by the anaesthetist but may be suitable for local or regional anaesthesia. Exercise tolerance is the best predictor of suitability.

Obesity

Obesity is associated with preoperative disease: hypertension, cardiac disease, diabetes, sleep apnoea and hiatus hernia. Intraoperative difficulty may be experienced with venous access, placing of local anaesthesia, intubation, airway control and hypoxaemia[40]. It also makes surgery difficult and predisposes to operative complications. It is amazing how often the easiest condition for surgeons to spot can escape their attention until they are struggling with the surgery.

In the past, obese patients were not considered suitable day cases because of delayed recovery associated with absorption of volatile anaesthetics into fat. This is less true of more modern anaesthetics: in obese patients with sleep apnoea, propofol for induction and maintenance was associated with better recovery and less postoperative hypoxaemia than thiopentone–isoflurane[41]. For body surface procedures, the use of the laryngeal mask in moderate obesity can avoid intubation in patients with difficult airways, provided there is no history of gastro-oesophageal reflux.

Obesity has been related to intraoperative complications in day surgery but only weakly to overnight admission[2,12,13]. If obese patients get through the operation uneventfully, it is illogical to keep them overnight.

How fat is too fat? The usual way to measure obesity is to use the body mass index (BMI; $kg\ m^{-2}$), and many DSUs restrict day surgery to those under BMI 30. There is no good evidence for choosing this figure; clinical experience in the DSUs in Oxford and Cambridge suggests that problems only begin to be significant at BMI >34.

However, the distribution of the fat is important. Increased waist measurement correlates well with BMI and is associated with increased cardiovascular disease[42]. Both BMI >30 and increased cardiovascular risk were related to a waist measurement of ≥102 cm in men and ≥88 cm in women and BMI ≥35 to 116 cm in men and 98 cm in women. Abdominal fat also causes difficulties with ventilation and may interfere with surgery, especially laparoscopy. Perhaps waist measurement might be a better predictor of perioperative problems than BMI – apples are worse than pears!

Preoperative preparation with H_2 antagonists and gastric prokinetic agents, such as ranitidine and metoclopramide, is useful in selected patients, especially if these can be given before admission to allow time to reach maximum effect[43].

> *Properly assessed, otherwise fit patients with BMI ≤34 are usually suitable for day surgery.*

Diabetes

Well-controlled non-insulin-dependent diabetics (NIDDM) do not cause problems in day surgery, but hypoglycaemic tablets must be omitted before surgery. Blood sugar must be within normal limits (6–10 mmol I^{-1}) without ketosis on urine testing, and the patient should be eating and drinking before discharge.

Insulin-dependent diabetics (IDDM) have not been shown to have more problems in day surgery[12] but, in practice, even with a well-controlled patient whose regime is organized before admission, the stress of surgery and the related events can upset the patient's diabetic control and make the stay in day surgery very labour intensive for the anaesthetist.

The association of diabetes with cardiovascular disease significantly increases the intraoperative risks[13]. Renal disease and autonomic dysfunction may also be present.

All diabetics should have their operations early in the day to allow time to sort out their diabetic control. Natof has described this as 'moving the sun in the sky' and has outlined his management approach[44] (*Table 2.3*).

Table 2.3. The management of IDDM patients for general anaesthesia in day surgery

Aim to return patient as soon as possible to usual diet and environment

Exclude young/brittle/ketotic diabetic patients
Consider local or regional anaesthesia ± minimal sedation
The anaesthetist <u>must</u> assess the patient before admission
Schedule as early as possible on day of surgery
Omit morning insulin and breakfast, and carry sugar in case of hypoglycaemia
Test blood sugar on arrival and at least once during recovery
IV glucose infusion if required until ready to eat
Choose a technique to minimize PONV
Resume normal regime as soon as possible after surgery, starting with the patient's usual morning insulin and breakfast even though it is later in the day (= 'moving the sun in the sky')

PONV, postoperative nausea and vomiting.

NIDDM and IDDM patients may be suitable for procedures under local anaesthesia, and preoperative fasting and alteration of their normal regime may be unnecessary.

> *Insulin-dependent diabetic patients may be suitable for day surgery, but need to be individually evaluated. They are time consuming to sort out and need planned perioperative management.*

Drug abuse and human immunodeficiency virus (HIV)-positive status

If otherwise fit, these patients may be suitable but should be carefully screened for other health risks. Of more concern are unrecognized infected patients, a problem shared with in-patient surgery. Universal precautions for all patients are essential.

Immunocompromised status

Organ transplant patients on immunosuppressant drugs and other patients with immune disorders (e.g. HIV-positive or leukaemia), who are otherwise well, are suitable for day surgery. This may be the best option for these patients to reduce the risk of hospital-acquired postoperative infection.

Drug history

Patients taking systemic steroids, monoamine oxidase inhibitors, anticoagulants, digoxin and other cardioactive drugs, such as antidysrhythmics, require individual evaluation to assess their general fitness in relation to the planned surgery and type of anaesthesia.

In the UK, recommendations are that combined oral contraceptives containing oestrogen should be stopped for 4 weeks before operations on the lower limb, especially if a tourniquet is to be used[45]. They need not be stopped for other types of day surgery. If they are not discontinued for lower-limb surgery, subcutaneous heparin prophylaxis should be considered, especially in patients with other risk factors for thromboembolism[46]. A protocol for thromboembolism prophylaxis is given in *Table 2.4*.

Hormone replacement therapy for the menopause and progesterone-only contraceptives need not be stopped before any type of surgery[47].

Which investigations are required?

Investigations are expensive and time consuming. Therefore, it is important to decide whether they are really needed. *Routine* preoperative investigations in asymptomatic patients are unnecessary. They have not been shown to affect management[48] and are often not available, or are disregarded, even if they are abnormal[49]. The majority of patients with abnormal investigations could have been predicted from the history and examination[48]. Abnormal tests were not found to influence cancellation, perioperative complications or unplanned overnight admission[48]. Ninety-six per cent of abnormal results were ignored by the anaesthetists and surgeons[49].

Wyatt *et al.*[50] compared patients having a standard battery of investigations (biochemistry, full blood count and urinalysis) with those in whom investigations were based on history and physical examination. The rate of cancellation was the same in both groups, and cancellation was more likely to be related to intercurrent illness, scheduling conflicts and other unpredictable factors.

> The avoidance of routine preoperative tests saved AU$89.60 per patient in a survey by Rudkin et al.[51] and US$397 per patient in a study by Golub et al.[49]. They may also be unnecessary as they seldom influence the patient's care.

Chest radiography

Most radiologists consider that routine chest radiography is unnecessary, even before major surgery. The Royal College of Radiologists[52] found that 26% of patients had their surgery before the report was available, and that the result of the chest radiography did not influence treatment. In asymptomatic patients with no relevant history, the chance

Table 2.4. Risk factors and venous thromboembolism prophylaxis

Risk factors – tick every box relevant to the patient

☐   Age >60
☐   Obesity (BMI >30 or >50% above ideal weight)
☐ ☐ Previous history of DVT or pulmonary embolus (2 risk factors)
☐   Pregnancy or oestrogen-containing oral contraceptives
☐   Preoperative immobility
☐   Malignancy
☐   Cardiac disease
☐   Expected procedure duration >60 min
☐   Pelvic surgery
☐   Laparoscopic surgery

☐   **Total number of risk factors**

Risk factors		Recommended prophylaxis
0–2		Early mobilization
3&4	low risk	Pneumatic calf compression **OR** Graduated compression stockings **OR** Low MW heparin s.c. 1–2 hours preoperatively & daily until mobile Early mobilization
5&6	moderate risk	Pneumatic calf compression **OR** Graduated compression stockings **AND** Low MW heparin s.c. 1–2 hours preoperatively & daily until mobile Early mobilization
>6	high risk	Graduated compression stockings **AND** Pneumatic calf compression **AND** Low MW heparin s.c. 1–2 hours preoperatively & daily until mobile Early mobilization

DVT, deep vein thrombosis; MW, molecular weight.
Reproduced with permission from R.A. Fitridge, Senior Lecturer in Vascular Surgery, University of Adelaide, Australia.

of an abnormal result which would affect the patient's management is extremely small[53,54].

> *If you think the patient needs chest radiography, he/she is almost certainly unfit for day surgery.*

ECGs
The incidence of ECG abnormalities increases with age[55]. However, even in patients over 75, the chance of finding a previously undiagnosed infarct was <0.5%. If this is found, the age of the infarct may be impossible to determine. Even abnormal rhythms, a cardiac risk factor[38], would almost certainly have been picked up on history and examination.

Johnson *et al.*[48] found that although abnormal ECGs were relatively common, the majority would have been predicted by the history, and that the findings were not relevant to the patient's management. Preoperative ECG abnormalities were not found to be predictive of adverse cardiovascular perioperative events in day surgery[56].

> *The indications for preoperative ECG are given in* Table 2.5. *Preoperative ECGs should be reviewed before the patient's admission. An automated diagnostic ECG machine may be used to highlight abnormalities needing review by the anaesthetist.*

Table 2.5. Indications for preoperative ECG[a]

Chest pain	Any history of heart disease in the past
Palpitations	Diabetes (insulin or non-insulin dependent)
Dyspnoea	Cardioactive drugs

Age over 60 and hypertension are indications for ECG in some but not all DSUs

[a]Some of these patients may already have been excluded from day surgery on the basis of history or blood pressure alone.

Full blood count or haemoglobin (Hb)
A routine Hb is only indicated where the history suggests that the patient has a risk of anaemia (e.g. menorrhagia, rectal bleeding or renal disease).

Routine preoperative testing showed that only 0.34% of patients in one study had Hb less than 11 g l^{-1} [57] and that this could have been predicted by the history[48].

> *Patients with chronic anaemia who are well hydrated and kept well oxygenated are probably safe if the Hb > 7 g l^{-1}* [58]. *This level of anaemia will result in a history of dyspnoea*[59].

Sickle test
Sickle testing is routine practice in individuals considered at risk (African, Asian and Mediterranean origin) but it has been challenged in *adults* because the chance of detecting a previously unidentified adult with sickle-cell disease is minimal, as these patients present in childhood with chronic haemolytic anaemia. The purpose of preoperative screening is therefore to identify those with sickle-cell trait. The value of this is controversial[60] and the at-risk population may be difficult to define because of ethnic mixing[61].

No sickling complications have been reported in sickle-cell trait patients for the past 15 years. It is suggested that this is due to improvements in anaesthetic drugs and monitoring techniques, and better perioperative hydration[62]. Conditions of extreme hypoxaemia, hypotension, acidosis and dehydration which precipitate sickling in patients with the trait are less likely to occur in day surgery practice.

The use of tourniquets in patients with the trait has been suggested to be safe provided that the limb is exsanguinated beforehand[63].

> *Patients with sickle-cell trait are suitable for day surgery. Preoperative sickle testing in adults is unnecessary.*

Creatinine/urea and electrolytes

These tests may be indicated in patients for general anaesthesia who are hypertensive, taking diuretics[64], or who have a history of renal disease. However, in many DSUs, patients with hypertension or taking diuretics are not routinely tested, and there are no reports of complications resulting from this.

Urinalysis

This test is cheap and simple and has been recommended as a routine preoperative investigation[65], but results may be ignored[66], and the chance of picking up a previously unsuspected disease is small. In the DSU at the Churchill Hospital (Oxford), routine urine testing in more than 30 000 patients has resulted in the cancellation of only one patient, for previously undiagnosed diabetes (J. Millar, unpublished results).

> *Do we continue to test urine because it is enshrined in nursing care?*

Which investigations should be carried out?

In general, *all* preoperative investigations should be determined by the patient's symptoms or by the procedure (e.g. Rhesus blood grouping before termination of pregnancy). It is more important to have an assessment process which detects symptoms requiring further investigation than to carry out an array of routine tests.

> *Routine investigations are not needed for asymptomatic day surgery patients.*

Why do patients fail to have their operation as planned?

There are many factors which may result in cancellation before surgery, some of which cannot be predicted, and some which can be prevented. Not all of these are related to the assessment of the patients' fitness (*Table 2.6*).

Table 2.6. Why do patients fail to have their operation?

Failure to identify those who are unfit for anaesthesia – most commonly, raised BP
Change in the surgical condition since booking for day surgery
Unpredictable reasons – upper respiratory tract infection, sudden change in the patient's condition
Organizational – staff shortage, overbooking of session
Patient factors – failure to attend, change of mind about operation

> *Cancelled operations are related not only to the method and exclusion criteria of pre-admission selection, but also to the type of surgery, the patients and the local population.*

References

1. **Warner MA, Shields SE, Chute CG.** Major morbidity and mortality within 1 month of ambulatory surgery and anesthesia. *J. Am. Med. Assoc.* 1993; **270**: 1437–1441.
2. **Duncan PG, Cohen MM, Tweed WA, et al.** The Canadian four-centre study of anaesthetic outcomes: III. Are anaesthetic complications predictable in day surgical practice? *Can. J. Anaesth.* 1992; **39**: 440–448.
3. **Jarrett PEM, Wallace M, Jarrett MED, et al.** Experience of a hospital hotel. *Ambulatory Surg.* 1996; **4**: 1–3.
4. **Fogg KJ, Saunders PRI.** Folly! The long distance day surgery patient. *Ambulatory Surg.* 1995; **3**: 209–210.
5. **Nygaard B.** Are travelling distances a barrier to day surgery? 1. Day Surgery in the World. *Proc. 1st Int. Congr. Amb. Surg.* 1995.
6. **Gabalski EC, Mattucci KF, Setezen M, et al.** Ambulatory tonsillectomy and adenoidectomy. *Laryngoscope* 1996; **106**: 77–80.
7. **Reiner SA, Sawyer WP, Clark KF, et al.** Safety of outpatient tonsillectomy and adenoidectomy. *Otolaryngol. Head Neck Surg.* 1990; **102**: 161–168.
8. **Singleton RJ, Rudkin GE, Osborne GA, et al.** Laparoscopic cholecystectomy as a day surgery procedure. *Anaesth. Intens. Care* 1996; **24**: 231–236.
9. **Arregui ME, Davis CJ, Arkush A, et al.** In selected patients outpatient laparoscopic cholecystectomy is safe and significantly reduces hospitalization charges. *Surg. Laparosc. Endosc.* 1991; **1**: 240–245.
10. **Kelly A, Griffith H, Jamjoom A.** Results of day case surgery for lumbar disc prolapse. *Br. J. Neurosurg.* 1994; **8**: 47–49.
11. **Keoghane SR, Millar JM, Cranston DW.** Is day case prostatectomy feasible? *Br. J. Urol.* 1995; **76**: 600–603.
12. **FASA.** Special study 1 (1986) 700 N. Fairfax Street, No 520, Alexandria, Virginia 221314, USA.
13. **Gold BS, Kitz DS, Lecky JH, et al.** Unanticipated admission to the hospital following ambulatory surgery. *J. Am. Med. Assoc.* 1989; **262**: 3008–3010.
14. **Meridy HW.** Criteria for selection of ambulatory surgical patients and guidelines for anesthetic management: a retrospective study of 1553 cases. *Anesth. Analg.* 1982; **61**: 921–926.
15. **Paix A, Rudkin GE, Osborne GA.** Ambulatory surgery complications and patient fitness. *Ambulatory Surg.* 1994; **2**: 166–170.
16. **Osborne G, Rudkin G.** Outcome after day-care surgery in a major teaching hospital. *Anaesth. Intens. Care* 1993; **21**: 822–827.
17. **Philip B.** Patients' assessment of ambulatory anesthesia and surgery. *J. Clin. Anesth.* 1992; **4**: 355–58.
18. **Wolters U, Wolf T, Stützer H, et al.** ASA classification and perioperative variables as predictors of postoperative outcome. *Br. J. Anaesth.* 1996; **77**: 217–222.
19. **Nehme AE.** Groin hernias in elderly patients. Management and prognosis. *Am. J. Surg.* 1983; **146**: 257–260.
20. **Williams-Russo P, Urquhart BL, Sharrock NE, et al.** Postoperative delirium: predictors and prognosis in elderly orthopedic patients. *J. Am. Geriatr. Soc.* 1992; **40**: 759–767.
21. **Bennett JA, Lingaraju N, Horrow JC, et al.** Elderly patients recover more rapidly from desflurane than from isoflurane anesthesia. *J. Clin. Anesth.* 1992; **4**: 378–381.
22. **Hollenberg M, Mangano DT, Browner WS, et al.** Predictors of postoperative myocardial ischemia in patients undergoing noncardiac surgery. *J. Am. Med. Assoc.* 1992; **268**: 205–209.
23. **Stone JG, Foex P, Sear JW, et al.** Risk of myocardial ischaemia during anaesthesia in treated and untreated hypertensive patients. *Br. J. Anaesth.* 1988; **61**: 675–679.
24. **Fahey TP, Peters TJ.** What constitutes controlled hypertension? Patient based comparison of hypertension guidelines. *Br. Med. J.* 1996; **313**: 93–96.
25. **Craft TM, Upton PM.** (1995) *Key Topics in Anaesthesia.* BIOS Scientific Publishers, Oxford. p. 118.
26. **Fee JPH, McCaughey W.** (1994) Preoperative preparation, premedication and concurrent drug therapy. In: *Anaesthesia* (Eds WS Nimmo, DJ Rowbotham, G Smith). Blackwell Scientific Publications, Oxford. p. 680.
27. **Goldman L, Caldera DL.** Risks of general anesthesia and elective operation in hypertensive patients. *Anesthesiology* 1979; **50**: 285–292.

28. **Glen SK, Elliott HL, Curzio JL,** *et al.* White-coat hypertension as a cause of cardiovascular dysfunction. *Lancet* 1996; **348**: 654–657.
29. **Allman KG, Muir A, Howell SJ,** *et al.* Resistant hypertension and preoperative silent myocardial ischaemia in surgical patients. *Br. J. Anaesth.* 1994; **73**: 574–578.
30. **Bedford RF, Feinstein B.** Hospital admission blood pressure: a predictor for hypertension following endotracheal intubation. *Anesth. Analg.* 1980; **59**: 367–370.
31. **McHugh P, Gill NP, Wyld R,** *et al.* Continuous ambulatory ECG monitoring in the perioperative period: relationship of preoperative status and outcome. *Br. J. Anaesth.* 1991; **66**: 285–291.
32. **Howell SJ, Sear YM, Yeates D,** *et al.* Hypertension, admission blood pressure and perioperative cardiovascular risk. *Anaesthesia* 1996; **51**: 1000–1004.
33. **Fleisher LA, Rosenbaum SH, Nelson AH,** *et al.* The predictive value of preoperative silent ischemia for postoperative ischemic cardiac events in vascular and nonvascular surgery patients. *Am. Heart J.* 1991; **122**: 980–986.
34. **Windsor A, French GWG, Sear JW,** *et al.* Silent myocardial ischaemia in patients undergoing transurethral prostatectomy. A study to evaluate risk scoring and anaesthetic technique. *Anaesthesia* 1996; **51**: 728–732.
35. **Stone JG, Foex P, Sear JW,** *et al.* Myocardial ischemia in untreated hypertensive patients: effect of a single small dose of a beta-adrenergic-blocking agent. *Anesthesiology* 1988; **68**: 495–500.
36. **Fleisher LA, Barash PG.** Preoperative cardiac evaluation for noncardiac surgery: a functional approach. *Anesth. Analg.* 1992; **74**: 586–598.
37. **Mangano DT, Browner WS, Hollenberg M,** *et al.* Long-term cardiac prognosis following noncardiac surgery. The Study of Perioperative Ischaemia Research Group. *J. Am. Med. Assoc.* 1992; **268**: 233–239.
38. **Goldman L, Caldera DL, Nussbaum SR,** *et al.* Multifactorial index of cardiac risk in noncardiac surgical procedures. *New Engl. J. Med.* 1977; **297**: 845–850.
39. **Committee on Safety of Medicines.** Avoid all NSAIDs in aspirin sensitive patients. *Curr. Prob. Pharmacovig.* 1993; **19**: 8.
40. **Shenkman Z, Shir Y, Brodsky JB.** Perioperative management of the obese patient. *Br. J. Anaesth.* 1993; **70**: 349–359.
41. **Hendolin H, Kansanen M, Koski E,** *et al.* Propofol–nitrous oxide versus thiopentone—isoflurane–nitrous oxide anaesthesia for uvulopalatopharyngoplasty in patients with sleep apnea. *Acta Anaesthiol. Scand.* 1994; **38**: 694–698.
42. **Han TS, van Leer EM, Seidell JC,** *et al.* Waist circumference action levels in the identification of cardiovascular risk factors: prevalence study in a random sample. *Br. Med. J.* 1995; **311**: 1401–1405.
43. **Lam AM, Grace DM, Manninen PH,** *et al.* The effects of cimetidine and ranitidine with and without metoclopramide on gastric volume and pH in morbidly obese patients. *Can. Anaesth. Soc. J.* 1986; **33**: 773–779.
44. **Natof HE.** (1990) Complications. In: *Anesthesia for Ambulatory Surgery* (Ed. BV Wetchler) J B Lippincott Company, Philadelphia, PA. pp. 454–456.
45. **British Medical Association and the Royal Pharmaceutical Society of Great Britain.** Combined oral contraceptives. *British National Formulary* 1996; **32**: 337.
46. **Thromboembolic Risk Factors (THRIFT) Consensus Group.** Risk of and prophylaxis for venous thromboembolism in hospital patients. *Br. Med. J.* 1992; **305**: 567–574.
47. **British Medical Association and the Royal Pharmaceutical Society of Great Britain.** Hormone replacement therapy and progesterone only contraceptives. *British National Formulary* 1996; **32**: 305 and 341.
48. **Johnson H, Knee-Ioli S, Butler TA,** *et al.* Are routine preoperative laboratory screening tests necessary to evaluate ambulatory surgical patients? *Surgery* 1988; **104**: 639–645.
49. **Golub R, Cantu R, Sorrento JJ,** *et al.* Efficacy of preadmission testing in ambulatory surgical patients. *Am. J. Surg.* 1992; **163**: 565–571.
50. **Wyatt WJ, Reed DN, Apelgren KN.** Pitfalls in the role of standardized preadmission laboratory screening for ambulatory surgery. *Am. Surg.* 1989; **55**: 343–346.
51. **Rudkin GE, Osborne GA, Doyle CE.** Assessment and selection of patients for day surgery in a public hospital. *Med. J. Aust.* 1993; **158**: 308–312.
52. **National Study by the Royal College of Radiologists.** Preoperative chest radiology. *Lancet* 1979; **2**: 83–86.

53. **Archer C, Levy AR, McGregor M.** Value of routine preoperative chest X-rays: a metanalysis. *Can. J. Anaesth.* 1993; **40**: 1022–1027.
54. **Rucker L, Frye EB, Staten MA.** Usefulness of screening chest roentgenograms in preoperative patients. *J. Am. Med. Assoc.* 1983; **250**: 3209–3211.
55. **Goldberger AL, O'Konski M.** Utility of routine electrocardiogram before surgery and on general hospital admission. *Ann. Intern. Med.* 1986; **105**: 552–557.
56. **Gold BS, Young ML, Kinman JL, *et al.*** The utility of preoperative electrocardiograms in the ambulatory surgical patient. *Arch. Intern. Med.* 1992; **152**: 301–305.
57. **Walton GM.** The cost benefit of routine pre-operative Hb investigations for oral surgery. *Br. Dent. J.* 1988; **165**: 406–407.
58. **National Institutes of Health Consensus Development Conference Statement** (1988) Preoperative red cell transfusion. **Vol 7**: 27–29 June.
59. **Shapiro MF, Greenfield S.** The complete blood count and leucocyte differential count. An approach to their rational application. *Ann. Intern. Med.* 1987; **106**: 65–74.
60. **Eichorn JH.** Pre-operative screening for sickle cell trait. *J. Am. Med. Assoc.* 1988; **259**: 907.
61. **Rogers ZR, Powars DR, Kinney TR, *et al.*** Non-black patients with sickle cell disease have African beta-s-gene cluster haplotypes. *J. Am. Med. Assoc.* 1989; **261**: 2991–2994.
62. **Wong E-M, Tillyer ML, Saunders PRI.** Pre-operative screening for sickle cell trait in adult day surgery; is it necessary? *Ambulatory Surg.* 1996; **4**: 41–45.
63. **Adu Gyamfi Y, Sankarankutty M, Marwa S.** Use of a tourniquet in patients with sickle cell disease. *Can. J. Anaesth.* 1993; **40**: 24–27.
64. **McCleane GJ.** Urea and electrolyte measurement in pre-operative surgical patients. *Anaesthesia* 1988; **43**: 413–415.
65. **Campbell IT, Gosling P.** Preoperative biochemical screening (Editorial). *Br. Med. J.* 1988; **297**: 803–804.
66. **Morgan AG.** Is routine urine testing in outpatient clinics useful? *Br. Med. J.* 1988; **297**: 1173.

CHAPTER 3

Assessment and preparation of adult day cases

J.M. Millar

Once the criteria for the selection and investigation of day case patients has been established, a system for ensuring that these criteria are met is needed. It is easy to pour resources into patient assessment without greatly improving outcome. An effective system targets those who need further investigation. Assessment systems depend on the patient population and the type of day surgery facility. The assessment process should be flexible – by addressing specific problems, patients may become suitable for day surgery. The aims of day surgery assessment are given in *Table 3.1*.

Table 3.1. Aims of assessment for day surgery

The patient should be:
Properly prepared for anaesthesia and surgery
Not cancelled on the day for a preventable reason
Safe to undergo the procedure
Able to go home safely

Why is assessment of patients for day surgery important?

Pre-admission assessment reduces preventable cancellation on the day of surgery[1-3]. Cancellations waste operating time and money, but, more importantly, distress patients.

Assessment should aim to improve the patient's condition and enable more patients to be day cases. Identification of problems in advance (e.g. high blood pressure (BP) or lack of overnight supervision) often means that these can be addressed so that the patient becomes suitable[4].

Effective assessment also speeds the admission process and saves time on the day of surgery. Assessing patients and gathering information or results on the day of surgery slows turnover and may result in cancellation[5].

Assessment should reduce overnight admission and/or perioperative morbidity[6]. There may be pressure to proceed with unfit or unprepared patients on the day of surgery and this may increase perioperative complications and unplanned overnight admission.

Assessment may improve non-attendance rates and patient compliance with pre- and postoperative instructions[7]. By involving the patient in this process at an early stage, the proposed date for surgery can be agreed, information given and any anxieties discussed[8,9].

Assessment may also reduce the medico-legal risk. This is unconfirmed but it is good practice to have a well organized and documented assessment system.

Setting selection criteria

Selection criteria need local agreement and co-operation from all the anaesthetists involved in day surgery. Wilson *et al.*[10] compared anaesthetists' opinions on patient fitness for surgical procedures and found that they varied according to the pessimism or optimism of the anaesthetist, but agreement could be achieved in 96% of cases. If anaesthetists disagree about criteria for suitability for day surgery, arrange for borderline patients to be assessed by the individual anaesthetist who will anaesthetize them.

Some DSUs and anaesthetists may be prepared to accept relatively less fit patients. These patients may require more anaesthetic input to assessment, and on the day of surgery, so selection criteria depend on how much effort you are prepared to invest in that patient's care; for example, insulin-dependent diabetics will require more medical management. The criteria may need to be more strict where the DSU is free standing, or if unplanned overnight patient admission is relatively difficult to arrange. However, it is mandatory to identify where and how to admit the inevitable few patients who are unfit to go home.

> *Agree on selection criteria, and publicize them widely. Send a copy to each surgeon, remembering that junior staff change. Post laminated copies in out-patient departments and clinics. Nurses can help, even if they are not actually assessing the patient formally. The more people who know the selection criteria, the better the chance of reducing unsuitable admissions. Keep it simple – long lists of obscure diseases will confuse rather than help (Table 3.2).*

Methods of patient assessment

The methods used to assess patients depend on the type of day surgery facility, and the fitness and geographical location of the patients they serve. Inner-city DSUs may need a different system from more rural hospitals where patients travel some distance or are seen at peripheral clinics. Patients in deprived inner-city areas may also have more health and social problems than rural areas. The type of surgery may also determine how intensive the assessment needs to be. For example, day case gynaecology patients are generally younger and fitter than those for day case urology.

A flexible filtering system should differentiate at an early stage those patients who need further investigation or assessment. This targets efforts and resources where they are needed. Patients who need minimal assessment and investigation should be quickly identified, so that neither the patient's nor the hospital's time is wasted (*Figure 3.1*).

Patient questionnaires

As is clear from the indications for preoperative investigations, the patient's medical history is the single most important feature in determining fitness for day surgery. A patient questionnaire identifies problems and helps the anaesthetist to quickly assess the patient on the day of surgery. It also provides a record. An example of a patient questionnaire is given in *Appendix 3.1*.

The questionnaire triages patients into those who are fit, those needing further assessment and those who can be immediately recognized as unsuitable[10]. Asymptomatic patients, in general, are fit.

> *However, a questionnaire is of no use if it is filed in the notes and ignored.*

Table 3.2. Day surgery criteria for surgeons

CRITERIA FOR ADULT PATIENT SELECTION
FOR DAY SURGERY UNDER GENERAL ANAESTHESIA

Social criteria
Responsible adult to escort home + supervise at home overnight
Lives within 1 hour's drive <u>maximum</u>
Reasonable social circumstances – consider stairs, telephone, toilet, heating, etc.

Physical fitness
Generally fit and ambulant
Not grossly obese (BMI >35)
The patient should be able to climb 1 flight of stairs

DO *NOT* BOOK PATIENTS WHO HAVE:

Cardiovascular disease – *poorly controlled hypertension* (BP >170/100)
                                angina, CCF or peripheral vascular disease
                                MI, TIA or CVA within last 6 months
                                symptomatic valvular disease

Respiratory disease – severe asthma or chest disease

Diabetes – insulin dependent or poorly controlled NIDDM

Renal or hepatic disease, alcoholism, narcotic addiction

Multiple sclerosis (advanced), myasthenia, severe cervical spondylosis

Severe psychiatric disease

DRUGS – DO *NOT* BOOK PATIENTS TAKING:

Anticoagulants	Antidysrhythmics
Digoxin	GTN
Monoamine oxidase inhibitors	?Oral contraceptive
Steroids	

Patients who do not meet these criteria may be suitable for day surgery
but need to be arranged with the anaesthetist

CCF, congestive cardiac failure; MI, myocardial infarct; TIA, transient ischaemic attack; CVA, cerebrovascular accident; NIDDM, non-insulin-dependent diabetes mellitus; GTN, glycerol trinitrate.

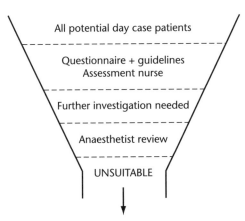

Figure 3.1. Filtering patients by the assessment process.

Who should screen the patient for day surgery? (Table 3.3)

It may appear a cheap and easy option to have the surgeon carry out the assessment at the time of arranging the surgery. However, unless surgeons are educated in what is appropriate from an anaesthetic point of view, surgeon selection may be little better than no assessment at all. This may be false economy, as the introduction of pre-admission assessment clinics has been demonstrated to reduce cancellations, investigations, overnight admissions and costs[1,11]. Macarthur *et al.*[12] reported that patients who attended a preoperative assessment clinic had a five times lower cancellation rate than those patients seen only in the surgeon's office.

Table 3.3. Who should screen the patient for day surgery?

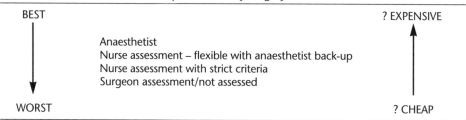

BEST		? EXPENSIVE
	Anaesthetist	
	Nurse assessment – flexible with anaesthetist back-up	
	Nurse assessment with strict criteria	
	Surgeon assessment/not assessed	
WORST		? CHEAP

The first stage in the assessment process is best carried out by trained nurses using a patient questionnaire, and a height/weight chart (*Figure 3.2*). They should also check BP. A nurse-led pre-admission clinic has been shown to reduce both preventable cancellations and doctors' workload[13]. Nurses are often better at recognizing problems related to the patient's home circumstances.

Rigid application of selection criteria with no flexibility for anaesthetic review may result in an unnecessarily restrictive policy for day surgery. Combining the questionnaire (*Appendix 3.1*) with structured assessment guidelines (*Appendix 3.2*) identifies investigations and any further action needed, and allows more patients to be booked as day cases.

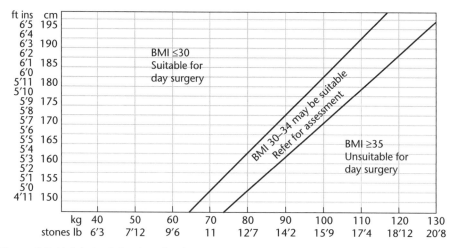

Figure 3.2. Height/weight chart for day case selection.

Computer programs have been used to administer questionnaires and guidelines, and are likely to be used more in future[14,15].

GPs may also become more involved in assessment, as they have easy access to patients' records, and have an interest in cost-effective care.

Referral to the anaesthetist
It is usually impractical, expensive and unnecessary for anaesthetists to assess every patient before admission[16], but there must be access to anaesthetic back-up. Most queries about fitness can be dealt with by reviewing the patient's history, often by telephone. Infrequently the anaesthetist may have to see the patient before admission to assess fitness, discuss the anaesthetic or allay anxiety.

Where should assessments be carried out?
Many DSUs specify that the patient must attend the DSU for assessment, and this can often be combined with the patient's out-patient visit. This interview is ideally carried out in the DSU, as patients can be shown the unit at the same time. However, if patients are initially seen by the surgeon at another site, they may find it inconvenient to travel or take time off work to attend the DSU. An assessment nurse can see patients at these other sites at the time of their initial consultation.

Telephone screening also works well for these patients, but contact is improved by calling in the evening[17]. The nurse assesses the patient using the questionnaire; BP check and any necessary tests are arranged with the GP or practice nurse. When the anaesthetist was telephoned by the patient, the number of preoperative tests requested was reduced[18] but this might prove difficult to organize in practice. Borderline cases can be asked to come to the DSU if further assessment is needed.

GPs now usually have the patient's information on computer, and this can be accessed by the practice personnel if further information about a patient is needed.

Following assessment, suitable patients can be given a date for their surgery, as well as information on the procedure, preoperative instructions and day surgery information. Unsuitable patients are referred back to the surgeon.

> However patients are screened, an anaesthetist should be identified to provide advice and further assessment.

When <u>should</u> the anaesthetist meet the patient?
Patient assessment by the anaesthetist before admission should only be needed for exceptional patients. Meeting the anaesthetist before admission has not been shown to be beneficial to the patient. Twersky *et al.* found that this did not reduce anxiety or perioperative problems, or increase satisfaction, compared with meeting the anaesthetist in the DSU on the day of admission[16]. Leigh *et al.* showed that anxiety was reduced by discussing the procedure with other informed hospital personnel, and he suggested the use of a patient information booklet[8].

However, it is unacceptable for the anaesthetist to meet the patient for the first time in the anaesthetic room or theatre. Problems may be missed, and this is not the time to discuss the anaesthetic. Anaesthetic assessment should be carried out after admission but before going to theatre, and sufficient time must be allowed for this assessment.

Before rejecting or postponing a patient for day surgery, clear benefits of in-patient surgery should be identified (*Table 3.4*).

Table 3.4. Questions to ask before rejecting a patient for day surgery

Can the procedure be carried out under local anaesthesia ± sedation?
Can the patient's condition be improved?
What benefit(s) would there be from admitting the patient to hospital pre- or postoperatively?
Would the patient be suitable for surgery if scheduled as an in-patient tomorrow? If so, what
   difference would this make?

> *The patient should meet the anaesthetist in the day surgery unit before going to
> theatre.*

The process is outlined in *Figure 3.3*. Each DSU should establish a system that fits its own situation and needs. Reasons for cancellations, delays and overnight admissions should be regularly reviewed to ensure that the process is effective.

> *If assessment is effective, few patients should be cancelled for predictable unfitness for
> surgery and anaesthesia, and treatment on the day should be smooth and efficient.*

Preparation of the patient for day surgery

Preparation of the patient is an important part of good day surgery practice. Patients may have their operations cancelled for other reasons than physical unfitness for surgery (*Table 3.5*). Good preparation and information in advance improves patient care[8] and the efficiency of the DSU[3].

Table 3.5. Reasons for postponed or cancelled operations unrelated to physical unfitness for anaesthesia

Inability to keep the appointment
Fear or anxiety about the procedure
Patient decided not to have surgery
Change in the surgical condition
Failure to arrange escort or overnight supervision
Failure to make suitable arrangements for time off work/child care
Failure to comply with NPO instructions
Failure to comply with instructions for medication
Failure to notify the DSU of acute medical conditions

NPO, *nil per os* or fasting.

What information should be given to the patient?

Date and time of surgery
If this is agreed with the patient in advance, there is a greater chance that the patient will keep the appointment. If notification is by post, then a prepaid return slip should be provided to make sure that the patient received the letter.

Escort and supervision
Patients need to be aware before admission that they will not have their surgery unless arrangements have been made for a suitable escort and overnight supervision. Because

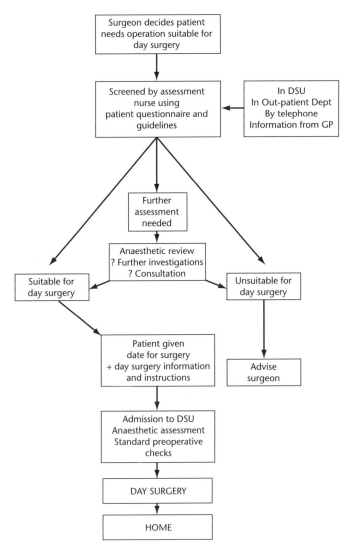

Figure 3.3. The assessment process.

of the reduced number of in-patient beds, the availability of an in-patient bed cannot be left to chance.

Fasting instructions
There is general agreement that fasting patients for long periods before surgery adds to morbidity and patient discomfort without improving safety[19,20]. Current recommendations are that solids should be stopped 6 hours before surgery, but clear fluids may be safely taken up to 2–3 hours before surgery. The volume allowed may be greater than initially supposed – free fluids[21] or 330 ml water[22] up to 2 hours before the procedure were not shown to affect residual gastric volume or pH.

Logistically, allowing patients to take oral fluids may be difficult to plan in day surgery unless the operating time can be predicted accurately. One option is to give the patient oral fluids in the DSU if the wait is going to be longer than 2 hours.

Medication instructions
In general, the recommendation should be to continue all regular medication as usual before surgery. This is particularly important for antihypertensive, anticonvulsant, steroid or bronchodilator drugs. The only patients who may need to be told *not* to take their regular medication are those taking oral hypoglycaemics, insulin, anticoagulants, diuretics or oestrogen-containing contraceptive pills. These patients may need to be reviewed by the anaesthetist to decide when the drugs should be discontinued.

Patients with hiatus hernia, significant oesophageal reflux or obesity may be given H_2 blockers to take the night before admission to reduce gastric acid[23,24]. Ranitidine 300 mg orally taken the night before has been found to be effective[23].

Driving after general anaesthesia or sedation
If not warned in advance, patients may drive themselves to the hospital and be tempted to drive home again after their operation. The time restriction on driving and operating machinery should be clearly stated on the information given to the patient (see also Chapter 16).

Pregnancy
Women should be warned to take adequate precautions against becoming pregnant before their surgery. This is particularly important in women having laparoscopy for investigation of infertility, who may not use contraception unless told to do so.

Routine pregnancy testing has not been found necessary, and patient history has been found to be sufficient[25]. However, this will not detect women in very early pregnancy who have not yet missed a menstrual period.

Pre-admission information on day surgery and the proposed procedure
Patients are likely to be less anxious if they know what will happen on the day of surgery and understand the procedure they are to have. It also allows them to make suitable arrangements about child care, work and activities. Warnings about expected levels of pain and morbidity may make the patient more, rather than less, able to cope, and have been found to improve patient satisfaction[26].

If the procedure is to be carried out under local or regional anaesthesia with or without sedation, this is a good time to discuss it with the patient. Protocols will be needed to help nurses identify patients and procedures where this is an option.

Information is ideally given in the DSU, where anxieties can be discussed and further help found if needed. It must be backed up with written information which is easy to read and understand[27] (*Tables 3.6* and *3.7*). If the patient cannot attend the DSU, information should be sent to back up telephone information. Occasional surveys should be carried out to discover if patients receive, read and understand what they have been sent or given. Videos and cassette tapes have also been used to provide information to patients.

> *Anaesthetic input into pre-admission information is important. Well-prepared and relaxed patients are easier to anaesthetize.*

Table 3.6. Pre-admission information

On the front – important information
Time and date of the operation
The need for an escort and taxi or car to go home (not public transport)
The need for supervision overnight or longer
Fasting instructions
Do not omit medication unless specifically requested to do so
Instructions not to drive or operate machinery for 24–48 hours[a]
Instructions for clothing, valuables and something to pass the time
Contact telephone number if unable or unfit to keep the appointment
For women, ring the day surgery unit if you think there is a possibility that you might be pregnant

Other information on the DSU and what will happen on the day
Map, parking and how to find the DSU
Nursing procedures before surgery
Anaesthetic assessment: pain, PONV, anxiety and needle phobia
Surgical: last minute questions and consent if not already signed
Description of the trip to theatre and the recovery process
Duration of stay and time for escort to come
Post-anaesthetic restrictions on driving, alcohol, taking decisions, etc.
Who to contact after discharge
Follow-up arrangements

Procedure-specific information
What the operation is, in simple, non-frightening terms ± diagrams/pictures
Preoperative preparation, e.g. shaving
Time required off work
Expected resumption of normal duties
Expected postoperative morbidity
When to seek advice – postoperative problems
Wound management, stitch removal and follow-up, if relevant

[a]The time depends on locally decided guidelines (Chapter 16).

Table 3.7. Dos and don'ts of written patient information

Give all instructions in written form (as well as verbal where possible)
Have versions available in appropriate languages
Keep them simple, succinct and to the point or patients may not read them
Use short sentences with active verbs and clear expressions
Use a friendly style but do not patronize
Avoid medical jargon, e.g. sublingual should be replaced with 'under your tongue'
Do not use slang words for body parts
Avoid jokes – they may not be funny to the patient
Be positive – say what should be done
Consider including 'questions that patients often ask about their surgery'
Co-ordinate procedure information with individual surgeon's practice
Layout and style should be attractive and easy to read, with bold headings
Put all the important points briefly on the front page
Make sure a contact telephone number is prominently displayed
Computers make information easy and cheap to update and personalize
Assess whether patients read, understand and approve of the information
Edit and review regularly

Is your assessment process working?

The reasons for patient non-attendance, cancellation of surgery and unplanned overnight admission should be reviewed to ensure that assessment is effective. However, equally importantly, the reasons for rejecting patients for day surgery should also be considered, to ensure that the criteria are not too exclusive. Patient satisfaction with the process should be audited. Did they find the assessment reassuring and informative, or too time consuming and inconvenient?

> *Patient assessment for day surgery should be a collaborative process which involves the surgeon, anaesthetist, nursing staff and the patient. Anaesthetic input into the process of assessing patients is imperative.*

References

1. **Pollard JB, Zboray AL, Mazze RI.** Economic benefits attributed to opening a preoperative evaluation clinic for outpatients. *Anesth. Analg.* 1996; **83**: 407–410.
2. **Hand R, Levin P, Stanziola A.** The causes of cancelled elective surgery. *Qual. Ass. Util. Rev.* 1990; **5**: 2–6.
3. **Conway JB, Goldberg J, Chung F.** Preadmission anesthesia consultation clinic. *Can. J. Anaesth.* 1992; **39**: 1051–1057.
4. **MacDonald JB, Dutton MJ, Stott DJ, et al.** Evaluation of preadmission screening of elderly patients accepted for major joint replacement. *Health Bull. Edinb.* 1992; **50**: 54–60.
5. **Boothe P, Finnegan BA.** Changing the admission process for elective surgery: an economic analysis. *Can. J. Anaesth.* 1995; **42**: 391–394.
6. **Macpherson DS, Lofgren RP.** Outpatient internal medicine preoperative evaluation: a randomized clinical trial. *Med. Care* 1994; **32**: 498–507.
7. **Banahan I, Quenby S, Stewart H, et al.** Preliminary evaluation of the effectiveness of a preoperative clinic for gynaecological surgery. *Br. J. Hosp. Med.* 1994; **52**: 535–538.
8. **Leigh JM, Walker J, Janaganathan P.** Effect of pre-operative anaesthetic visit on anxiety. *Br. Med. J.* 1977; **2**: 987–989.
9. **Rutten CL, Gubbels JW, Smelt WL, et al.** [Outpatient preoperative examination by the anaesthesiologist. II. Patient satisfaction]. *Ned. Tijdschr. Geneeskd.* 1995; **139**: 1032–1036.
10. **Wilson ME, Williams NB, Baskett PJF, et al.** Assessment of fitness for surgical procedures and the variability of anaesthetists' judgments. *Br. Med. J.* 1980; **280**: 509–512.
11. **Rutten CL, Post D, Smelt WL.** [Outpatient preoperative examination by the anaesthesiologist. I. Fewer procedures and preoperative hospital days.] *Ned. Tijdschr. Geneeskd.* 1995; **139**: 1028–1032.
12. **Macarthur AJ, Macarthur C, Bevan JC.** Preoperative assessment clinic reduces day surgery cancellations (abstract). *Anesthesiology* 1991; **75**: A1109.
13. **Koay CB, Marks MJ.** A nurse led pre-admission clinic for elective ENT surgery – the first eight months. *Ann. R. Coll. Surg. Engl.* 1996; **78**: 15–19.
14. **Blackwell Science.** Day Surgery Server. Osney Mead, Oxford OX2 0EL.
15. **Calcius Systems Ltd.** Daynamics. Ash Corner, Walters Ash, High Wycombe, Buckinghamshire HP14 4UD.
16. **Twersky RS, Lebovits AH, Lewis M, et al.** Early anesthesia evaluation of the ambulatory surgical patient: does it really help? *J. Clin. Anesth.* 1992; **4**: 204–207.
17. **Patel RI, Hanallah RS.** Preoperative screening for pediatric ambulatory surgery: evaluation of a telephone questionnaire method. *Anesth. Analg.* 1992; **75**: 258–261.
18. **Germond M, Narchi P, Mahiou P, et al.** [A traditional anesthesia consultation or a 'telephone interview' within the framework of ambulatory surgery.] *Cah. d'Anesthésiol.* 1993; **41**: 459–461.
19. **Scarr M, Maltby JR, Jani K, et al.** Volume and acidity of residual gastric fluid after oral fluid ingestion before elective ambulatory surgery. *Can. Med. Assoc. J.* 1989; **141**: 1151–1154.
20. **Strunin L.** How long should patients fast before surgery? Time for new guidelines (editorial). *Br. J. Anaesth.* 1993; **70**: 1–3.

21. **Phillips S, Hutchinson S, Davidson T.** Preoperative drinking does not affect gastric contents. *Br. J. Anaesth.* 1993; **70**: 6–9.
22. **Greenfield SM, Webster GJM, Brar AS, et al.** Assessment of residual gastric volume and thirst in patients who drink before gastroscopy. *Gut* 1996; **39**: 360–362.
23. **Gallagher EG, White M, Ward S, et al.** Prophylaxis against acid aspiration syndrome. Single oral dose of H_2-antagonist on the evening before elective surgery. *Anaesthesia* 1988; **43**: 1011–1014.
24. **Lam AM, Grace DM, Manninen PH, et al.** The effects of cimetidine and ranitidine with and without metoclopramide on gastric volume and pH in morbidly obese patients. *Can. Anaesth. Soc. J.* 1986; **33**: 773–779.
25. **Malviya S, D'Errico C, Reynolds P, et al.** Should pregnancy testing be routine in adolescent patients prior to surgery? *Anesth. Analg.* 1996; **83**: 854–858.
26. **Vallerand WP, Vallerand AH, Heft M.** The effects of postoperative preparatory information on the clinical course following third molar extraction. *J. Oral Maxillofac. Surg.* 1994; **52**: 1165–1170.
27. **Kitching JB.** Patient information leaflets – the state of the art. *J. R. Soc. Med.* 1990; **83**: 298–300.

Adult Day Surgery Assessment Questionnaire for General Anaesthesia

You may be able to have your operation as a day case.
To help us plan your treatment, please answer the following questions.

Can an adult take you home by car or taxi after your operation ?   Yes ☐   No ☐

Is there a responsible and physically fit adult to look after you
for the first night after your operation?   Yes ☐   No ☐

Would it take you less than 1 hour to get home
from the hospital/DSU   Yes ☐   No ☐

Do you suffer from or have you ever suffered from

Heart disease or a heart murmur	Yes ☐	No ☐
High blood pressure	Yes ☐	No ☐
Chest pains or angina	Yes ☐	No ☐
Stroke	Yes ☐	No ☐
Asthma	Yes ☐	No ☐
Chronic cough or bronchitis	Yes ☐	No ☐
Too breathless to climb 1 flight stairs	Yes ☐	No ☐
Diabetes	Yes ☐	No ☐
Epilepsy	Yes ☐	No ☐
Kidney problems	Yes ☐	No ☐
Jaundice	Yes ☐	No ☐
Heartburn or hiatus hernia	Yes ☐	No ☐
Bleeding problems	Yes ☐	No ☐
Any other diseases	Yes ☐	No ☐

If you answered YES to any of these questions, please tell us about it
....

Are you taking any tablets, pills, inhalers or medicine?   Yes ☐   No ☐
If yes, please list them
....

Have you any allergies (including drug allergies)?   Yes ☐   No ☐
If yes, please list them
....

Do you smoke? If YES, how many per day ....   Yes ☐   No ☐

Do you have false, capped, crowned or loose teeth?   Yes ☐   No ☐

Have you had any operations or anaesthetics before?   Yes ☐   No ☐
If yes, please list
....

Were there any problems? If so please give details
....

Have any of your family had problems with anaesthetics?   Yes ☐   No ☐

If so, what were the problems?   Yes ☐   No ☐
....

Appendix 3.1. Patient questionnaire.

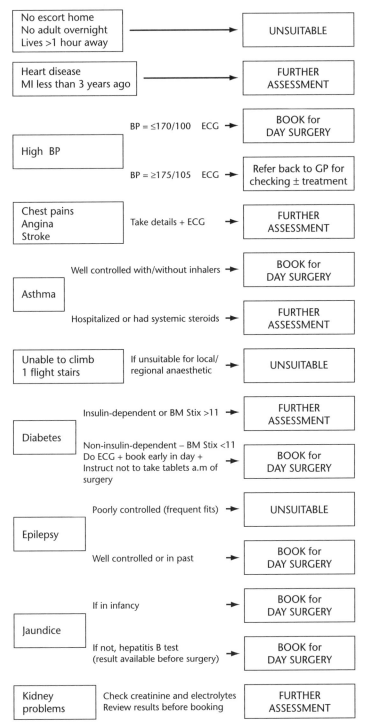

Appendix 3.2. Day surgery assessment guidelines for patients having general anaesthesia (continued over page).

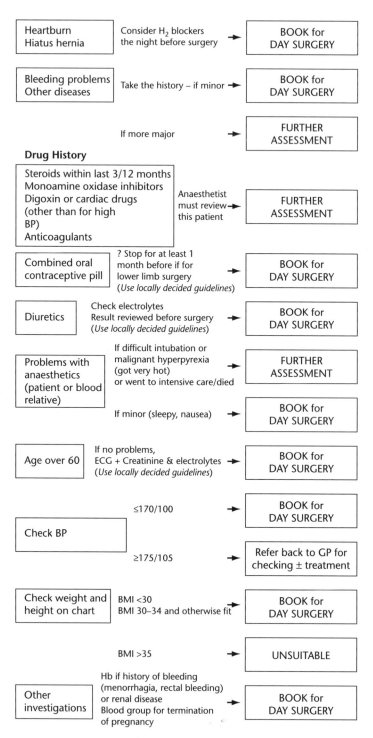

Heartburn Hiatus hernia	Consider H$_2$ blockers the night before surgery →	BOOK for DAY SURGERY
Bleeding problems Other diseases	Take the history – if minor →	BOOK for DAY SURGERY
	If more major →	FURTHER ASSESSMENT

Drug History

Steroids within last 3/12 months Monoamine oxidase inhibitors Digoxin or cardiac drugs (other than for high BP) Anticoagulants	Anaesthetist must review → this patient	FURTHER ASSESSMENT
Combined oral contraceptive pill	? Stop for at least 1 month before if for lower limb surgery (*Use locally decided guidelines*) →	BOOK for DAY SURGERY
Diuretics	Check electrolytes Result reviewed before surgery (*Use locally decided guidelines*) →	BOOK for DAY SURGERY
Problems with anaesthetics (patient or blood relative)	If difficult intubation or malignant hyperpyrexia (got very hot) or went to intensive care/died →	FURTHER ASSESSMENT
	If minor (sleepy, nausea) →	BOOK for DAY SURGERY
Age over 60	If no problems, ECG + Creatinine & electrolytes → (*Use locally decided guidelines*)	BOOK for DAY SURGERY
Check BP	≤170/100 →	BOOK for DAY SURGERY
	≥175/105 →	Refer back to GP for checking ± treatment
Check weight and height on chart	BMI <30 BMI 30–34 and otherwise fit →	BOOK for DAY SURGERY
	BMI >35 →	UNSUITABLE
Other investigations	Hb if history of bleeding (menorrhagia, rectal bleeding) or renal disease Blood group for termination of pregnancy →	BOOK for DAY SURGERY

Appendix 3.2. Continued.

CHAPTER 4

Premedication in adult day surgery

J.M. Millar

Premedication is often considered unnecessary in day surgery but may contribute to the quality or safety of the anaesthetic. Premedication in this context is drugs given in the DSU before the patient goes to surgery rather than given intravenously (IV) immediately before induction of anaesthesia. In most DSUs this also implies that premedication is given orally, or perhaps rectally, as IV administration is usually logistically difficult. The time available preoperatively for these drugs to be effective is a limiting factor (*Table 4.1*).

Table 4.1. Possible indications for premedication in day surgery

Anxiolysis and sedation
Reduction of risk factors for acid reflux and aspiration
Antiemesis
Analgesia for venepuncture and postoperative pain
Other drugs, e.g. asthma prophylaxis

Sedation and anxiolysis

Sedative premedication is usually omitted in day case patients in the belief that day surgery does not merit anxiolysis and that prolonged recovery times after sedation may delay discharge[1]. Both of these may not be true[2].

Day case patients do experience anxiety – 19% of patients in Mackenzie's study would have liked something to relieve their anxiety[3], particularly if they were young, female, were having their first general anaesthetic or had had a previous unpleasant anaesthetic experience. Certain types of surgery may also be associated with more anxiety – for example, breast lumpectomy, oral surgery or adult circumcision.

Good preoperative information and reassurance will calm the majority of patients, who settle down after arrival, and do not need anxiolysis. However, the anaesthetist and nursing staff should attempt to identify patients who do need it. The preoperative visit by the anaesthetist on the day of surgery should be used to assess anxiety and reassure the patient. Preoperative sedation should be offered to those who are very anxious. There is little evidence that mild sedation does delay discharge[4], and premedication may reduce the anaesthetic doses required at induction[5].

In the ward setting, oral premedication is indicated. IV sedatives should not be given to unmonitored patients. For extremely anxious patients who are identified before admission, oral anxiolytics may be given to take at home before coming to the DSU.

However, once patients are given sedative premedication they require nursing surveillance, may need to lie down, and may not be able to walk to theatre, so there are practical and cost considerations.

Drugs used for preoperative day case sedation are usually short-acting benzodiazepines, most commonly midazolam and temazepam. Midazolam (15 mg PO) and temazepam (20 mg PO) both reduce anxiety. Although midazolam may be more anxiolytic, it has also been associated with greater delay in recovery[6,7], and its amnesic properties may make recall of postoperative instructions difficult[8]. Midazolam, 7.5 mg PO, did not reduce anxiety compared with 15 mg but still impaired psychomotor performance postoperatively[9].

Temazepam, 10 mg or 20 mg, have both been shown to reduce anxiety; the larger dose is more anxiolytic, but may delay recovery more[4,10].

Alternative drugs that have been used for preoperative sedation are beta-blockers[11], oral clonidine or short-acting narcotics given transmucosally, but these have other side-effects and are better avoided.

> *Anxious patients who do not respond to reassurance should be given temazepam 10 mg PO. Exceptionally 20 mg may be required.*

Prophylaxis against acid reflux and aspiration

Although regurgitation and aspiration are extremely rare in day case patients, they have been shown, in theory, to be at greater risk than in-patients, perhaps because of the effects of stress and anxiety on gastric emptying[12]. Manchikanti showed that 76–88% of day cases had gastric pH <2.5 and 52–60% had resting gastric volumes >25 ml, both of which are considered risk factors in the aspiration of stomach contents[13,14] (*Table 4.2*).

Table 4.2. Risk factors for acid reflux and aspiration in day surgery

Higher resting gastric volumes and lower gastric pH in day cases
Anxiety
Hiatus hernia or symptomatic gastric reflux
Obesity
Early pregnancy
Laparoscopy

Gynaecological patients may be at extra risk. Patients in early pregnancy may have delayed gastric emptying[15,16] and reduced lower oesophageal sphincter tone[17] which is further reduced in the lithotomy position[18]. Laparoscopy is associated with high intra-abdominal pressure as well as the head-down lithotomy position, and regurgitation has been reported[19,20].

There are other indications for routine acid aspiration prophylaxis. Obesity has an association with hiatus hernia and gastric reflux, and overweight patients are recognized to be at greater risk because of slowed gastric emptying and lower gastric pH[21].

Ranitidine, given as 50–100 mg IV or 150 mg PO, has been demonstrated to be more effective in reducing the risk factors in aspiration compared with sodium citrate[16], cimetidine[22,23], famotidine[24] or omeprazole[24,25]. Ranitidine, 150 mg PO, has been shown to be effective after 60 minutes[26]; 300 mg is not significantly better than 150 mg[27]. Larger doses, 300 mg PO given the night before surgery and on arrival, were found to reduce significantly both PONV and time to discharge[28].

The addition of metoclopramide to ranitidine premedication does not further reduce the risk factors[29] but may increase lower oesophageal barrier pressure[30] and contribute to postoperative antiemesis[31].

Ingestion of fluid up to 3 hours preoperatively does not seem to increase or decrease gastric volume or pH, with or without ranitidine[32–34].

> *Ranitidine 150 mg PO, with or without metoclopramide 10 mg PO, given 60 min preoperatively provides reliable prophylaxis against acid reflux and aspiration. It should be given to patients at increased risk of acid reflux, and considered for every patient.*

Antiemesis

If opioid premedication is avoided, there is usually no need to include antiemetics as part of premedication, as these can be given if needed with the general anaesthetic. The possible benefits of ranitidine and metoclopramide in reducing PONV have been referred to above.

Analgesia

It may be advantageous to give oral NSAIDs for postoperative pain as premedication, particularly if the operation is of short duration, as this allows time for them to be effective when the patient wakes[35–38].

Preoperative NSAIDs should not be given before operations associated with increased bleeding[39], or to patients with a history of peptic ulcer or renal disease. In normal patients, ranitidine may reduce the gastrointestinal effects of NSAIDs on an empty stomach[40].

Oral preparations also tend to be cheaper than parenteral, an added advantage. Although rectal diclofenac is well absorbed, persuading patients to self-administer it preoperatively may not be easy in cultures where the rectal route is not popular. Enteric-coated diclofenac is absorbed from the duodenum[41], so combining it with a prokinetic drug such as metoclopramide may help to speed up absorption if a soluble preparation is not used.

Even adults may be anxious about venepuncture, and a sympathetic preoperative visit will detect this. The application to the venepuncture site of EMLA® cream (lignocaine 2.5% and prilocaine 2.5% in a eutectic mixture) 60 minutes preoperatively, or Ametop® (amethocaine 4% gel) 35 minutes preoperatively[42], reduces pain.

Other drugs

It is often useful to give asthmatics an extra dose of their usual bronchodilator or nebulized salbutamol 1 hour preoperatively or on arrival. Anxiety can provoke wheeze in some asthmatics.

Different surgical specialities may have requirements for preoperative drugs, for instance prostaglandins for termination of pregnancy[43] or antibiotics before urological procedures.

> *Premedication may have a place in day surgery in reducing anxiety, the risk of acid reflux and pain. It should be given soon after arrival if it is to be effective before surgery.*

References

1. **Shafer A, White PF, Urquhart ML,** *et al.* Outpatient premedication: use of midazolam and opioid analgesics. *Anesthesiology* 1989; **71**: 495–501.
2. **White PF.** Pharmacology and clinical aspects of preoperative medication. *Anesth. Analg.* 1986; **65**: 963–974.
3. **Mackenzie JW.** Day case anaesthesia and anxiety. A study of anxiety profiles amongst patients attending a Day Bed Unit. *Anaesthesia* 1989; **44**: 437–440.
4. **Obey PA, Ogg TW, Gilks WR.** Temazepam and recovery in day surgery. *Anaesthesia.* 1988; **43**: 49–51.
5. **Redfern N, Stafford MA, Hull CJ.** Incremental propofol for short procedures. *Br. J. Anaesth.* 1985; **57**: 1178–1182.
6. **Hargreaves J.** Benzodiazepine premedication in minor day-case surgery: comparison of oral midazolam and temazepam with placebo. *Br. J. Anaesth.* 1988; **61**: 611–616.
7. **Nightingale JJ, Norman J.** A comparison of midazolam and temazepam for premedication of day case patients. *Anaesthesia* 1988; **43**: 111–113.
8. **Philip BK.** Hazards of amnesia after midazolam in ambulatory surgical patients. *Anesth. Analg.* 1987; **66**: 97.
9. **Raybould D, Bradshaw EG.** Premedication for day case surgery. A study of oral midazolam. *Anaesthesia* 1987; **42**: 591–595.
10. **Bailie R, Christmas L, Price N,** *et al.* Effects of temazepam premedication on cognitive recovery following alfentanil–propofol anaesthesia. *Br. J. Anaesth.* 1989; **63**: 68–75.
11. **Mackenzie JW, Bird J.** Timolol: a sedative anxiolytic premedicant for day cases. *Br. Med. J.* 1989; **298**: 363–364.
12. **Ong BY, Palhniuk RJ, Cumming M.** Gastric volume and pH in outpatients. *Can. Anaesth. Soc. J.* 1978; **25**: 36–39.
13. **Manchikanti L, Roush JR.** Effect of preanesthetic glycopyrrolate and cimetidine on gastric fluid pH and volume in outpatients. *Anesth. Analg.* 1984; **63**: 40–46.
14. **Manchikanti L, Canella MG, Hohlbein LJ,** *et al.* Assessment of effect of various modes of premedication on acid aspiration risk factors in outpatient surgery. *Anesth. Analg.* 1987; **66**: 81–84.
15. **Levy DM, Williams OA, Magides AD,** *et al.* Gastric emptying is delayed at 8-12 week's gestation. *Br. J. Anaesth.* 1994; **73**: 237–238.
16. **Duffy BL, Woodhouse PC, Schramm MD,** *et al.* Ranitidine prophylaxis before anaesthesia in early pregnancy. *Anaesth. Intens. Care* 1984; **13**: 29–32.
17. **Brock-Utne JG, Dow TGB, Dimopoulos GE,** *et al.* Gastric and lower oesophageal sphincter (LOS) pressures in early pregnancy. *Br. J. Anaesth.* 1981; **53**: 381–384.
18. **Jones MJ, Mitchell RWD, Hindocha N,** *et al.* The lower oesophageal sphincter in the first trimester of pregnancy: comparison of supine with lithotomy positions. *Br. J. Anaesth.* 1988; **61**: 475–476.
19. **Duffy BL.** Regurgitation during pelvic laparoscopy. *Br. J. Anaesth.* 1979; **51**: 1089–1090.
20. **Roberts CJ, Goodman NW.** Gastro-oesophageal reflux during elective laparoscopy. *Anaesthesia* 1990; **45**: 1009–1011.
21. **Vaughan RW, Bauer S, Wise L.** Volume and pH of gastric juice in obese subjects. *Anesthesiology* 1975; **43**: 686–689.
22. **Stock JL, Sutherland AD.** The role of H_2 receptor antagonist premedication in pregnant day care patients. *Can. Anaesth. Soc. J.* 1985; **32**: 463–467.
23. **Lam AM, Grace DM, Manninen PH,** *et al.* The effects of cimetidine and ranitidine with and without metoclopramide on gastric volume and pH in morbidly obese patients. *Can. Anaesth. Soc. J.* 1986; **33**: 773–779.
24. **Boulay K, Blanlœil Y, Bourveau M,** *et al.* Effects of oral ranitidine, famotidine, and omeprazole on gastric volume and pH at induction and recovery from general anaesthesia. *Br. J. Anaesth.* 1994; **73**: 475–478.
25. **Nishina K, Mikawa K, Maekawa N,** *et al.* A comparison of lansoprazole, omeprazole, and ranitidine for reducing preoperative gastric secretion in adult patients undergoing elective surgery. *Anesth. Analg.* 1996; **82**: 832–836.
26. **Escolano F, Sierra P, Ortiz JC,** *et al.* The efficacy and optimum time of administration of ranitidine in the prevention of the acid aspiration syndrome. *Anaesthesia* 1996; **51**: 182–184.

27. **Vinik HR, Covarrubias S.** Ranitidine – role of dose and time for prophylaxis of perioperative acid aspiration. *Anesthesiology* 1990; **73:** A13.

28. **Kraynack BJ, Bates MF.** Antiemetic action of ranitidine in out-patient laparoscopy under propofol–isoflurane anesthesia. *Anesthesiology* 1990; **73:** A14.

29. **Maltby JR, Elliott RH, Warnell I,** *et al.* Gastric fluid volume and pH in elective surgical patients: triple prophylaxis is not superior to ranitidine alone. *Can. J. Anaesth.* 1990; **37:** 650–655.

30. **Brock-Utne JG, Rubin J, Welman S,** *et al.* The action of commonly used antiemetics on the lower oesophageal sphincter. *Br. J. Anaesth.* 1978; **50:** 295–298.

31. **Miller CD, Anderson WG.** Silent regurgitation in day case gynaecological patients. *Anaesthesia* 1988; **43:** 321–323.

32. **Maltby JR, Reid CR, Hutchinson A.** Gastric fluid volume and pH in elective inpatients. Part II: Coffee or orange juice with ranitidine. *Can. J. Anaesth.* 1988; **35:** 16–19.

33. **Hutchinson A, Maltby JR, Reid CR.** Gastric fluid volume and pH in elective patients. Part I: Coffee or orange juice versus overnight fast. *Can. J. Anaesth.* 1988; **35:** 12–15.

34. **Scarr M, Maltby JR, Jani K,** *et al.* Volume and acidity of residual gastric fluid after oral fluid ingestion before elective ambulatory surgery. *Can. Med. Assoc. J.* 1989; **141:** 1151–1154.

35. **Bunnemann L, Thorshauge H, Herlevesen P,** *et al.* Analgesia for outpatient surgery: placebo versus naproxen sodium (a non-steroidal anti-inflammatory drug) given before or after surgery. *Eur. J. Anaesthesiol.* 1994; **11:** 461–464.

36. **Rosenblum M, Weller RS, Conard PL,** *et al.* Ibuprofen provides longer lasting analgesia than fentanyl after laparoscopic surgery. *Anesth. Analg.* 1991; **73:** 255–259.

37. **Code WE, Yip RW, Browne ME,** *et al.* Preoperative naproxen sodium reduces postoperative pain following arthroscopic knee surgery. *Can. J. Anaesth.* 1994; **41:** 98–101.

38. **Gillberg LE, Harsten AS, Stahl LB.** Preoperative diclofenac reduces post-laparoscopy pain. *Can. J. Anaesth.* 1993; **40:** 406–408.

39. **Thiagarajan J, Bates S, Hitchcock M,** *et al.* Blood loss following tonsillectomy in children. A blind comparison of diclofenac and papaveretum. *Anaesthesia* 1993; **48:** 132–135.

40. **Swift GL, Heneghan M, Williams GT,** *et al.* Effect of ranitidine on gastroduodenal mucosal damage in patients on long-term non-steroidal anti-inflammatory drugs. *Digestion* 1989; **44:** 86–94.

41. **Todd PA, Sorkin EM.** Diclofenac sodium. A reappraisal of its pharmacodynamic and pharmacokinetic properties, and therapeutic effect. *Drugs* 1988; **35:** 244–285.

42. **McCafferty DF, Woolfson AD.** New patch delivery system for percutaneous local anaesthesia. *Br. J. Anaesth.* 1993; **71:** 370–374.

43. **MacKenzie IZ, Fry A.** Prostaglandin E_2 pessaries facilitate first trimester aspiration termination. *Br. J. Obstet. Gynaecol.* 1981; **88:** 1033–1037.

CHAPTER 5

General anaesthesia for adult day surgery

J.M. Millar

Good general anaesthesia is fundamental to the success and feasibility of much of day surgery practice. The impact of anaesthetic side-effects may be disproportionate to the invasiveness of the procedure, and this may be a limiting factor in expanding day surgery. The move to increasing day surgery, with longer and more complex operations, depends on patients being fit to go home after the procedure. The popularity of day surgery is not increased by patients who feel unwell after discharge and who may have to contact their general practitioner (GP). Patient satisfaction is an increasingly important issue for anaesthetists[1].

How can we judge the best day surgery anaesthetic?

The outcomes on which the ideal general anaesthetic for day surgery may be judged are often difficult to define and measure (*Table 5.1*). Rapid immediate recovery may not equate with good outcome later on, although the length of time spent in the recovery room is important if it means that throughput is slowed down or more nurses are needed[2]. Time spent in first-stage recovery may be related more to PONV and/or pain, rather than to slow wake up[3]. Postoperative nausea and vomiting (PONV) and other morbidity such as dizziness and sleepiness are important measures, as these increase time to discharge[4], and the rates of overnight admission and re-admission[5,6].

Table 5.1. Outcome measures of day surgery anaesthesia

Immediate recovery – time to eye opening, date of birth, etc.
Time spent in first-stage recovery/recovery room/PACU
Incidence of PONV
Other postoperative morbidity (pre- and postdischarge)
Time to discharge
Unplanned overnight admission and re-admission
The ability to carry out longer or more major day case surgery
Patient satisfaction
Return to normal activity
Cost effectiveness

PACU, postanaesthesia care unit.

Even time to discharge may not be an accurate measure of anaesthetic outcome, as it can be affected by other factors, such as surgical complications or time for escorts to arrive[7]. Furthermore, discharge criteria may be observer-dependent and subjective, so patients may not be sent home in comparable states of recovery in different studies.

Patient satisfaction and longer-term recovery are more difficult to assess and cost. In general, patient satisfaction is high after day surgery[8,9], but designing questionnaires which evaluate this accurately is difficult[1,10].

Although the cost of the anaesthetic agents is important, in terms of the overall cost of the day surgery stay, the amounts involved are small. Provided that improved outcome can be demonstrated[11], and that drugs are used with good indications, there may be little to gain from a reduction in the anaesthetic budget at an increased cost to the DSU or hospital as a whole[12,13]. Methods available to cost the outcomes of day surgery are not yet sufficiently sophisticated or accurate, whereas it is easy to calculate the price of anaesthetic drugs.

The interpretation of what is the ideal anaesthetic for day surgery therefore depends on the value placed on the different outcomes. For example, studies showing significant differences in PONV between two different anaesthetic techniques assessed both techniques as being equally suitable for day surgery[14–16]. This makes a judgement that PONV, which distresses patients[17], is not important in the selection of an anaesthetic technique for day surgery, an opinion which should not be accepted.

> *Quality of recovery is more important than speed of recovery. An anaesthetic technique may be subjectively or objectively assessed depending on the value assigned to a particular outcome measure.*

The ideal anaesthetic for day surgery

The qualities of the ideal anaesthetic for day surgery are given in *Table 5.2*. The individual drugs used for induction, maintenance, analgesia and muscle relaxation, and their effects in combination, need to be considered. The role of IV fluids may also be important.

Table 5.2. The ideal day surgery anaesthetic

Overall safety with little cardiovascular and respiratory depression
Rapid, smooth induction
Good operating conditions
Fast turnover facilitated
Rapid immediate recovery, allowing shortened recovery room stays
Low rates of PONV
Low rates of other postoperative morbidity – especially dizziness or sleepiness
Rapid return to normal psychomotor state with minimal hangover effect
Reliable and prompt discharge home

Induction agents

Propofol

Propofol has established itself as the intravenous induction agent of choice[18,19] in day surgery, because of its ease of use and rapid, clear-headed recovery with few side-effects. In short procedures, where recovery may be less influenced by the choice of maintenance agent, propofol has been shown to have a low incidence of postoperative morbidity, especially PONV, and shorten time to street fitness and discharge when compared with thiopentone and enflurane[20] or with methohexitone[21].

Patients have reported improved subjective recovery for up to 24 hours postoperatively after propofol when compared with thiopentone–enflurane[20] or thiopentone alone[22]. This is confirmed by other studies where patients assessed the quality of their recovery. In the study of Jakobssen *et al.*[23], propofol–fentanyl anaesthetics were considered by patients to offer the best quality of recovery compared with thiopentone or methohexitone with fentanyl or propofol in combination with ketamine[23].

Prevention of pain on injection with propofol
Propofol may cause quite severe pain on injection, particularly if small veins or slow speed of injection are used[24]. A variety of strategies for reducing this have been tried[24–27] (*Table 5.3*). The only methods that have abolished pain completely are the use of the antecubital vein[24] and the addition of 2 ml lignocaine 2% (40 mg) to propofol 200 mg[25]. The stability of the propofol emulsion has been shown to be affected by adding more than 20 mg lignocaine to 200 mg propofol and by delay between mixing and administration[28]. This is not known to cause problems in practice.

Table 5.3. Strategies for reducing pain on injection with propofol

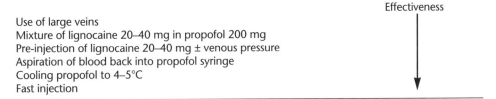

	Effectiveness
Use of large veins	
Mixture of lignocaine 20–40 mg in propofol 200 mg	
Pre-injection of lignocaine 20–40 mg ± venous pressure	
Aspiration of blood back into propofol syringe	
Cooling propofol to 4–5°C	
Fast injection	

However, these methods may be inappropriate if propofol is administered by syringe driver as part of an infusion technique. Pre-treatment with 2 ml lignocaine 2% plus temporary venous occlusion was not significantly different from mixing it with propofol in the study of Johnson *et al.*[25], so using it as a pre-injection or to prime the infusion line, combined with venous pressure, may be a satisfactory alternative.

> *Lignocaine 20–40 mg, either added to propofol 200 mg just before injection, or pre-injected before propofol, deals with pain on injection satisfactorily.*

Propofol and epilepsy
The relationship of propofol to postoperative convulsions, and its use in epileptic patients, remains unclear. By 1992, the Committee for the Safety of Medicines had received 170 reports of convulsions or involuntary movements after propofol[29]. The situation is confused by propofol's ability to produce cortical depression and an isoelectric EEG[30], reports of its success in treating refractory status epilepticus[31] and its reduction of seizure duration in electroconvulsive therapy[32]. Epileptiform activity in epileptic patients monitored by electroencephalography was not triggered by propofol[33,34].

> *Cochran* et al. *have commented that it seems sensible to avoid the use of propofol in patients who are known to be at risk of developing seizures, but who are on no preventative treatment, or where epilepsy is poorly controlled, or where anticonvulsant medication has been omitted[35].*

Co-induction

The combination of different induction agents, usually midazolam with propofol, is termed co-induction. The aim may be to improve haemodynamic stability, to reduce the amount of propofol used or to produce sedation or amnesia.

As a sole induction agent, midazolam has slower recovery than propofol, even when reversed by flumazenil[36]. Small doses (0.03–0.06 mg kg^{-1}) of midazolam given with propofol and alfentanil[37] reduced the propofol required, and did not prolong time to discharge, but immediate recovery was delayed. Larger doses of midazolam delay recovery even more[38].

The benefits of flumazenil to reverse midazolam are short lived, and resedation appears after 60–90 minutes, so early discharge may be inadvisable[39,40].

> *No significant benefits of co-induction in day surgery have been demonstrated, apart from modest savings in propofol usage.*

Maintenance

While the place of propofol for induction is well established, the optimal drug for maintenance of anaesthesia is less well defined, particularly since the introduction of the newer, less soluble, volatile agents, desflurane and sevoflurane (*Table 5.4*).

Table 5.4. Characteristics of volatile agents used in day surgery in adults

	Blood/gas coefficient	MAC in $O_2 \pm$ air (%)
Desflurane	0.42	6
Sevoflurane	0.63	2
Isoflurane	1.46	1.2
Enflurane	1.90	1.6
Halothane	2.4	0.75

Adapted from Jones[41].
MAC, minimal alveolar concentration.

Halothane

Although cheap, this has virtually disappeared from day surgery practice, due to its prolonged recovery[42] and anxiety about its hepatotoxic effects[43]. Sevoflurane is likely to replace it for gaseous induction in children[44].

Enflurane and isoflurane

These give faster recovery than halothane[42,45,46]. However, there may be little to choose between enflurane and isoflurane in terms of speed of recovery and incidence of PONV[38,47–50]. Of the two, enflurane may be preferable[47,48].

Desflurane

This is the volatile agent with the lowest solubility and fastest immediate recovery time, but time to discharge and PONV are similar to isoflurane[51] or sevoflurane[52]. Desflurane's pungency may cause coughing, salivation and laryngospasm[15], making smooth anaesthesia difficult in unpremedicated, spontaneously breathing patients. Mood scores were better after isoflurane than desflurane[53] and a high incidence of emergence delirium has been reported[54]. These characteristics, together with PONV[55], may detract from the predicted popularity of desflurane for day surgery.

Sevoflurane

This is a more clinically acceptable volatile agent. It is well tolerated even at light levels of anaesthesia and may even be used for gaseous induction in adults[56,57]. Despite rapid early recovery, it has not been shown to reduce time to discharge after laparoscopy compared with isoflurane[6], and its incidence of PONV is similar to that of isoflurane[58]. Compared with desflurane, its early recovery is slightly slower[52].

The main disadvantage of volatile agents in day surgery is the incidence of PONV, which is similar for all the current volatile agents[6,51–53]. This has a greater effect on the quality of recovery than small improvements in wake up times, and it may delay or prevent discharge[6,59]. Neither desflurane nor sevoflurane has been demonstrated to shorten time to discharge compared with isoflurane or propofol maintenance. Both are expensive.

> *All currently available volatile anaesthetic agents have similar levels of PONV which affect quality of recovery more than small differences in wake up times.*

Propofol maintenance

Unlike other induction agents[60], propofol is suitable for maintenance of anaesthesia (*Table 5.5*). This is discussed in Chapter 7.

Table 5.5. Propofol maintenance in day surgery

Advantages	Possible limitations
Good intraoperative control	Worries about awareness
No risk of malignant hyperpyrexia	Interpatient variability of blood level
Reduction of PONV	Equipment – syringe pumps, etc.
Patients feel better	Infection if asepsis not maintained
Faster, more reliable discharge home	Cost

Propofol is considered to be antiemetic[61,62], but its beneficial effects on PONV may be lost or reduced by using volatile agents for maintenance in long procedures[16]. When enflurane or halothane were used for maintenance in longer operations, no difference could be found in recovery with propofol induction compared with methohexitone[63] or thiopentone[16,64]. However, after day case oral surgery procedures lasting 2–4 hours, recovery was improved, with less PONV and faster discharge, using maintenance with propofol compared with isoflurane[65].

Immediate recovery after enflurane and isoflurane is comparable with propofol maintenance; after desflurane[55,66] and sevoflurane[67], wake-up is similar or slightly faster than propofol. Dexter and Tinker's[68] meta-analysis of times to obeying commands and discharge after desflurane, isoflurane or propofol maintenance showed fastest early recovery with desflurane, and fastest discharge with propofol. Quality of recovery and PONV were not considered.

However, time to discharge is often delayed or prevented by volatile-related PONV[55,59]. In day case laparoscopies[55], desflurane/nitrous oxide maintenance significantly prolonged time to discharge because of its high incidence of PONV (80%) compared with propofol maintenance (20%). The addition of ondansetron 4 mg to the desflurane anaesthetic reduced the incidence of PONV to 40%, and the discharge time to that of propofol, but at increased cost. More patients were admitted overnight in both the desflurane groups.

The benefits of total intravenous anaesthesia (TIVA) may be more difficult to demonstrate in operations and patients where PONV is not common. Propofol and isoflurane were equally suitable for maintenance in out-patient arthroscopy, where no patient in either group had PONV[70].

The good quality of recovery after TIVA may also be due to euphoria and a feeling of well being. No study which has looked for it has failed to find that patients report feeling better after propofol anaesthesia[20,23,71–73].

> *Propofol for both induction <u>and</u> maintenance of anaesthesia improves the quality of recovery, particularly where PONV is common.*

Nitrous oxide

Nitrous oxide is cheap, has analgesic properties and reduces the requirements for other anaesthetics. Its use is controversial. Do patients or operating department personnel suffer from its use and has it any beneficial effects?

Nitrous oxide has been found to increase PONV in some studies[74,75] but not in others[50,76,77]. Two meta-analyses[78,79] have concluded that nitrous oxide *does* increase emesis in susceptible patients and operations associated with PONV.

However, these meta-analyses mainly considered studies using thiopentone/volatile anaesthesia. Studies where propofol was used for induction and/or maintenance of anaesthetic have not shown a significant increase in PONV with nitrous oxide[80,81].

Nitrous oxide has been implicated in adverse effects in theatre personnel, but the only prospective study[82] has not reported a significant occupational health risk associated with the use of inhalation anaesthetics[83]. Despite significant anaesthetic pollution, Stollery *et al.* were unable to demonstrate any psychomotor impairment in anaesthetists working in theatre[84].

Omitting nitrous oxide increases the doses of other anaesthetic drugs used[85], and this may increase side-effects and cost. It also makes the anaesthetic more difficult to control[86]. Tramer *et al.*[79] considered that the risk of awareness under anaesthesia outweighed the benefits of omitting nitrous oxide.

> *Nitrous oxide reduces the risk of awareness, and the amount and cost of other anaesthetic drugs required. PONV may not be increased if it is used with propofol for maintenance of anaesthesia.*

Perioperative opioids

Morphine

In day surgery morphine is accompanied by unacceptable levels of emesis, sedation, delay in discharge and unplanned overnight admission[87–91]. Its long duration outlasts the antiemetic effects of propofol, so that PONV may increase later in recovery[62,72,92] (see also Chapter 9).

Alfentanil and fentanyl

In contrast, these shorter-acting opioids may improve recovery by reducing propofol requirements and providing intraoperative analgesia without increasing PONV[20,93,94], although this has been disputed[95,96]. Alfentanil and fentanyl increased PONV when used with thiopentone, despite the inclusion of droperidol[97].

Various studies have compared the addition of alfentanil (7–15 μg kg^{-1}) or fentanyl (0.75–1.5 μg kg^{-1}) to propofol anaesthesia and there may be little to choose between the two analgesics. Alfentanil has faster onset and may reduce the induction dose of propofol more, but the analgesic effects of fentanyl may be longer lasting[93].

Alfentanil infusions have been used with propofol for TIVA, but large doses of alfentanil may be inappropriate for day surgery[98–100].

Remifentanil

This new ultra-short-acting opioid has yet to be evaluated in day surgery. Its speed of onset is similar to that of alfentanil and its potency similar to fentanyl. Recovery is rapid because of its breakdown by blood and tissue esterases, so infusion is needed[101]. Concerns remain about its short-lived postoperative analgesia[102].

Muscle relaxants

The need for muscle relaxants has been greatly reduced by the introduction of the laryngeal mask airway (LMA) which is discussed in Chapter 6, but they still have a place in day surgery. The ideal neuromuscular blocking agent would have rapid onset and short duration, and would preferably not require reversal with neostigmine (*Table 5.6*). The newer, non-depolarizing muscle relaxants have gone some way to meet this ideal, but at a financial cost which may not be reflected in the outcome to the patient. An extra minute taken to intubate is probably unimportant in overall patient care.

Table 5.6. The ideal day surgery neuromuscular blocking agent

Minimal risk of anaphylaxis, morbidity and mortality
Rapid onset
Short duration
No necessity to reverse
Or easily reversed after short time interval
Inexpensive

Suxamethonium

Suxamethonium should be avoided wherever possible. It carries serious risks of anaphylaxis (44% of all anaesthetic-related anaphylaxis[103]), prolonged apnoea due to pseudocholinesterase deficiency and malignant hyperpyrexia. However, its major disadvantage in day surgery is postoperative myalgia, which is worse in young, ambulant female patients[104]. This appears the day after surgery and may be disregarded by anaesthetists, but not by patients. Compared with alfentanil used to facilitate intubation[105], suxamethonium greatly increased the incidence and severity of muscle pain. However, muscle pain may still occur after laparoscopy, even if no suxamethonium has been given[106].

Pre-treatment with non-depolarizing neuromuscular blockers is unreliable and not totally effective in reducing muscle pain[107,108]. Pretreatment with oral aspirin[109] or IM diclofenac[110] has been shown to reduce, but not abolish, the incidence and severity.

With shorter-acting and safer non-depolarizing muscle relaxants now available, the only indication for suxamethonium in day surgery is the patient at risk of acid aspiration because of hiatus hernia or symptomatic gastric reflux. Even this may be challenged, as rapid sequence intubation may be as fast with rocuronium, the non-depolarizing agent with the fastest onset.

Rocuronium 0.6 mg kg^{-1} with thiopentone or propofol gave intubating conditions comparable with suxamethonium when alfentanil 20 µg kg^{-1} was included as part of the induction technique[111], and fewer maintenance boluses were needed[112]. Because of suxamethonium's short duration, repeated boluses which may cause bradycardia may be required, or a non-depolarizing muscle relaxant may be used subsequently. There seems little point in incurring the risks of suxamethonium when intubating conditions are similar with a non-depolarizing agent which may be required anyway. Suxamethonium will continue to have a place for rapid intubation in emergency situations, however.

> *In day cases, suxamethonium should be reserved for those patients who have a significant risk of acid reflux and aspiration, or for emergency situations.*

Non-depolarizing neuromuscular blocking agents

The older, non-depolarizing muscle relaxants, tubocurare, alcuronium and pancuronium, are inappropriate for day surgery because of their slow onset, long duration and side-effects. If a muscle relaxant is necessary, the choice is between the newer neuromuscular blockers (*Table 5.7*).

Table 5.7. Suitable neuromuscular agents for day surgery

Atracurium:	slower onset, may not need reversal, histamine release
Cisatracurium:	similar to atracurium, but less histamine release
Vecuronium:	slower onset and longer duration, lower dose (0.6 mg kg^{-1}) may be satisfactory for shorter procedures
Mivacurium:	slower inset but short duration, may not need reversal
Rocuronium:	fast onset, duration similar to vecuronium, expensive

Atracurium. This has an onset time of 2–3 minutes, which may be reduced by increasing the dose. After 35–45 minutes, it may not need reversal with neostigmine, but it can be difficult to reverse after shorter operations[113]. **Cisatracurium** is similar in action to atracurium but has less histamine release[114]. It has not been studied in day case patients.

Vecuronium. This is slightly slower in onset than atracurium, and although its duration is longer, clinically it can prove easier to reverse after short procedures. In low doses for laparoscopy, vecuronium 0.06 mg kg^{-1} and atracurium 0.3 mg kg^{-1} provided similar intubating conditions but neuromuscular recovery was faster with vecuronium[113]. Other studies have shown little difference between vecuronium and atracurium in day case laparoscopies using these doses[115,116].

Bradycardia has been associated with vecuronium[117], and, to a lesser extent, atracurium, used for operations with vagal stimulation, such as laparoscopy[115]. Routine glycopyrrolate seems to be effective[118] and should be considered when these drugs are used in situations where vagal stimulation can be expected.

Mivacurium. This is slower in onset, but is destroyed by plasma cholinesterases so has a short action which may not need reversal[112], although residual block has been reported where reversal was not used[119]. It was not considered to offer any advantage over suxamethonium in out-patient laparoscopies[120].

Rocuronium. This is currently the non-depolarizing agent with the shortest onset of action[121]. A dose of 0.6 mg kg^{-1} seems to offer reasonably fast intubating conditions without long duration of action. Rocuronium was compared with atracurium and vecuronium for day case dental surgery[122]. Intubating conditions at 60 seconds were better with rocuronium and spontaneous recovery was faster. Intubation within 45 seconds was achieved when doses of 0.9 mg kg^{-1} were given with alfentanil 20 μg kg^{-1} and propofol[123].

Reversal of neuromuscular block

Failure to reverse neuromuscular block, even with mivacurium, may result in residual block[119]. However, glycopyrrolate/neostigmine mixture has been implicated in increasing PONV compared with no reversal[124] or with atropine/neostigmine[125].

Glycopyrrolate may be preferable to atropine, to avoid central cholinergic effects. Atropine crosses the blood–brain barrier and may cause short-term memory deficit[126] or delayed arousal[127], which were not seen with glycopyrrolate.

It has been suggested[128,129] that edrophonium may speed reversal of neuromuscular block with non-depolarizing agents, but this has not been confirmed by other studies[130,131]. Reports that it may be associated with less postoperative emesis[124,130] have also not been confirmed[132].

Are muscle relaxants necessary?

Muscle relaxants may be unnecessary if they are required only for intubation, and not for the surgical technique. Alfentanil and propofol gave good or excellent intubating conditions in 86% of patients, provided that sufficient propofol was given to cause jaw relaxation[105]. This was better than propofol alone[133] or with lignocaine[134], which have also been used to intubate without muscle relaxants.

From this, it could be predicted, and seems true in clinical practice, that induction with propofol and short-acting opioids, particularly alfentanil, probably obscures minor differences in onset with muscle relaxants.

If rapid onset is desirable, rocuronium is the best choice; mivacurium has the shortest duration but, in general, if muscle relaxation is needed, vecuronium 0.6 mg kg^{-1} will give satisfactory conditions without the histamine release of atracurium. For day surgery, smaller doses may be sufficient, particularly with propofol and alfentanil, and may shorten its duration of action[122,135].

> *Expensive new muscle relaxants are difficult to justify. Small differences in speed of onset or offset may make little clinical difference.*

Intravenous fluids in day surgery

The routine administration IV fluids in day surgery is controversial and it is common practice to omit them for minor procedures.

In patients having minor operations who were anaesthetized with thiopentone and halothane[136], 2 litres IV reduced drowsiness, dizziness, headache and thirst, and, subjectively, these patients felt better, especially if they had experienced anaesthetic

Table 5.8. Planning the anaesthetic for adult day surgery

	Consider
Premedication	
Anxious patient?	Temazepam premedication
Obese or pregnant	
Symptomatic reflux	Ranitidine ± metoclopramide PO
Laparoscopy	
Analgesia	
Painful operation?	NSAID – PO premedication or IV/PR intraoperatively
	Local/regional analgesia if possible
Induction	
Induction agent	Propofol usually
Opioid	
short procedure?	Alfentanil
longer/more painful procedure?	Fentanyl
Airway	
Intubation not needed	LMA or face mask
Rapid sequence – acid aspiration risk	Suxamethonium
Fast onset	Rocuronium
Short action	Mivacurium
Otherwise, cheap and satisfactory	Vecuronium 0.6 mg kg^{-1}
Reversal if needed	Neostigmine + glycopyrrolate
Maintenance	
Patient with history of PONV	Propofol maintenance
Procedure associated with PONV	? omit N_2O
Long procedure	IV fluids
Otherwise	
cheap, longer immediate recovery	Enflurane or isoflurane
expensive, faster immediate recovery but same incidence of PONV	Desflurane or sevoflurane

recovery problems previously. However, this study used an anaesthetic which would not be the first choice for day surgery now.

With propofol alone, or with isoflurane or enflurane, improvements in recovery with IV fluids may be more difficult to demonstrate, particularly in short procedures lasting less than 20 minutes[137–139], where only modest benefits, if any, could be shown.

However, in patients given propofol and isoflurane anaesthesia for mainly minor gynaecological surgery lasting 30 minutes, Yogendran *et al.*[140] did report less thirst, drowsiness, dizziness and nausea after 20 ml kg^{-1} isotonic electrolyte solution IV, although time to discharge was not shortened. They concluded that fluids were beneficial in reducing postoperative morbidity.

IV fluids may be less important if preoperative fluid fasting is reduced as is currently recommended. However, although drinking 150–1000 ml clear fluids 1.5–2.5 hours preoperatively did not increase the risk of acid aspiration, neither did it appear to have a major effect on recovery from short operations[141,142].

There may be advantages in giving IV fluids to patients having longer or more invasive procedures such as laparoscopy, or to those who have been fluid restricted for long periods, or in hot weather. Reduction of thirst may be useful if it reduces the need for early oral fluids, which can provoke vomiting.

> *IV fluids may be useful in reducing postoperative morbidity. They are inexpensive and should be considered for more invasive or prolonged day surgery procedures.*

Choosing the best anaesthetic for day surgery

All the issues discussed above need to be considered in planning the anaesthetic for day surgery for a particular patient or a particular operation. Combining different drugs may result in a better outcome than after one drug alone. The factors influencing decisions are outlined in *Table 5.8*. Although cost effectiveness is important, the cost and inconvenience of a poor recovery may greatly exceed the price of the anaesthetic drugs.

> *Planning the anaesthetic by considering the requirements of the patient and the operation, and selecting best available drugs to achieve this, improves the quality of recovery and outcome after day surgery.*

References

1. **Klock PA, Roizen MF.** More or better – educating the patient about the anesthesiologists's role as perioperative physician. *Anesth. Analg.* 1996; **83:** 671–672.
2. **Marais ML, Maher MW, Wetchler BW, et al.** Reduced demands on recovery room resources with propofol (Diprivan) compared with thiopental–isoflurane. *Anesthesiol. Rev.* 1989; **16:** 29–40.
3. **Twersky RS, Lebovits AH, Lewis M, et al.** Early anesthesia evaluation of the ambulatory surgical patient: does it really help? *J. Clin. Anesth.* 1992; **4:** 204–207.
4. **Cardosa M, Rudkin GE, Osborne GA.** Outcome from day-case knee arthroscopy in a major teaching hospital. *Arthroscopy* 1994; **10:** 624–629.
5. **Ramon C, Pelegri D, Turon E, et al.** [Selection criteria used in 1,310 patients in ambulatory major surgery.] *Rev. Esp. Anesthesiol. Reanim.* 1993; **40:** 234–237.
6. **Eriksson H, Haasio J, Korttila K.** Recovery from sevoflurane and isoflurane anaesthesia after outpatient gynaecological laparoscopy. *Acta Anaesthesiol. Scand.* 1995; **39:** 377–380.
7. **Chung F.** Recovery pattern and home-readiness after ambulatory surgery. *Anesth. Analg.* 1995; **80:** 896–902.
8. **Philip BK.** Patients' assessment of ambulatory anesthesia and surgery. *J. Clin. Anesth.* 1992; **4:** 355–358.
9. **Osborne GA, Rudkin GE.** Outcome after day-care surgery in a major teaching hospital. *Anaesth. Intens. Care* 1993; **21:** 822–827.
10. **Cohen G, Forbes J, Garraway M.** Can different patient satisfaction survey methods yield consistent results? Comparison of three surveys. *Br. Med. J.* 1996; **313:** 841–844.
11. **Wetchler BV.** Economic impact of anesthesia decision making; they pay the money, we make the choice. *J. Clin. Anesth.* 1992; **4:** 20S–24S.
12. **Hitchcock M, Rudkin GE.** The real cost of total intravenous anaesthesia: cost versus price. *Ambulatory Surg.* 1995; **3:** 43–48.
13. **Sung Y-F, Reiss N, Tillette T.** The differential cost of anesthesia and recovery with propofol–nitrous oxide anesthesia versus thiopental sodium–isoflurane–nitrous oxide anesthesia. *J. Clin. Anesth.* 1991; **3:** 391–394.
14. **Rapp SE, Conhan TJ, Pavlin DJ, et al.** Comparison of desflurane with propofol on outpatients undergoing orthopedic surgery. *Anesth. Analg.* 1992; **75:** 572–579.
15. **Lebenbom-Mansour MH, Pandit SH, Kothary SP, et al.** Desflurane versus propofol anesthesia: a comparative analysis in outpatients. *Anesth. Analg.* 1993; **76:** 936–941.
16. **Ding Y, Fredman B, White PF.** Recovery following outpatient anesthesia: use of enflurane versus propofol. *J. Clin. Anesth.* 1993; **5:** 447–450.

17. **Orkin F.** What do patients want? – Preferences for immediate postoperative recovery. *Anesth. Analg.* 1992; **74:** S225.

18. **White PF.** Studies of desflurane in outpatient anesthesia. *Anesth. Analg.* 1992; **75:** S47–S54.

19. **Heath PJ, Kennedy DJ, Ogg TW,** *et al.* Which induction agent for day surgery? A comparison of propofol, thiopentone, methohexitone and etomidate. *Anaesthesia* 1988; **43:** 365–368.

20. **Millar JM, Jewkes CF.** Recovery and morbidity after day case anaesthesia. A comparison of propofol with thiopentone–enflurane with and without alfentanil. *Anaesthesia* 1988; **43:** 738–743.

21. **Doze VA, Westphal LM, White PF.** Comparison of propofol with methohexital for outpatient anesthesia. *Anesth. Analg.*1986; **65:** 1189–1195.

22. **Sanders LD, Clyburn PA, Rosen M,** *et al.* Propofol in short gynaecological procedures. Comparison of recovery over two days with propofol or thiopentone as sole anaesthetic agent. *Anaesthesia* 1991; **46:** 451–455.

23. **Jakobsson J, Oddby E, Rane K.** Patient evaluation of four different combinations of intravenous anaesthetics for short outpatient procedures. *Anaesthesia* 1993; **48:** 1005–1007.

24. **Scott RPF, Saunders DA, Norman J.** Propofol: clinical strategies for preventing the pain of injection. *Anaesthesia* 1988; **43:** 492–494.

25. **Johnson RA, Harper NJN, Chadwick S,** *et al.* Pain on injection of propofol. Methods of alleviation. *Anaesthesia* 1990; **45:** 439–442.

26. **McCirrick A, Hunter S.** Pain on injection: the effect of injectate temperature. *Anaesthesia* 1990; **45:** 434–444.

27. **McDonald DS, Jameson P.** Injection pain with propofol. Reduction with aspiration of blood. *Anaesthesia* 1996; **51:** 878–880.

28. **Lilley EMM, Isert PR, Carasso ML,** *et al.* The effect of the addition of lignocaine on propofol emulsion stability. *Anaesthesia* 1996; **51:** 815–818.

29. **The Committee on Safety of Medicines.** Propofol and delayed convulsions. *Current Problems* 1992; **35:** 2.

30. **Smith M, Smith SJ, Scott CA,** *et al.* Activation of the electrocorticogram by propofol during surgery for epilepsy. *Br. J. Anaesth.* 1996; **76:** 499–502.

31. **Mackenzie SJ, Kapadia F, Grant IS.** Propofol infusion for control of status epilepticus. *Anaesthesia* 1990; **45:** 1043–1045.

32. **Avramov MN, Huain MM, White PF.** The comparative effects of methohexital, propofol, and etomidate, for electroconvulsive therapy. *Anesth. Analg.* 1995; **81:** 596–602.

33. **Ebrahim ZY, Schubert A, Van Ness P,** *et al.* The effect of propofol on the electroencephalogram of patients with epilepsy. *Anesth. Analg.* 1994; **78:** 275–279.

34. **Cheng MA, Tempelhoff R, Silbergeld DL,** *et al.* Large-dose propofol alone in adult epileptic patients: electrocorticographic results. *Anesth. Analg.* 1996; **83:** 169–174.

35. **Cochran D, Price W, Gwinnutt CL.** Unilateral convulsion after induction of anaesthesia with propofol. *Br. J. Anaesth.* 1996; **76:** 570–572.

36. **Norton AC, Dundas CR.** Induction agents for day-case anaesthesia. A double blind comparison of propofol and midazolam antagonised by flumazenil. *Anaesthesia* 1990; **45:** 198–203.

37. **Elwood T, Huchcroft S, MacAdams C.** Midazolam coinduction does not delay discharge after very brief propofol anaesthesia. *Can. J. Anaesth.* 1995; **42:** 114–118.

38. **Shultz RE, Richardson DD, Nespeca JA.** Comparison of recovery times of isoflurane and enflurane as a sole anesthetic agent for outpatient oral surgery. *Anesth. Prog.* 1989; **36:** 13–14.

39. **Ghouri AF, Ruiz MA, White PF.** Effect of flumazenil on recovery after midazolam and propofol sedation. *Anesthesiology* 1994; **81:** 333–339.

40. **Philip BK, Simpson TH, Hauch MA,** *et al.* Flumazenil reverses sedation after midazolam induced general anaesthesia in ambulatory surgery patients. *Anesth. Analg.* 1990; **71:** 371–376.

41. **Jones RM.** Desflurane and sevoflurane: inhalation anaesthetics for this decade? *Br. J. Anaesth.* 1990; **65:** 527–536.

42. **Storms LH, Stark AH, Calverley RK,** *et al.* Psychological functioning after halothane or enflurane anesthesia. *Anesth. Analg.* 1980; **59:** 245–249.

43. **Inman WH, Mushin WW.** Jaundice after repeated exposure to halothane: a further analysis of reports to the Committee on Safety of Medicines. *Br. Med. J.* 1978; **2:** 1455–1456.

44. **Black A, Sury MRJ, Hemington L,** *et al.* A comparison of the induction characteristics of sevoflurane and halothane in children. *Anaesthesia* 1996; **51:** 539–542.

45. **Stanford BJ, Plantevin OM, Gilbert JR.** Morbidity after day case gynaecological surgery. Comparison of enflurane with halothane. *Br. J. Anaesth.* 1979; **51:** 1143–1145.
46. **Davison LA, Steinhelber JC, Eger EI,** *et al.* Psychological effects of halothane and isoflurane anesthesia. *Anesthesiology* 1975; **43:** 313–324.
47. **Tracey JA, Holland AJC, Unger L.** Morbidity in minor gynaecological surgery: a comparision of halothane, enflurane and isoflurane. *Br. J. Anaesth.* 1982; **54:** 1213–1215.
48. **Carter JA, Dye AM, Cooper GM.** Recovery from day-case anaesthesia. The effect of different anaesthetic agents. *Anaesthesia* 1985; **40:** 545–548.
49. **Hovorka J, Korttila K, Erkola O.** Nausea and vomiting after general anaesthesia with isoflurane, enflurane or fentanyl in combination with nitrous oxide and oxygen. *Eur. J. Anaesthesiol.* 1988; **5:** 177–182.
50. **Muir JJ, Warner MA, Offord KP,** *et al.* Role of nitrous oxide and other factors in postoperative nausea and vomiting: a randomized and blinded prosective study. *Anesthesiology* 1987; **66:** 513–518.
51. **Ghouri AF, Bodner M, White PF.** Recovery profile after desflurane–nitrous oxide versus isoflurane–nitrous oxide in outpatients. *Anesthesiology* 1991; **74:** 419–424.
52. **Nathanson MH, Fredman B, Smith I,** *et al.* Sevoflurane versus desflurane for outpatient anesthesia: a comparison of maintenance and recovery profiles. *Anesth. Analg.* 1995; **81:** 1186–1190.
53. **Gupta A, Kullander M, Ekberg K,** *et al.* Anaesthesia for day care arthroscopy – a comparison between desflurane and isoflurane. *Anaesthesia* 1996; **51:** 56–62.
54. **Davis PJ, Cohen IT, McGowan FX,** *et al.* Recovery characteristics of desflurane versus halothane for maintenance of anesthesia in pediatric ambulatory patients. *Anesthesiology* 1994; **80:** 298–302.
55. **Eriksson H, Korttila K.** Recovery profile after desflurane with or without ondansetron compared with propofol in patients undergoing outpatient gynaecological laparoscopy. *Anesth. Analg.* 1996; **82:** 533–538.
56. **Sloan MH, Conard PF, Karsunky PK,** *et al.* Sevoflurane versus isoflurane: induction and recovery characteristics with single-breath inhaled inductions of anesthesia. *Anesth. Analg.* 1996; **82:** 528–532.
57. **Yurino M, Kimura H.** Vital capacity rapid inhalational induction technique: comparison of sevoflurane and halothane. *Can. J. Anaesth.* 1993; **40:** 440–443.
58. **Frink EJ, Malan TP, Atlas M,** *et al.* Clinical comparison of sevoflurane and isoflurane in healthy patients. *Anesth. Analg.* 1992; **74:** 241–245.
59. **Raftery S, Sherry E.** Total intravenous anaesthesia with propofol and alfentanil protects against postoperative nausea and vomiting. *Can. J. Anaesth.* 1992; **39:** 37–40.
60. **Kashtan H, Edelist G, Mallon J,** *et al.* Comparative evaluation of propofol and thiopentone for total intravenous anaesthesia. *Can. J. Anaesth.* 1990; **37:** 170–176.
61. **Borgeat A, Wilder-Smith OHG, Saiah M,** *et al.* Subhypnotic doses of propofol possess direct antiemetic properties. *Anesth. Analg.* 1992; **74:** 539–541.
62. **McCollum JSC, Milligan KR, Dundee JW.** The antiemetic effect of propofol. *Anaesthesia* 1988; **43:** 239–240.
63. **Valanne J, Korttila K.** Comparison of methohexitone and propofol (Diprivan) for induction of enflurane anaesthesia in outpatients. *Postgrad. Med. J.* 1985; **61:** 138–143.
64. **Sanders LD, Isaac PA, Yeomans WA,** *et al.* Propofol induced anaesthesia. Double blind comparison of recovery after anaesthesia induced by propofol or thiopentone. *Anaesthesia* 1989; **44:** 200–204.
65. **Valanne J.** Recovery and discharge of patients after long propofol infusion vs isoflurane anaesthesia for ambulatory surgery. *Acta Anaesthesiol. Scand.* 1992; **36:** 530–533.
66. **Van Hemelrijck J, Smith I, White PF.** Use of desflurane for outpatient anesthesia. *Anesthesiology* 1991; **75:** 197–203.
67. **Fredman B, Nathanson MH, Smith I,** *et al.* Sevoflurane for outpatient anesthesia: a comparison with propofol. *Anesth. Analg.* 1995; **81:** 823–828.
68. **Dexter F, Tinker JH.** Comparisons between desflurane and isoflurane or propofol on time to following commands and time to discharge. A meta-analysis. *Anesthesiology* 1995; **83:** 77–82.
69. **Gan TJ, Ginsberg B, Grant AP,** *et al.* Double-blind, randomized comparison of ondansetron and intraoperative propofol to prevent postoperative nausea and vomiting. *Anesthesiology* 1996; **85:** 1036–1042.
70. **Zuurmond WWA, Van Leeuwen L, Helmers JHJH.** Recovery from propofol infusion as the main agent for outpatient arthroscopy. *Anaesthesia* 1987; **42:** 356–359.

71. **Korttila K, Ostman PL, Faure E,** *et al.* Randomised comparison of outcome after propofol–nitrous oxide or enflurane–nitrous oxide in operations of long duration. *Can. J. Anaesth.* 1989; **36:** 651–657.

72. **Marshall CA, Jones RM, Bajorek PK,** *et al.* Recovery characteristics using isoflurane or propofol for maintenance of anaesthesia. *Anaesthesia* 1992; **47:** 461–466.

73. **Kalman SH, Jensen AG, Ekberg K,** *et al.* Early and late recovery after major abdominal surgery. Comparison between propofol anaesthesia with and without nitrous oxide and isoflurane anaesthesia. *Acta Anaesthiol. Scand.* 1993; **37:** 730–736.

74. **Lonie DS, Harper NJN.** Nitrous oxide anaesthesia and vomiting. The effect of nitrous oxide on the incidence of vomiting following gynaecological laparoscopy. *Anaesthesia* 1986; **41:** 703–707.

75. **Alexander G, Skupski JN, Brown EM.** The role of nitrous oxide in postoperative nausea and vomiting. *Anesth. Analg.* 1984; **63:** 175.

76. **Jensen AG, Prevedoros H, Kullman E,** *et al.* Peroperative nitrous oxide does not influence recovery after laparoscopic cholecystectomy. *Acta Anaesthesiol. Scand.* 1993; **37:** 683–686.

77. **Taylor E, Feinstein R, White PF,** *et al.* Anesthesia for laparoscopic cholecystectomy. Is nitrous oxide contraindicated? *Anesthesiology* 1992; **76:** 541–543.

78. **Hartung J.** Twenty four of twenty seven studies show a greater incidence of emesis associated with nitrous oxide than with alternative anesthetics. *Anesth. Analg.* 1996; **83:** 114–116.

79. **Tramer M, Moore A, McQuay H.** Omitting nitrous oxide in general anaesthesia: meta-analysis of intraoperative awareness and postoperative emesis in randomized controlled trials. *Br. J. Anaesth.* 1996; **76:** 186–193.

80. **Sukhani R, Lurie J, Jabamoni R.** Propofol for ambulatory gynecologic laparoscopy: does omission of nitrous oxide alter postoperative sequelae and recovery? *Anesth. Analg.* 1994; **78:** 831–835.

81. **Sengupta P, Plantevin OM.** Nitrous oxide and day case laparoscopy: effects on nausea, vomiting and return to normal activity. *Br. J. Anaesth.* 1988; **60:** 570–573.

82. **Spence AA.** Environmental pollution by inhalation anaesthetics. *Br. J. Anaesth.* 1987; **59:** 96–103.

83. **Halsey MJ.** (1996) Occupational exposure to inhalation anaesthetics. In: *Anaesthesia Rounds.* The Medicine Group (Education) Ltd, Abingdon, Oxon, UK; for Zeneca Pharmaceticals. p. 5.

84. **Stollery BT, Broadbent DE, Lee WR,** *et al.* Mood and cognitive functions in anaesthetists working in actively scavenged operating theatres. *Br. J. Anaesth.* 1988; **61:** 446–455.

85. **Davidson JAH, Macleod AD, Howie JC,** *et al.* Effective concentration 50 for propofol with and without 67% nitrous oxide. *Acta Anaesthesiol. Scand.* 1993; **37:** 458–464.

86. **de Grood PMRM, Harbers JBM, van Egmond J,** *et al.* Anaesthesia for laparoscopy. A comparison of five techniques including propofol, etomidate, thiopentone and isoflurane. *Anaesthesia* 1987; **42:** 815–823.

87. **Weinstein MS, Nicolson SC, Schreiner MS.** A single dose of morphine sulfate increases the incidence of vomiting after outpatient surgery in children. *Anesthesiology* 1994; **81:** 572–577.

88. **Vijay V, King TA.** Postoperative intramuscular opiates in day surgery. *J. One Day Surg.* 1995; **4:** 6–7.

89. **Cade L, Kakulas P.** Ketorolac or pethidine for analgesia after elective laparoscopic sterilization. *Anaesth. Intens. Care* 1995; **23:** 158–161.

90. **McGuire DA, Sanders K, Hendricks SD.** Comparison of ketorolac and opioid analgesics in postoperative ACL reconstruction outpatient pain control. *Arthroscopy* 1993; **9:** 653–661.

91. **Schofield NM, White JB.** Interrelations among children, parents, premedication, and anaesthetists in paediatric day surgery. *Br. Med. J.* 1989; **299:** 1371–1375.

92. **Oddby-Muhrbeck E, Jakobsson J, Andersson L,** *et al.* Postoperative nausea and vomiting. A comparison between intravenous and inhalation anaesthesia in breast surgery. *Acta Anaesthesiol. Scand.* 1994; **38:** 52–56.

93. **Jakobsson J, Davidson S, Andreen M,** *et al.* Opioid supplementation to propofol anaesthesia for outpatient abortion: a comparison between fentanyl and alfentanil. *Acta Anaesthesiol. Scand.* 1991; **35:** 767–770.

94. **Lindholm P, Helbo-Hansen HS, Jensen B,** *et al.* Effects of fentanyl or alfentanil as supplement to propofol anaesthesia for termination of pregnancy. *Acta Anaesthesiol. Scand.* 1994; **38:** 545–549.

95. **Moffat AC, Murray AW, Fitch W.** Opioid supplementation during propofol anaesthesia. The effects of fentanyl or alfentanil anaesthesia in day case surgery. *Anaesthesia* 1989; **44:** 644–647.

96. **Bagshaw ON, Singh P, Aitkenhead AR.** Alfentanil in day case anaesthesia. Assessment of a single dose on the quality of anaesthesia and recovery. *Anaesthesia* 1993; **48:** 476–481.

97. **White PF, Coe V, Shafer A,** *et al.* Comparison of alfentanil with fentanyl for outpatient anaesthesia. *Anesthesiology* 1986; **64**: 99–106.

98. **Vuyk J, Hennis PJ, Burm AGL,** *et al.* Comparison of midazolam and propofol in combination with alfentanil for total intravenous anaesthesia. *Anesth. Analg.* 1990; **71**: 645–650.

99. **Roberts FL, Dixon J, Lewis GT,** *et al.* Induction and maintenance of propofol anaesthesia. A manual infusion scheme. *Anaesthesia* 1988; **43** (Suppl.): 14–17.

100. **Shafer SL, Varvel JR.** Pharmacokinetics, pharmacodynamics, and rational opioid selection. *Anesthesiology* 1991; **74**: 53–63.

101. **Glass PSA, Hardman D, Kamiyama Y,** *et al.* Preliminary pharmacokinetics and pharmacodynamics of an ultra-short-acting opioid: remifentanil (G187084B). *Anesth. Analg.* 1993; **77**: 1031–1040.

102. **Dershwitz M, Randel GI, Roscow CE,** *et al.* Initial clinical experience with remifentanil, a new opioid metabolized by esterases. *Anesth. Analg.* 1995; **81**: 619–623.

103. **Laxenaire MC, Moneret-Vautrin DA, Widmer S,** *et al.* [Anesthetics responsible for anaphylactic shock. A French multicenter study.] *Ann. Fr. Anesth. Reanim.* 1990; **9**: 501–506.

104. **Churchill-Davidson HC.** Suxamethonium chloride and muscle pains. *Br. Med. J.* 1954; **74** (i): 74–75.

105. **Alcock R, Peachey T, Lynch M,** *et al.* Comparison of alfentanil with suxamethonium in facilitating nasotracheal intubation in day-case anaesthesia. *Br. J. Anaesth.* 1993; **70**: 34–37.

106. **Zahl K, Apfelbaum JL.** Muscle pain occurs after outpatient laparoscopy despite the substitution of vecuronium for succinylcholine. *Anesthesiology* 1989; **70**: 408–411.

107. **Bennetts FE, Khalil KI.** Reduction of postsuxamethonium pain by pretreatment with four non depolarising agents. *Br. J. Anaesth.* 1981; **53**: 531–535.

108. **Mingus ML, Herlich A, Eisencraft JB.** Attenuation of suxamethonium myalgias. Effect of midazolam and vercuronium. *Anaesthesia* 1990; **45**: 834–837.

109. **McLoughlin C, Nesbitt GA, Howe JP.** Suxamethonium induced myalgia and the effect of pre-operative administration oral aspirin. *Anaesthesia* 1988; **43**: 565–567.

110. **Kahraman S, Ercan S, Aypar U,** *et al.* Effect of preoperative i.m. administration of diclofenac on suxamethonium induced myalgia. *Br. J. Anaesth.* 1993; **71**: 238–241.

111. **Sparr HJ, Giesinger S, Ulmer H,** *et al.* Influence of induction technique on intubating conditions after rocuronium in adults: comparison with rapid sequence induction using thiopentone and suxamethonium. *Br. J. Anaesth.* 1996; **77**: 339–342.

112. **Tang J, Joshi GP, White PF.** Comparison of rocuronium and mivacurium to succinylcholine during outpatient laparoscopic surgery. *Anesth. Analg.* 1996; **82**: 994–998.

113. **Bailey DM, Nicholas AD.** Comparison of atracurium and vecuronium during anaesthesia for laparoscopy. *Br. J. Anaesth.* 1988; **61**: 557–559.

114. **Lepage J-Y, Malinovsky J-M, Malinge M,** *et al.* Pharmacodynamic dose–response and safety study of cisatracurium (51W89) in adult surgical patients during N_2O–O_2–opioid anesthesia. *Anesth. Analg.* 1996; **83**: 823–829.

115. **Raynes MA, Chisholm R, Woolner DF,** *et al.* A clinical comparison of atracurium and vecuronium in women undergoing laparoscopy. *Anaesth. Intens. Care* 1987; **15**: 310–316.

116. **Kong KL, Cooper GM.** Recovery of neuromuscular function and postoperative morbidity following blockade by atracurium, alcuronium and vecuronium. *Anaesthesia* 1988; **43**: 450–453.

117. **Inoue K, el-Banayosy A, Stolarski L,** *et al.* Vecuronium induced bradycardia following induction of anaesthesia with etomidate or thiopentone, with or without fentanyl. *Br. J. Anaesth.* 1988; **60**: 10–17.

118. **Cozanitis DA, Pouttu J, Rosenberg PH.** Bradycardia associated with the use of vecuronium. A comparative study with pancuronium with and without glycopyrronium. *Anaesthesia* 1987; **42**: 192–194.

119. **Bevan DR, Kahwaji R, Ansermino JM,** *et al.* Residual block after mivacurium with or without edrophonium reversal in adults and children. *Anesthesiology* 1996; **84**: 362–367.

120. **Poler SM, Watcha MF, White PF.** Mivacurium as an alternative to succinylcholine during outpatient laparoscopy. *J. Clin. Anaesth.* 1992; **4**: 127–133.

121. **Magorian T, Flannery KB, Miller RD.** Comparison of rocuronium, succinylcholine, and vecuronium for rapid-sequence induction of anesthesia in adult patients. *Anesthesiology* 1993; **80**: 1411–1412.

122. **Chetty MS, Pollard BL, Wilson A,** *et al.* Rocuronium bromide in dental day case surgery – a comparison with atracurium and vecuronium. *Anaesth. Intens. Care* 1996; **24**: 37–41.

123. **Crul JF, Vanbelleghem V, Buyse L, et al.** Rocuronium with alfentanil and propofol allows intubation within 45 seconds. *Eur. J. Anaesthesiol. Suppl.* 1995; **11:** 111–112.

124. **Ding Y, Fredman B, White PF.** Use of mivacurium during laparoscopic surgery: effect of reversal drugs on postoperative recovery. *Anesth. Analg.* 1995; **80:** 450–454.

125. **Salmenperä M, Kuoppamäki R, Salmenperä A.** Do anticholinergic agents affect the occurrence of postoperative nausea? *Acta Anaesthesiol. Scand.* 1992; **36:** 445–448.

126. **Simpson KH, Smith RJ, Davies LF.** Comparison of the effects of atropine and glycopyrrolate on cognitive function following general anaesthesia. *Br. J. Anaesth.* 1987; **59:** 966–969.

127. **Baraka A, Yared JP, Karam AM, et al.** Glycopyrrolate–neostigmine and atropine–neostigmine mixtures affect postanesthetic arousal times differently. *Anesth. Analg.* 1980; **59:** 431–434.

128. **Devcic A, Munshi CA, Gandhi SK, et al.** Antagonism of mivacurium neuromuscular block: neostigmine versus edrophonium. *Anesth. Analg.* 1995; **81:** 1005–1009.

129. **Bevan JC, Tousignant C, Stephenson C, et al.** Dose responses for neostigmine and edrophonium as antagonists of mivacurium in adults and children. *Anesthesiology* 1996; **84:** 354–361.

130. **Watcha MF, Safavi FZ, McCulloch DA, et al.** Effect of antagonism of mivacurium-induced neuromuscular block on postoperative emesis in children. *Anesth. Analg.* 1995; **80:** 713–717.

131. **Naguib M, Abdulatif M, al-Ghamdi A.** Dose–response relationships for edrophonium and neostigmine in antagonism of rocuronium bromide (Org 9426)-induced neuromuscular blockade. *Anesthesiology* 1993; **79:** 739–745.

132. **Huang CH, Wang MJ, Susetio L, et al.** Comparison of the combined effects of atropine and neostigmine with atropine and edrophonium on the occurrence of postoperative nausea and vomiting. *Ma Tsui Hsueh Tsa Chi* 1993; **31:** 113–116.

133. **Keaveny JP, Kneel PJ.** Intubation under induction doses of propofol. *Anaesthesia* 1988; **43** (Suppl.): 80–81.

134. **Mulholland D, Carlisle RJT.** Intubation with propofol augmented with intravenous lignocaine. *Anaesthesia* 1991; **46:** 312–313.

135. **Pearce AC, Williams JP, Jones RM.** Atracurium for short surgical procedures in day patients. *Br. J. Anaesth.* 1984; **56:** 973–976.

136. **Keane PW, Murray PF.** Intravenous fluids in day surgery. Their effect on recovery from anaesthesia. *Anaesthesia* 1986; **41:** 635–637.

137. **Spencer EM.** Intravenous fluids in minor gynaecological surgery. Their effect on postoperative morbidity. *Anaesthesia* 1988; **43:** 1050–1051.

138. **Cook R, Anderson S, Riseborough M, et al.** Intravenous fluid load and recovery. A double-blind comparison in gynaecological patients who had day-case laparoscopy. *Anaesthesia* 1990; **45:** 826–830.

139. **Ooi LG, Goldhill DR, Griffiths A, et al.** I.V. fluids and minor gynaecological surgery: effect on recovery from anaesthesia. *Br. J. Anaesth.* 1992; **68:** 576–579.

140. **Yogendran S, Asokumar B, Cheng DCH, et al.** A prospective randomized double-blinded study of the effect of intravenous fluid therapy on adverse outcomes in outpatient surgery. *Anesth. Analg.* 1995; **80:** 682–686.

141. **Goodwin AP, Rowe WL, Ogg TW, et al.** Oral fluids prior to day surgery. The effect of shortening the pre-operative fluid fast on postoperative morbidity. *Anaesthesia* 1991; **46:** 1066–1068.

142. **Gilbert SS, Easy WR, Fitch WW.** The effect of pre-operative oral fluids on morbidity following anaesthesia for minor surgery. *Anaesthesia* 1995; **50:** 79–81.

CHAPTER 6

The laryngeal mask airway (LMA)

M. Hitchcock

The laryngeal mask airway (LMA) has changed clinical practice in day case anaesthesia, often replacing endotracheal intubation[1]. Since its introduction in 1988, the LMA has gained widespread popularity amongst day case anaesthetists. It is now used more often than endotracheal tubes in modern day surgery units, even in operations that traditionally have been thought to require endotracheal intubation[2].

Sizes and types

As with any innovation, the LMA has undergone a series of developments. It is now available in sizes ranging from 1 to 5. The size of the appropriate LMA is determined by the size of the patient, the patient's weight being a useful guide (*Table 6.1*).

Table 6.1. Suggested size LMA according to patient weight

Size	Patient weight
1	6.5 kg
2	6.5–20 kg
2.5	20–30 kg
3	>30 kg child and adult female
4	Large female and adult male
5	Large adult male

The reinforced LMA

LMAs are also available with a narrower, reinforced tube section which is resistant to kinking. These are commonly used in head and neck, ENT and dental surgery and the prone position.

The intubating LMA

More recently, Kapila *et al.* have published a preliminary assessment of the intubating laryngeal mask airway (ILMA)[3]. This new prototype incorporates a shorter, wider metal stem with a handle, which allows the passage of an endotracheal tube of up to 9 mm. Using this device, the authors found that they were able to successfully intubate the trachea, at the first or second attempt, in 92% of patients. The place of this type of LMA in day surgical practice is yet to be determined.

The new prototype LMA

Brain *et al.* have described the preliminary evaluation of a new prototype LMA (pLMA)[4]. This device incorporates a second trumpet-shaped mask which rests on the upper oesophageal sphincter and a second cuff mounted on the dorsal surface to increase the seal pressure of the glottic mask and provide a firm anchor for the oesophageal mask. This has potential advantages over the standard LMA in terms of isolation of the oesophagus and higher leak pressures. These developments require further assessment.

Advantages of the LMA

The LMA offers a number of advantages to the day case anaesthetist (*Table 6.2*).

Table 6.2. Advantages of the LMA

Quick and easy to insert
Insertion does not require muscle relaxants
Less increase in intraocular pressure
Less coughing on emergence
Less sore throat
Faster turnaround time
Tolerated at light planes of anaesthesia
Allows 'hands-free' anaesthesia
Avoids tracheal intubation where this might be difficult
Less desaturation on emergence

Quick and easy to insert

Compared with the endotracheal tube, the insertion technique is simple and usually requires no additional equipment[5]. The use of stylets and skids have been described to aid LMA insertion[6,7] but these are seldom required. Brimacombe, in a personal series of 1500 LMA insertions, demonstrated a success rate at the first attempt at insertion of 95.5%, with an overall failure rate of 0.4% after three attempts[5]. This success rate at initial insertion relates to the use of the standard LMA. Greater difficulty is often experienced with the reinforced LMA which is less rigid, although a similar learning curve exists.

Requires no neuromuscular blocking drugs[8]

This avoids the morbidity associated with the depolarizing neuromuscular blockers and the increased risk of postoperative nausea and vomiting associated with the use of anticholinesterase drugs to reverse the effects of the non-depolarizing relaxants. The absence of the need for muscular relaxants renders the use of the LMA inherently safer. Brimacombe and Berry suggest that if insertion of the LMA is found to be difficult, despite an adequate dose of induction agent, the administration of muscle relaxants will not improve conditions for insertion[9].

> *The LMA is associated with greater haemodynamic stability and minimal increase in intraocular pressure on insertion[10,11].*

Associated with less coughing on emergence from anaesthesia[12]
Coughing and straining can be particularly harmful following eye and ENT surgery. The LMA is well tolerated at light levels of anaesthesia and can be left *in situ* until the return of protective reflexes, when it can be removed without coughing. Several studies have demonstrated that the use of the LMA is associated with improved oxygen saturation levels during emergence[13,14].

Associated with a lower incidence of sore throat
While several factors probably affect the incidence of sore throat in day case patients, the method of airway management used is a major cause. The published incidence of sore throat following day surgery in intubated patients varies between 28% and 47%, compared with 7% using the LMA and 10% in patients managed with a face mask and oropharyngeal airway[15]. With 3% of intubated day case patients still complaining of sore throat 24 hours after surgery compared with 0% of patients in the face mask and LMA groups, this is a significant advantage. While the incidence of sore throat associated with use of the LMA appears to decrease with the increased clinical experience of the person inserting the LMA, such an advantage has not been clearly demonstrated in children. The use of the LMA produces less voice change than the use of an endotracheal tube[16]. For patients who use their voice professionally, this can be extremely important.

Allows faster turnaround time
The LMA can be inserted rapidly following induction of anaesthesia, the depth of anaesthesia required being a little deeper than that necessary to insert a Guedel airway.
　As it is tolerated at lighter planes of anaesthesia than the endotracheal tube[17], the LMA permits spontaneous respiration without coughing, breath-holding and laryngospasm, and without the respiratory depression secondary to the deeper planes of anaesthesia required to tolerate an endotracheal tube. The transition from controlled to spontaneous respiration is therefore very much easier and can be achieved more rapidly.
　Patients should be awake and can have their LMA removed at the end of their day case procedure. While this is the ideal, spontaneously breathing patients can safely be cared for, by competent recovery staff, with an LMA still *in situ*. For operations where there is a risk of laryngospasm during emergence, due to blood or mucus, this practice of more gradual undisturbed recovery with an LMA still in place may actually be safer.

Allows 'hands free' anaesthesia
The day case anaesthetist has to observe the patient, record respiratory and cardiovascular parameters, make adjustments to the anaesthetic technique, administer drugs and tilt the operation table. All these things can be done during face mask anaesthesia but are considerably easier when using the LMA.

Ease of use in patients with difficult airways
The LMA may provide a better airway than the face mask in difficult patients, and avoids the need for endotracheal intubation in those patients in whom this would be difficult[18]. The ease of insertion is unrelated to anatomical features used to predict or score difficult intubation. It is valuable as a rescue device where difficult intubation has not been predicted.

Disadvantages of the LMA

The safe use of the LMA requires that its limitations relative to other forms of airway management are recognized (*Table 6.3*).

Table 6.3. Disadvantages of the LMA

The LMA does not protect the airway from regurgitated stomach contents
Leak pressures are lower using the LMA, resulting in lost tidal volume in patients with increased
  airway resistance or decreased compliance
This 'lost' tidal volume may be forced into the stomach

No protection from refluxed stomach contents

There is not the same degree of mechanical isolation of the respiratory tract with the LMA as that achieved by endotracheal intubation. However, the LMA has now been used in millions of patients yet the incidence of clinically apparent regurgitation and aspiration is low, between 0.08 and 0.2%, figures similar to that with the face mask and the endotracheal tube[19–22]. While oesophageal reflux may be more likely using the LMA than the face mask[23], a phenomenon related to the decrease in lower oesophageal sphincter (LOS) tone, the incidence of aspiration is influenced by a number of factors, not least of which is the protection afforded by the upper oesophageal sphincter[24].

The LMA is unsafe for use in patients with gastro-oesophageal reflux. Patients will say they suffer from indigestion, which may mean that they suffer from a range of symptoms from very occasional indigestion, after certain foods eaten late at night, to almost constant reflux on laying flat. This requires careful questioning at the preoperative assessment but, in general, postural reflux on bending or lying flat is of greater concern.

> *Exclude the use of the LMA with any suspicion of reflux of gastric contents not precipitated by food. When considering the severity of reflux symptoms, if a face mask is contraindicated, so is the LMA.*

Lower seal pressures than the endotracheal tube

The LMA is unsuitable for controlled ventilation in patients requiring high inflation pressures due to loss of ventilatory volume. The mean pressure at which leak occurs has been found to be 17 cmH_2O[25]. One study found that a leak of inspiratory tidal volume was present at each inflation pressure used (15, 20, 25 and 30 cmH_2O), and that at an inflation pressure of only 15 cmH_2O, a mean leak of 13% was calculated[26]. However, Cork *et al.* could find no difference when comparing controlled ventilation using the LMA or endotracheal tube, although anaesthetists tended to choose smaller tidal volumes, faster respiratory rates and lower anaesthetic concentrations when using the LMA, thus reflecting their awareness of the limitations of this airway[12].

Greater incidence of gastric insufflation during controlled ventilation

The use of the LMA for controlled ventilation in patients requiring high inflation pressures may result in any leaked inspiratory volume being forced into the stomach. Devitt *et al.*[26] demonstrated that as ventilatory pressure increased from 15 to 20 cmH_2O, so the incidence of gastric insufflation increased from 2.1 to 35.4%. However, other investigators have found no difference in the volume of gas aspirated from the stomach after ventilation using the LMA or endotracheal tube[27].

Contraindications to the use of the LMA

The use of the LMA in day case anaesthesia is only justifiable if it is as safe as other methods of airway management and is associated with less morbidity. Before the general and specific indications for the use of the LMA are discussed, the general contraindications to the use of the LMA must be considered (*Table 6.4*).

Table 6.4. Contraindications to the use of the LMA

Patient factors
Do NOT use LMAs in patients who:
    are not adequately fasted
    have a history of decreased gastric motility, gastro-oesophageal reflux or hiatus hernia
    are of BMI above 34
    have decreased lung compliance or require increased airway pressures

Surgical factors
Do NOT use LMAs for operations on the head and neck or involving a shared airway where the surgeon concerned:
    is unaware of its use
    doesn't understand its limitations
    is unhappy to work with or around it

BMI, body mass index.

> *The use of the LMA is safe provided such use is confined to properly selected patient and operative groups.*

General indications for use

It has been stated that the LMA is simply a hands-free alternative to the use of a face mask, and therefore should only be used in situations where a face mask would otherwise have been utilized. However, the LMA, with all its advantages, can be a safe and superior alternative to endotracheal intubation for several day case operations.

Duration of surgery

Whether or not to use the LMA for the majority of day case operations will be decided by the length of time the operation is expected to take. For rapid, short-duration operations, such as suction termination of pregnancy or hysteroscopy, the use of an LMA may add to the total anaesthetic time and confer little overall benefit. As different surgeons take differing amounts of time to perform the same operation, the skill and speed of the surgeon is a factor that the anaesthetist must bear in mind. The LMA can be used safely in long day case procedures, which rarely last more than 2 hours.

Access to the airway

The LMA is useful for operations where access to the head and neck by the anaesthetist is limited. Again, the expected duration of surgery is a contributory factor in the decision to use an LMA. For brief head operations such as the insertion of grommets, the use of the LMA may be unnecessary, whereas for longer operations, typically squint surgery, the use of the LMA offers significant advantages.

The LMA in specific day surgery procedures

Laparoscopy

The LMA has proved itself to be a safe and efficient method of airway maintenance for laparoscopy[28–30]. For the use of the LMA in laparoscopy to be safe, the surgeon must:

- be quick. An uncomplicated laparoscopy or laparoscopic sterilization should take no longer than 30 minutes;
- require no more than an average of 3 litres of gas intra-abdominally, limiting the intra-abdominal pressure to below 15 mmHg;
- require no more than a 15–20° head-down tilt.

Brimacombe and Berry[28] state that for use of the LMA in day case laparoscopy, the 'rule of 15s' should apply, i.e. no longer than 15 minutes' duration, no more than 15 mmHg intra-abdominal pressure and no more than 15° head-down tilt. In the UK, 40% of anaesthetists now use the LMA for day case gynaecological laparoscopy[2].

The use of the LMA during laparoscopic cholecystectomy is generally not recommended. Patients for this type of surgery commonly suffer from indigestion with varying degrees of reflux, and tend to have higher BMIs. In addition, laparoscopic cholecystectomy may take over an hour to perform, and has a fairly high incidence of surgically related complications[31]. Laparoscopic cholecystectomy is an example of the type of operation where the LMA has few advantages over the endotracheal tube, and where its disadvantages are more prominent.

The lateral and prone positions

Many day case operations on the back of the body can be performed with the patient in the lateral position. The LMA can be useful in such cases where airway management is awkward. For those day case operations which can only be performed with the patient in the prone position, the reinforced LMA has been used successfully, both with spontaneous and controlled ventilation[32]. McCaughey and Bhanumurthy have even claimed some advantages from inserting the LMA with the patient prone[33]. However, unless the surgery will be very brief it seems wise to use only controlled ventilation in such circumstances, and unless this can be achieved at modest inflation pressures while in the supine position it should not be attempted with the patient prone. It should also be possible to return the patient to the lateral position fairly rapidly if airway or ventilation problems occur.

ENT and oral surgery

ENT and oral surgery combine limited access to the head and neck and the need for protection of the airway from contamination with blood and mucus from above. Seal pressures obtainable with a correctly positioned LMA average 17 cmH$_2$O[25]. Thus for blood or any other fluid to enter the larynx it must be present in large volumes above the mask or be under considerable pressure. Several studies have demonstrated that the reinforced LMA protects the airway from contamination during adenotonsillectomy, wisdom teeth extraction and a variety of other operations for which tracheal intubation has previously been considered mandatory[34–36].

In such operations the reinforced LMA is usually preferred as its tube section is longer and narrower, allowing it to be less intrusive and more easily fixed, and it resists compression and kinking by gags (and surgeons). Some controversy exists as to whether or not a throat pack is required in these situations. Studies have shown that they are not needed and may increase the incidence and severity of postoperative sore throat. Initially the use of a throat pack may be beneficial in convincing your surgeon of the advantages of the LMA. However, it must not be used as an excuse to be careless with haemostasis or suction clearance of mucus.

Ophthalmic surgery

While the use of the LMA in patients breathing spontaneously is widely established, the use of the LMA in controlled ventilation is less generally practised. Many ophthalmic day surgery operations require controlled ventilation and muscle relaxation. The LMA has been shown to be a suitable alternative to endotracheal intubation for these operations[30]. In addition, the LMA has several advantages of particular relevance to ophthalmic surgery. Use of the reinforced LMA does not interfere with surgical access, and its insertion does not cause large increases in intraocular pressure. Transition between controlled and spontaneous respiration is smoother, reducing turnaround time, and its removal causes less coughing[37]. The use of the LMA for intraocular surgery should be accompanied by controlled ventilation and the use of neuromuscular blocking drugs, whose effect should be carefully monitored. Also the adequacy of ventilation, in terms of tidal volume and end-tidal CO_2 levels, must be assessed before commencing surgery, and should be achievable with modest inflation pressures[38].

Insertion of the LMA

The method of inserting the LMA is well described in the LMA manual[39], although there are several variations in common use[40]. Brimacombe, who has published his experience of thousands of LMA insertions, has stated that all anaesthetists should adopt a standard method of insertion to facilitate study of the LMA[5] (*Table 6.5*).

Table 6.5. Key points for insertion of LMA

No force is required. If you have to use force then something is wrong, usually the position of the head or the depth of anaesthesia. Lifting the jaw will improve the position for insertion
No matter how careful you are, multiple attempts will cause trauma[41], so limit yourself to three attempts
Remember, there are patients in whom it seems impossible to place an LMA correctly. Accept failure graciously
The most common reason for failing to insert an LMA is due to inadequate depth of anaesthesia. Swallowing is a good indication of inadequate depth of anaesthesia

Intravenous agents are not all the same with respect to providing suitable conditions for ease of LMA insertion[42]. Thiopentone heightens the sensitivity of laryngeal reflexes and deeper levels of anaesthesia are required, although the ease of insertion of the LMA with thiopentone can be modified by the addition of fentanyl and midazolam[43]. This combination provides equally satisfactory conditions for LMA insertion as those produced by propofol and fentanyl, at 65% of the cost. The majority of studies have concluded that the laryngeal reflex suppression produced by propofol makes it the agent of choice[44].

Bite blocks

These are recommended by the user manual. While it is true that a small minority of patients will bite the LMA during emergence from anaesthesia, this is no more of a problem with the LMA than with an endotracheal tube. The authors do not use bite blocks routinely.

> *If you use bite blocks with endotracheal tubes, then use them with LMAs.*

Removal of the LMA

The user manual states that the LMA should be left *in situ* and with the cuff still inflated until the patient awakes. Morris and Marjot[45] have shown that reducing the volume in the cuff by 50%, so that the cuff pressure falls below the pharyngeal mucosa perfusion pressure of 22 mmHg, results in a significant reduction in measured expiratory volume. Some anaesthetists and recovery staff deflate the cuff completely before the patient awakes, which may result in partial airway obstruction or inadequate ventilation, and this practice should be avoided.

> *Removal of the LMA with the cuff still inflated removes most of any pooled secretions above the LMA. This does no harm and may offer some advantages.*

The optimum time to remove an LMA, rather like the endotracheal tube, is either when the patient is still relatively deeply anaesthetized or is awake. Varughese *et al.*[46] have shown that removal of the LMA in children is less problematic if performed with the patient still deeply anaesthetized. However, Williams and Bailey[13] found that following operations in which blood and mucus are still likely to be present in the mouth and upper pharynx, leaving the LMA *in situ* and with the cuff still fully inflated, is the safer option.

Overall, in patients with an LMA *in situ* in recovery, who have a clear airway and normal oxygen saturation levels, the LMA should be left in place and the airway left undisturbed. This is even more important if blood and mucus are likely to be present following ENT or dental surgery, where patients should be turned into the left lateral head-down position, still with the LMA *in situ*.

> *If the patient is well oxygenated and has a clear airway, leave the LMA alone until the patient is awake. This is safer and is less likely to be associated with coughing, aspiration of blood or mucus, or laryngospasm.*

Cost effectiveness of the LMA

Any change in day case anaesthetic practice may have cost implications due to the high throughput in most day surgery units, and the widespread use of the LMA is a good example. The cost effectiveness of the LMA is influenced by a number of factors, mainly the number of times it can be re-used. While this can approach 200–250[47], in the UK the manufacturer's guarantee is limited to 40 uses. However, significant monetary savings, relative to endotracheal intubation, are associated with the use of the LMA for day case patients, even when the LMA is re-used only 40 times[48].

> *The LMA is cost effective if re-used 40 times.*

The place of the laryngeal mask in day case anaesthesia is already well established. However, the use of the LMA has recognized limitations with regard to protection of the airway from aspiration of stomach contents and ventilation of patients with decreased lung compliance or increased airways resistance. Such limitations may be overcome in the future with the latest LMA prototype[4]. Provided that a few simple conditions are met regarding patient characteristics and the conditions of surgery, the LMA is a safe, cost-effective and advantageous method of airway management in day case patients.

> *The LMA has significant advantages in many day case operations and, provided that its limitations are recognized, it is safe and associated with less morbidity.*

References

1. **Hitchcock M, Ogg TW.** A quality assurance initiative in day case surgery: general considerations. *Ambulatory Surg.* 1994; **2**: 181–192.
2. **Akhtar TM, Shankar RK, Street MK.** Is Guedel's airway and facemask dead ? *Today's Anaesthetist* 1994; **9**: 56–58.
3. **Kapila A, Addy EV, Verghese C, et al.** Intubating laryngeal mask airway: a preliminary assessment of performance. *Br. J. Anaesth.* 1995; **75**: 228–229.
4. **Brain AIJ, Verghese C, Strube P, et al.** A new laryngeal mask prototype. Preliminary evaluation of seal pressures and glottic isolation. *Anaesthesia* 1995; **50**: 42–48.
5. **Brimacombe J.** Analysis of 1500 laryngeal mask uses by one anaesthetist in adults undergoing routine anaesthesia. *Anaesthesia* 1996; **51**: 76–80.
6. **Philpott B, Renwick M.** An introducer for the flexible laryngeal mask airway. *Anaesthesia* 1993; **48**: 174.
7. **Harding JB.** A 'skid' for easier insertion of the laryngeal mask airway. *Anaesthesia* 1993; **48**: 80.
8. **Pennant JH, White PF.** The laryngeal mask airway. Its uses in anaesthesiology. *Anesthesiology* 1993; **79**: 144–163.
9. **Brimacombe J, Berry A.** Neuromuscular block and the insertion of the laryngeal mask airway. *Br. J. Anaesth.* 1993; **71**: 166–167.
10. **Fujii Y, Tanaka H, Toyooka H.** Circulatory responses to laryngeal mask airway insertion or tracheal intubation in normotensive and hypertensive patients. *Can. J. Anaesth.* 1995; **42**: 32–36.
11. **Barclay K, Wall T, Wareham H, et al.** Intra-ocular pressure changes in patients with glaucoma. Comparison between the laryngeal mask airway and tracheal tube. *Anaesthesia* 1994; **49**: 159–162.
12. **Cork RC, Depa RM, Standen JR.** Prospective comparison of the use of the laryngeal mask airway and endotracheal tube for ambulatory surgery. *Anesth. Analg.* 1994; **79**: 719–727.
13. **Williams PJ, Bailey PM.** Comparison of the reinforced laryngeal mask airway and tracheal intubation for adenotonsillectomy. *Br. J. Anaesth.* 1993; **70**: 30–33.
14. **Cros AM, Boudey C, Esteben D, et al.** Intubation vs laryngeal mask. Incidence of desaturations and spasms during adenoidectomy. *Anesthesiology* 1993; **79**: A1155.
15. **Alexander CA, Leach AB.** Incidence of sore throats with the laryngeal mask. *Anaesthesia* 1989; **44**: 791.
16. **Lee SK, Hong KH, Choe H, et al.** Comparison of the effects of the laryngeal mask airway and endotracheal intubation on vocal function. *Br. J. Anaesth.* 1993; **71**: 648–650.
17. **Wilkins CJ, Cramp PGW, Staples J.** Comparison of the anaesthetic requirements for tolerance of laryngeal mask airway and endotracheal tube. *Anesth. Analg.* 1992; **75**: 794–797.
18. **Sarma VJ.** The use of a laryngeal mask airway in spontaneously breathing patients. *Acta Anaesthesiol. Scand.* 1990; **34**: 669–672.
19. **Blake DW, Dawson P, Donnan G, et al.** Propofol induction for laryngeal mask airway insertion: dose requirement and cardio-respiratory effects. *Anaesth. Intens. Care* 1992; **20**: 479–483.
20. **Verghese C, Smith TG, Young E.** Prospective survey of the use of the laryngeal mask airway in 2359 patients. *Anaesthesia* 1993; **48**: 58–60.
21. **Brimacombe J, Berry A.** The laryngeal mask airway – the first ten years. *Anaesth. Intens. Care* 1993; **21**: 225–226.

22. **Brimacombe JR, Berry A.** The incidence of aspiration associated with the laryngeal mask airway: a meta-analysis of published literature. *J. Clin. Anesth.* 1995; **7**: 297–305.

23. **Owens TM, Robertson P, Twomey C,** *et al.* The incidence of gastro-oesophageal reflux with the laryngeal mask: a comparison with the face mask using oesophageal lumen pH electrodes. *Anesth. Analg.* 1995; **80**: 980–984.

24. **Joshi GP, Morrison SG, Okonwo NA,** *et al.* Continuous hypopharyngeal pH measurements in spontaneously breathing anaesthetised outpatients: laryngeal mask airway versus tracheal intubation. *Anesth. Analg.* 1996; **82**: 254–257.

25. **Brodrick PM, Webster NR, Nunn JF.** The laryngeal mask airway: a study of 100 patients during spontaneous breathing. *Anaesthesia* 1989; **44**: 238–241.

26. **Devitt JH, Wenstone R, Noel AG,** *et al.* The laryngeal mask airway and positive-pressure ventilation. *Anesthesiology* 1994; **80**: 550–555.

27. **Graziotti P, Murphy D.** Is a nasogastric tube useful when ventilating through the laryngeal mask airway? *Anaesth. Intens. Care* 1992; **20**: 108.

28. **Brimacombe J, Berry A.** Airway management during gynaecological laparoscopy – is it safe to use the laryngeal mask airway? *Ambulatory Surg.* 1995; **3**: 65–70.

29. **Swann DG, Spens H, Edwards SA,** *et al.* Anaesthesia for gynaecological laparoscopy – a comparison between the laryngeal mask airway and tracheal intubation. *Anaesthesia* 1993; **48**: 431–434.

30. **Verghese C, Brimacombe JR.** Survey of laryngeal mask airway usage in 11,910 patients: safety and efficacy for conventional and nonconventional usage. *Anesth. Analg.* 1996; **82**: 129–133.

31. **Singleton RJ, Rudkin GE, Osborne GA,** *et al.* Laparoscopic cholecystectomy as a day surgery procedure. *Anaesth. Intens. Care* 1996; **24**: 231–236.

32. **Milligan KA.** Laryngeal mask in the prone position. *Anaesthesia* 1994; **49**: 449.

33. **McCaughey W, Bhanmurthy S.** Laryngeal mask placement in the prone position. *Anaesthesia* 1993; **48**: 1104.

34. **Goodwin APL, Ogg TW, Lamb WT,** *et al.* The reinforced laryngeal mask airway in dental day surgery. *Ambulatory Surg.* 1993; **1**: 31–35.

35. **Quinn AC, Samaan A, McAteer EM** *et al.* The reinforced laryngeal mask airway for dento-alveolar surgery. *Br. J. Anaesth.* 1996; **77**: 185–188.

36. **Brimacombe J, Berry A.** The laryngeal mask airway for ENT, head and neck surgery. *J. Otolaryngol.* in press.

37. **Holden R, Morsman D, Butler J,** *et al.* The laryngeal mask airway and intra-ocular surgery. *Anaesthesia* 1992; **47**: 445–446.

38. **Brimacombe J, Berry A.** The laryngeal mask airway and intra-ocular surgery. *Anaesthesia* 1993; **48**: 827.

39. **Brain AIJ.** (1991) *The Intravent Laryngeal Mask Instruction Manual,* 2nd Edn. Intravent, Henley on Thames, UK.

40. **Brimacombe J, Berry A.** Insertion of the laryngeal mask airway – a prospective study of four techniques. *Anaesth. Intens. Care* 1993; **21**: 89–92.

41. **Mckinney B, Grigg R.** Epiglottitis after anaesthesia with a laryngeal mask. *Anaesth. Intens. Care* 1995; **23**: 618–619.

42. **Brown GW, Patel N, Ellis FR.** Comparison of propofol and thiopentone for laryngeal mask insertion. *Anaesthesia* 1991; **46**: 771–772.

43. **Bapat P, Joshi RN, Yound E,** *et al.* Comparison of propofol versus thiopentone with midazolam or lidocaine to facilitate laryngeal mask insertion. *Can. J. Anaesth.* 1996; **43**: 564–568.

44. **Scanlon P, Carey M, Power M,** *et al.* Patient response to laryngeal mask insertion after induction of anaesthesia with propofol or thiopentone. *Can. J. Anaesth.* 1993; **40**: 816–818.

45. **Morris GN, Marjot R.** Laryngeal mask airway performance: effect of cuff deflation during anaesthesia. *Br. J. Anaesth.* 1996; **76**: 456–458.

46. **Varughese A, McCulloch D, Lewis M,** *et al.* Removal of the laryngeal mask airway (LMA) in children: awake or deep? *Anesthesiology* 1994; **81**: A1321.

47. **Leach A, Alexander C.** The laryngeal mask airway: a new concept – an overview. *Eur. J. Anesthesiol.* 1991; **4** (Suppl.): 19–31.

48. **Macario A, Chang P, Stempel DB,** *et al.* A cost analysis of the laryngeal mask airway for elective surgery in adult outpatients. *Anesthesiology* 1995; **83**: 250–257.

CHAPTER 7

Total intravenous anaesthesia (TIVA)

M. Hitchcock

Total intravenous anaesthesia (TIVA) involves the induction and maintenance of balanced anaesthesia using the IV route alone. The success of a TIVA regime depends on the drugs used: Schuttler *et al.*[1] stated that drugs used in this way should guarantee, besides a lack of major side-effects, a reasonable degree of control over their main pharmacodynamic effects, which is dependent on their pharmacokinetic behaviour. TIVA has been described using many IV agents, but the cumulative properties of drugs such as thiopentone limit their use in day surgery[2]. The only anaesthetic agent currently suitable for use for TIVA in day case anaesthesia is propofol, which will be discussed in this chapter.

Induction with propofol may be followed by maintenance with intermittent boluses or variable-rate infusions of propofol. To achieve balanced anaesthesia with minimal side-effects, it is necessary to combine propofol with short-acting opioid analgesics by bolus or infusion or local/regional anaesthesia, and/or muscle relaxants. Small doses of hypnotics such as midazolam may be included, usually as a bolus at induction. Nitrous oxide may or may not be included in TIVA.

Why use TIVA?

Although recovery is improved after propofol used for induction compared with thiopentone, these advantages are maximized when propofol is also used for maintenance (*Table 7.1*).

Table 7.1. Advantages of TIVA with propofol

Rapid early recovery
Reduced PONV
Improved subjective recovery
Rapid control of the depth of anaesthesia
No risk of triggering malignant hyperpyrexia
Less theatre and recovery pollution

PONV, postoperative nausea and vomiting.

Rapid early recovery
TIVA has been shown to produce high-quality, rapid recovery[3–6]. Early recovery has been shown to be improved compared with isoflurane[7], recovery room stays are shortened[8], and patients are ready to be discharged sooner[3,8]. This may be even more apparent after day case operations of longer duration[7].

Compared with the new volatile agents, desflurane and sevoflurane, early recovery times following TIVA may be similar or slightly longer[9,10], but later recovery is little different, with similar times to discharge[9,11].

Reduced PONV
The use of TIVA is associated with a low incidence of PONV, even after procedures which predispose to a high incidence[12,13]. This has led to the proposition that propofol has intrinsic antiemetic activity[14]. TIVA has been demonstrated to be more effective than ondansetron in reducing PONV following breast surgery, and may be more cost effective[15,16]. Both desflurane and sevoflurane have the same high incidence of PONV as the other volatile agents, and significantly increase PONV compared with TIVA[17,18]. This has more impact on time to discharge than rapid immediate recovery, and results in delayed recovery and increased overnight admssion[19].

Improved subjective recovery
Patients have reported improved subjective recovery and well-being for up to 24 hours postoperatively after TIVA with propofol compared with other anaesthetics[3,20,21]. In contrast, rapid awakening from desflurane anaesthesia has been associated with emergence delirium, and poorer mood scores compared with isoflurane[22,23].

> *While immediate recovery may be faster after the new volatile agents, they are associated with more postoperative morbidity, especially PONV, and time to discharge is similar or delayed compared with TIVA with propofol[24].*

Rapid control of the depth of anaesthesia
IV maintenance of anaesthesia has the advantage of allowing rapid control of the depth of anaesthesia, which is independent of the patient's minute ventilation or equilibration with functional residual capacity and anaesthetic circuit deadspace.

Avoidance of trigger agents for dangerous events
The use of propofol for maintenance avoids the risk of triggering malignant hyperthermia, and it has an excellent safety record in porphyria[25-27], making TIVA an acceptable anaesthetic for the day case patient.

Less theatre pollution
In the UK, the use of inhalational anaesthetics is subject to the Control of Substances Hazardous to Health (COSHH) regulations[28]. While scavenging of volatile anaesthetics is now commonplace in theatre, it is often minimal or non-existent in recovery rooms. However, although scavenging may not be as effective as predicted[29,30], there is little evidence that chronic exposure to anaesthetic agents is harmful[31].

> *TIVA using air/oxygen avoids theatre, recovery and environmental pollution.*

Barriers to the use of TIVA

TIVA, despite its advantages, is still not widely used for day case anaesthesia. This may be due to a failure to appreciate its benefits, although other factors may be equally important (*Table 7.2*).

Table 7.2. Perceived barriers to the use of TIVA

Lack of familiarity and training in the technique
Need for special equipment and time-consuming set-up
Concern about the risk of awareness
Concern about cost

Unfamiliarity with principles and concepts

TIVA is a technique with which many anaesthetists are unfamiliar. Anaesthetic maintenance has traditionally been taught using volatile agents, although the pharmacokinetics and dynamics involved in the use of TIVA are as readily comprehensible as those of inhalational agents. With the expansion of day surgery, there is a need to train anaesthetists in techniques which improve outcome. TIVA is also a useful technique in many circumstances outside day surgery, and should be part of every anaesthetist's repertoire[32].

Requirement for special equipment

Although inhalational anaesthesia requires specialized and often expensive delivery and monitoring equipment, this is usually readily available in most operating theatres. TIVA can be performed with intermittent bolus doses of propofol, but infusion pumps are necessary for longer procedures. Modern pumps now incorporate many features that make the technique of TIVA relatively simple. The desirable features of infusion pumps for TIVA are given in *Table 7.3*. Like other equipment, infusion pumps must be checked before use.

Table 7.3. Desirable features of syringe pumps

Construction
Simplicity in display and design
Compatible with a range of syringes
Easy set-up and syringe insertion
Prolonged rechargeable battery life
Mains power alternative
Robust
Lightweight

Functionality
Accurate
Single-handed bolus facility
Wide range of infusion rates
Ability to pre-set bolus/induction dose and rate
Minimum number of key presses to change parameters
Clear displays of rate and total volume infused

Alarms
Visual and auditory
Pump not infusing
Syringe almost empty
Empty
High pressure (occlusion)
Low pressure (disconnection)

To make giving infusions simpler, the latest infusion pumps incorporate a computer, programed with a pharmacokinetic model for propofol. These 'target-controlled infusion (TCI) devices' are set up using patient data, such as weight and age, and automatically adjust the infusion rate of propofol to maintain a set target blood propofol concentration.

Prefilled syringes of propofol are now available so that the effort involved in setting up pumps for TIVA is reduced.

Worries about awareness

Unfamiliarity with TIVA is the main reason for concern about awareness, although some studies have suggested that day case anaesthesia itself, irrespective of the technique utilized, may be associated with an incidence of awareness of 9%, in unpremedicated day case patients[33]. Awareness has been reported with all anaesthetic techniques: constant clinical observation of the patient is essential. Sandin and Nordstrom[34] described five cases of awareness during TIVA using propofol, and found that physiological parameters, such as heart rate and blood pressure, were useful in predicting awareness in four out of five patients. The incidence of awareness in this study compared very favourably with that quoted for inhalational agents[35].

> *It would appear that assessing the depth of anaesthesia is, in reality, no more or less difficult with TIVA than with volatile agents.*

Inter-patient variability in propofol requirements may be another cause for concern. It is apparent in unparalysed patients that considerably higher infusion rates may be required to prevent reaction to painful stimuli than those used in published infusion regimes. An appreciation of the factors that can affect the EC_{50} (the effective concentration at which 50% of patients do not respond to a painful stimulus) of propofol and experienced gained in non-paralysed patients should alleviate some of these concerns[36].

> *Awareness is no more or less likely using TIVA than with any other form of anaesthetic maintenance.*

Cost

TIVA is often regarded as expensive and not sufficiently superior to other cheaper forms of anaesthesia to justify its increased cost. As the cost of maintenance of anaesthesia with propofol may be 2–4 times more than maintenance with the cheaper volatile agents, the widespread use of TIVA in day surgery units with large throughputs would have far-reaching financial implications[37].

However, the cost of anaesthetic drugs is small compared with the overall cost of an operation[37], and it is misleading to consider only the cost of the drugs utilized. The quality of anaesthesia can influence the incidence of postoperative morbidity, unanticipated admission, patient satisfaction and even the workload imposed on community medical services[38]. When these additional costs are also included in the overall analysis, the increased cost of TIVA compared with volatile anaesthesia may be justified if it improves outcome and reduces unit costs[39]. TIVA has been shown to be cost effective compared with volatile anaesthesia when overall costs are considered, and may actually be cheaper when used for operations of less than 30 minutes' duration[40].

While the cost of patient outcome may be difficult to calculate, the price of anaesthetic drugs utilized is simple to obtain. In addition, although TIVA may result in a reduction in overall costs, this will not be apparent in a system with segregated budgets, so that there will always be an incentive to use cheaper drugs regardless of outcome. While cost will always be an issue, it should not be the prime determinant of any quality anaesthetic service, as the morbidity associated with inferior anaesthetic techniques may not only have significant financial implications, but may decrease the perceived quality of service.

> *Cost of TIVA with propofol can be offset by the improvement in the quality of recovery and outcome. TIVA for day case patients is good value for money for the reduction in PONV alone.*

Pharmacokinetics

Detailed pharmacokinetics are beyond the scope of this book, but some understanding of them is needed to use TIVA effectively. A number of complex infusion schemes have been described to enable a constant blood level of propofol to be achieved. These are all based on the 'BET' (bolus, elimination, transfer) principle which has been shown to be effective for other anaesthetics and analgesics[41,42].

- A loading dose (*bolus*) is required to fill the initial volume of distribution of the drug.
- The final infusion rate should equal the clearance (*elimination*) of the drug.
- An interim infusion scheme is necessary to match the redistribution (*transfer*) of the drug from the central volume of distribution to peripheral sites.

Clinical factors affecting infusion regimes

Several clinical variables affect the induction dose and infusion rate of propofol required for anaesthesia (*Table 7.4*).

Table 7.4. Factors affecting the induction dose and infusion rate of TIVA

Patient factors
Age
Weight
ASA status
Anxiety

Anaesthetic factors
Premedication
Supplementary drugs: benzodiazepines, opioids, nitrous oxide
Dose and rate of injection of induction dose
Effective local or regional anaesthesia

Surgical factors
Degree of surgical stimulation
Depth of anaesthesia required
Duration of infusion

Patient factors
Age. Children and younger patients require increased doses of propofol for both induction and maintenance compared with older patients[43], who have a reduced initial volume of distribution and total clearance.

Weight. Sear has shown that an infusion regime based on an average body weight of 70 kg, would provide clinically adequate anaesthesia for patients within the weight range 60–90 kg[44]. Infusion regimes based on lean body mass may be more appropriate[45].

ASA status. Sick patients are very sensitive to all anaesthetics, often due to slow circulation which delays time to effector site concentration. Slower induction and lower infusion rates should be used, titrated to clinical response.

Anxiety. Anxious patients may require higher induction doses of propofol. Once anaesthesia is achieved, infusion rates required for maintenance of anaesthesia may also be increased.

Anaesthetic factors
Premedication. The use of oral premedication in day case patients is not common practice. Published infusion regimes have usually been described for premedicated patients; both benzodiazepines and opioid premedication will reduce the required infusion rates[46,47].

> *Unpremedicated day case patients will require higher propofol induction doses and infusion rates.*

Opioids. Propofol and opioids given together act synergistically to reduce induction dose and infusion rate. Alfentanil infusion is commonly used with TIVA because of its rapid time to effector site concentration, short elimination half-life and context-sensitive half-time, although the large doses used may be inappropriate for day surgery[48]. Fentanyl 1–3 µg kg^{-1} is useful given as a bolus to provide intraoperative and some postoperative analgesia in day surgery procedures. The blood concentration of opioid at the end of anaesthesia also affects the propofol concentration at which the patient wakes up: the greater the plasma opioid concentration at the end of anaesthesia, the lower the propofol concentration must fall before the patient awakes[48].

Remifentanil, the new short-acting opioid (see Chapter 5), has been used successfully with TIVA to reduce propofol requirements[49]. As its blood concentration falls extremely rapidly, wake-up is correspondingly rapid, although analgesia is equally rapidly terminated.

Hypnotics. Midazolam has been used to provide amnesia and reduce the induction dose of propofol[50,51]. Co-induction using propofol and midazolam may decrease the subsequent infusion rate of propofol required, and although initial recovery may be delayed, time to discharge is unaffected[52].

Speed and dose used for induction. The dose of propofol required to induce anaesthesia is a useful guide to the infusion rates required for maintenance, provided that it is given slowly.

The 'Bristol' infusion regime[53,54], which is commonly quoted (see *Table 7.5*), uses an induction dose of 1 mg kg^{-1} given slowly. This does not reflect the clinical practice of many anaesthetists, and if an induction dose of 2.5–3 mg kg^{-1} or more is given fairly rapidly, the blood concentration may overshoot the level needed to achieve anaesthesia before the effector site concentration (i.e. brain concentration) has had time to catch up. It may therefore be possible to reduce the initial maintenance infusion rate.

Nitrous oxide. The use of nitrous oxide to supplement TIVA has been shown to affect propofol requirements[36], 67% nitrous oxide reduces the measured EC_{50} by 33%.

Surgical stimulus

The depth of anaesthesia required during a day case operation often varies[55]. Infusion rates should be increased, or a bolus of propofol or analgesic given before particularly stimulating events.

The pre-emptive use of effective local anaesthesia may mean that the propofol infusion rate can be markedly reduced to sedation levels of about 3 mg kg^{-1} $hour^{-1}$, so enabling rapid recovery.

These factors mean that unswerving adherence to any TIVA infusion regime in the day case patient could result in either excessive or inadequate levels of anaesthesia. Infusion regimes are only a guide. The depth of anaesthesia at any given infusion rate must be continually assessed and adjustments made based on the patient's response to the surgical procedure[55].

A popular and clinically useful propofol infusion regime for adults, designed to give a blood propofol concentration of 3 µg ml^{-1}, is given in *Table 7.5*. Temazepam premedication, analgesic supplementation with 3 µg kg^{-1} of fentanyl and nitrous oxide were also used[53].

Table 7.5. A common infusion regime

Premedication	Temazepam 20 mg PO
Induction	Propofol 1 mg kg^{-1} Fentanyl 3 µg kg^{-1}
Maintenance	Propofol 　10 mg kg^{-1} $hour^{-1}$ for the first 10 minutes 　8 mg kg^{-1} $hour^{-1}$ for the subsequent 10 minutes 　6 mg kg^{-1} $hour^{-1}$ thereafter Nitrous oxide 67% in oxygen

Opioids by infusion or intermittent boluses?

TIVA requires some form of analgesic supplementation for the majority of day case operations. Intraoperatively this is commonly provided by the use of either alfentanil or fentanyl. When propofol and alfentanil infusions are used together in TIVA, the effect of each is potentiated[56]. However the use of opioids by infusion while attractive, especially in the case of the newer drugs such as remifentanil, requires the use of separate infusion pumps and the consideration of a new set of pharmacokinetics[57]. Intermittent bolus doses of opioids, on the other hand, are very familiar to most anaesthetists, are not markedly inferior to opioid infusions, and allow the level of analgesia to be more readily titrated to clinical need. However remifentamil may require infusion.

> *The use of opioid infusions to supplement TIVA is unnecessary in day surgery. Use intermittent bolus doses to cover painful stimuli.*

Should you use nitrous oxide as part of TIVA?

Nitrous oxide is cheap, widely available, and provides some degree of anaesthesia and analgesia. Despite a recent paper claiming that 24 out of 27 papers found an increased incidence of PONV associated with the use of nitrous oxide[58], its use to supplement TIVA has been shown to decrease the requirement for propofol, decrease the duration of immediate recovery and not produce any significant increase in the incidence of PONV[59].

> *The use of nitrous oxide to supplement TIVA is not essential, but may provide some benefits. Its use has been recommended to avoid the risk of awareness.*

Maintenance of anaesthesia by infusion or intermittent boluses?

For short procedures of less than 10 minutes, boluses of propofol are satisfactory, and save the effort of setting up an infusion. For longer procedures, infusion produces a more stable level of anaesthesia and permits 'hands-free' anaesthesia but may be associated with increased drug wastage if less than 20 ml is required for maintenance.

How to gain confidence in the use of TIVA

- If possible, work with someone experienced in using TIVA.
- Begin by using TIVA in straightforward, spontaneously breathing cases. Initially avoid using TIVA in children and in operations on the head and neck. Gynaecological dilatation and curettage or hysteroscopy are ideal.
- Use a dedicated IV cannula for the propofol infusion, sited so that it can be seen at all times.
- If infusing propofol into a line also being used for IV fluids, use a non-return valve to prevent the propofol going into the fluid and not the patient. Be aware that, depending on the distance from the patient that the propofol enters the line, the rate of fluid administration can affect the rate of delivery of propofol to the patient.
- Use an infusion pump specifically designed for the purpose.
- There is no need to use premedication unless otherwise indicated. However, initially at least, supplement TIVA with the use of nitrous oxide.
- Following induction of anaesthesia with a bolus of propofol sufficient to lose the eyelash reflex, usually 3+ mg kg^{-1}, and alfentanil 3–7 µg kg^{-1} or fentanyl 1–1.5 µg kg^{-1}, commence the propofol infusion at 10 mg kg^{-1} hour^{-1} (i.e. 1 ml kg^{-1} hour^{-1}) until the procedure begins. A bolus of alfentanil or fentanyl may be given prior to incision depending on the time since the initial dose.
  (i) If the patient moves in response to surgery or is clinically 'light', give a bolus of propofol, remembering that there will be a time lag until its effect is seen.
  (ii) If no response occurs, decrease the infusion rate to 6 mg kg^{-1} hour^{-1} (i.e. infusion rate in ml hour^{-1} = 0.6 × weight in kg).
  (iii) Initially, stop the infusion at the end of surgery and observe the time to awakening. With experience the infusion can be stopped earlier.

Target-controlled infusion (TCI)

With a TCI pump, all the calculations are performed by the built-in computer pre-programed with a pharmacokinetic model for propofol. At present these pumps will only work in this way if used with bar-coded pre-filled syringes of propofol. The anaesthetist enters the patient's weight and age, and the target blood propofol concentration required. The pump automatically delivers the induction dose and infusion rate needed to maintain this level. The target blood level set, the infusion rate and the calculated blood concentration reached are all displayed.

What target blood concentration?
- For induction of anaesthesia: target concentration = 4–8 μg ml^{-1} in patients under 55 years of age.
- For maintenance: target concentration = 3–6 μg ml^{-1} depending on the amount of supplementary analgesia used.
- For awakening: the concentration is generally between 1 and 2 μg ml^{-1}.

The use of TCI pumps enables the anaesthetist to maintain a stable blood propofol concentration without the manual adjustments to infusion rates required in non-computerized pumps. However TIVA is given, the anaesthetist must continually assess the depth of anaesthesia. Changing the depth of anaesthesia is achieved by changing the target concentration set, similar to using a conventional vaporizer for volatile agents. The advantages of TCIs are shown in *Table 7.6*.

Table 7.6. Advantages of TCIs

Simple to use
Removes the need for calculations
Displays calculated blood level of propofol
Displays decreasing blood level calculated from end of TCI
Compensates for interrupted infusion
Produces stable anaesthesia
Predictable control of the depth of anaesthesia

Points to remember
- Target concentration relates to *blood concentration* and not effector site (brain) concentration. There is a time lag of between 2 and 3 minutes between an increase in blood concentration and the maximum effect on the brain[60]. Failure to take this into consideration can to lead to overdose, particularly at induction of anaesthesia. Slow induction allows titration to effect, and usually achieves anaesthesia with smaller doses of propofol.
- *Time to awakening* depends on the blood concentration at which the infusion has been maintained. The higher the concentration, the longer to wake up. 'Context-sensitive half-time' has been used to take account of the variable processes of redistribution and elimination between compartments with duration of infusion[61]. It is the time required for the plasma drug concentration to fall by 50% after stopping the infusion. The context-sensitive half-time for propofol is short compared with that of other anaesthetic drugs for infusions of longer duration because propofol returned to the central compartment is metabolized rapidly. This makes it particularly suitable for TIVA in day surgery.
- Due to inter-patient variability in propofol pharmacokinetics and pharmacodynamics, there can be no single target concentration that will produce satisfactory anaesthesia in all patients. The target concentration required to induce anaesthesia is a useful guide to maintenance requirements but the depth of anaesthesia must be continually assessed and the target concentration adjusted accordingly.

The development of TCI devices may overcome the main obstacle to the more widespread use of TIVA in day case surgery, that is, unfamiliarity with the concepts and techniques involved. These new pumps are as easy to use as vaporizers, and should encourage wider use of TIVA.

> *TIVA has advantages over maintenance with volatile anaesthesia for day surgery. Its cost may be offset by its excellent recovery and freedom from postoperative morbidity, particularly in operations where this is expected to be significant. TIVA may be cost effective in day surgery.*

References

1. **Schuttler J, Kloos S, Schwilden H, et al.** Total intravenous anaesthesia with propofol and alfentanil by computer-assisted infusion. *Anaesthesia* 1988; **43**: 2–7.
2. **Kashtan H, Edelist G, Mallon J, et al.** Comparative evaluation of propofol and thiopentone for total intravenous anaesthesia *Can. J. Anaesth.* 1990; **37**: 170–176.
3. **Millar JM, Jewkes CF.** Recovery and morbidity after day case anaesthesia. A comparison of propofol with thiopentone–enflurane anaesthesia with and without alfentanil. *Anaesthesia* 1988; **43**: 738–743.
4. **Cork RC, Scipione P, Vonesh MJ, et al.** Propofol infusion vs thiopental/isoflurane for outpatient anaesthesia. *Anesthesiology* 1988; **69** (Suppl.): 3A; A563.
5. **Yung-Fong S, Freniere S, Tillette T, et al.** Comparison of propofol and thiopental anaesthesia in outpatient surgery: Speed of recovery. *Anesthesiology* 1988; **69** (Suppl.): 3A; A562.
6. **Korttila K, Faure E, Apfelbaum J, et al.** Recovery from propofol vs thiopental/isoflurane in patients undergoing outpatient anaesthesia. *Anesthesiology* 1988; **69** (Suppl.): 3A; A564.
7. **Valanne J.** Recovery and discharge of patients after long propofol infusion vs isoflurane anaesthesia for ambulatory surgery. *Acta Anaesthesiol Scand.* 1992; **36**: 530–533.
8. **Siler JN, Horrow JC, Rosenberg H.** Propofol reduces prolonged outpatient PACU stay. *Anesthesiol. Rev.* 1994; **11**: 129–132.
9. **Van Hemelrijck J, Smith I, White PF.** Use of desflurane for outpatient anaesthesia: a comparison with propofol and nitrous oxide. *Anesthesiology* 1991; **75**: 197–203.
10. **Dubin SA, Huang S, Martin E.** Multicentre comparative study evaluating sevoflurane versus propofol in anaesthesia maintenance and recovery in adult outpatients. *Anesthesiology* 1994; **81**: A2.
11. **Pregler J, Stead SW, Beatie CD.** Return of cognitive functions after sevoflurane and propofol general anaesthesia. *Anesthesiology* 1994; **81**: A1.
12. **Weir PM, Munro HM, Reynolds PI, et al.** Propofol infusion and the incidence of emesis in paediatric outpatient strabismus surgery. *Anesth. Analg.* 1993; **76**: 760–764.
13. **Korttila K, Ostman P, Faure E et al.** Randomised comparison of recovery after propofol–nitrous oxide versus thiopentone–isoflurane–nitrous oxide anaesthesia in patients undergoing ambulatory surgery. *Acta Anaesthesiol. Scand.* 1990; **34**: 400–403.
14. **Borgeat A, Wilder-Smith OHG, Sariah M, et al.** Subhypnotic doses of propofol possess direct antiemetic properties *Anesth. Analg.* 1992; **74**: 536–540.
15. **Gan TJ, Ginsberg B, Grant AP, et al.** Double-blind, randomised comparison of ondansetron and intraoperative propofol to prevent postoperative nausea and vomiting. *Anesthesiology* 1996; **85**: 1036–1042.
16. **Hitchcock M, Ogg TW.** Antiemetics in laparoscopic surgery. *Br. J. Anaesth.* 1994; **72**: 608.
17. **Rapp SE, Conahan TJ, Pavlin DJ, et al.** Comparison of desflurane with propofol in outpatients undergoing peripheral orthopaedic surgery. *Anesth. Analg.* 1992; **75**: 572–579.
18. **Huang S, Wong CH, Yang JC, et al.** Comparison of emergence and recovery times between sevoflurane and propofol as maintenance in adult outpatient surgery. *Anesthesiology* 1994; **81**: A6.
19. **Eriksson H, Korttila K.** Recovery profile after desflurane with or without ondansetron compared with propofol in patients undergoing outpatient gynaecological laparoscopy. *Anesth. Analg.* 1996; **82**: 533–538.
20. **Jakobsson J, Oddby E K.** Patient evaluation of four different combinations of intravenous anaesthetics for short outpatient procedures. *Anaesthesia* 1993; **48**: 1005–1007.

21. **Kalman SH, Jensen AG, Ekberg K, et al.** Early and late recovery after major abdominal surgery. Comparison between propofol anaesthesia with and without nitrous oxide and isoflurane anaesthesia. *Acta Anaesthesiol. Scand.* 1993; **37**: 730–736.
22. **Davis PJ, Cohen IT, Mcgowan FX, et al.** Recovery characteristics of desflurane versus halothane for maintenance of anaesthesia in paediatric ambulatory patients. *Anesthesiology* 1994; **80**: 298–302.
23. **Gupta A, Kullander M, Ekberg K, et al.** Anaesthesia for day-care arthroscopy. A comparison between desflurane and isoflurane. *Anaesthesia* 1996; **51**: 56–62.
24. **Apfelbaum JL, Lichtor JL, Lane BS, et al.** Awakening, clinical recovery, and psychomotor effects after desflurane and propofol anaesthesia. *Anesth. Analg.* 1996; **83**: 721–725.
25. **Khan KJ, Cooper GM.** Propofol and malignant hyperthermia: a case for day case anaesthesia? *Anaesthesia* 1993; **48**: 455–456.
26. **Elcock D, Norris A.** Elevated porphyrins following propofol anaesthesia in acute intermittent porphyria. *Anaesthesia* 1994; **49**: 957–958.
27. **Harrison GG, Meissner PN, Hift RJ.** Anaesthesia for the porphyric patient. *Anaesthesia* 1993; **48**: 417–421.
28. **Glass DC, Hall AJ, Harrington JM.** (1989) *The Control of Substances Hazardous to Health: Guidance for Initial Assessment in Hospitals.* HMSO, London.
29. **Armstrong PJ, Spence AA.** Long term exposure of anaesthetic personnel. *Clin. Anaesthesiol.* 1993; **7**: 915–935.
30. **Wood C, Ewen A, Goresky G.** Exposure of operating room personnel to nitrous oxide during paediatric anaesthesia *Can. J. Anaesth.* 1992; **32**: 682–686.
31. **Halsey MJ.** Occupational exposure to inhalational anaesthetics. *Anaesthetic Rounds* 1996. The Medicine Group (Education) Ltd, Abingdon, Oxon, UK.
32. **Phillips AS.** Total intravenous anaesthesia with propofol or inhalational anaesthesia with isoflurane for major abdominal surgery. *Anaesthesia* 1996; **51**: 1055–1059.
33. **Bitner RL.** (1983) Awareness during anaesthesia. In: *Complications in Anesthesiology* (Eds FK Orkin, LH Cooperman). JB Lippincott Co., Philadephia, PA. p. 349.
34. **Sandin R, Nordstrom O.** Awareness during total IV anaesthesia. *Br. J. Anaesth.* 1993; **71**: 782–787.
35. **Ghoneim MM, Block RI.** Learning and consciousness during general anaesthesia. *Anesthesiology* 1992; **76**: 279–305.
36. **Davidson JAH, Macleod AD, Howie JC, et al.** Effective concentration 50 for propofol with and without 67% nitrous oxide. *Acta Anaesthesiol. Scand.* 1993; **37**: 458–464.
37. **Macario A, Vitez TS, Dunn B, et al.** Where are the costs in perioperative care? Analysis of hospital costs and charges for inpatient surgical care. *Anesthesiology* 1995; **83**: 1138–1144.
38. **Ratcliffe F, Lawson R, Millar J.** Day-case laparoscopy revisited: have postoperative morbidity and patient acceptance improved? *Health Trends* 1994; **26**: 47–49.
39. **Bulpitt CJ, Fletcher AE.** Economic assessments in randomised controlled trials. *Med. J. Aust.* 1990; **153** (Suppl.): S16–19.
40. **Hitchcock M, Rudkin G.** The real cost of total intravenous anaesthesia: cost versus price. *Ambulatory Surg.* 1995; **3**: 43–48.
41. **Wagner JG.** A safe method for rapidly achieving plasma concentration plateaux. *Clin. Pharmacol. Ther.* 1974; **16**: 691–697.
42. **Vaughan DP, Tucker GT.** General theory for rapidly establishing steady state drug concentrations using two consecutive constant rate infusions. *Eur. J. Clin. Pharmacol.* 1975; **9**: 235–238.
43. **Hannallah RS, Baker SB, Casey W, et al.** Propofol: effective dose and induction characteristics in unpremedicated children. *Anesthesiology* 1991; **74**: 217–219.
44. **Sear JW.** (1991) Should propofol infusion rate be related to body weight? In: *Focus on Infusion: Intravenous Anaesthesia* (Ed. C Prys-Roberts). Current Medical Literature, London. pp.100–101.
45. **Chassard D, Berrada K, Bryssine B, et al.** Influence of body compartments on propofol induction dose in female patients. *Acta Anaesthesiol. Scand.* 1996; **40**: 889–891.
46. **Turtle MJ, Cullen P, Prys-Roberts C, et al.** Dose requirements of propofol by infusion during nitrous oxide anaesthesia in man: II. Patients premedicated with lorazepam. *Br. J. Anaesth.* 1987; **59**: 283–287.
47. **Spelina KR, Coates DP, Monk CR, et al.** Dose requirements of propofol by infusion during nitrous oxide anaesthesia in man: I. Patients predicated with morphine sulphate. *Br. J. Anaesth.* 1886; **58**: 1080–1084.

48. **Vuyk J, Griever GER, Engbers FHM** *et al.* Alfentanil modifies the concentration–effect relationships of propofol during induction of anaesthesia. *Anesthesiology* 1994; **81:** A402.
49. **Fragen RJ.** Implications of the use of remifentanil on patient outcomes. *Eur. J. Anaesthesiol.* 1995; **10** (Suppl.): 75–76.
50. **Gonzalez-Arrieta ML, Juarez Melendez , Silva Hernandez J,** *et al.* Total intravenous anaesthesia with propofol vs. propofol/midazolam in oncology patients. *Arch. Med. Res.* 1995; **26:** 75–78.
51. **The J, Short TG, Wong J,** *et al.* Pharmacokinetic interactions between midazolam and propofol: an infusion study. *Br. J. Anaesth.* 1994; **72:** 62–65.
52. **Elwood T, Huchcroft S, MacAdams C.** Midazolam coinduction does not delay discharge after very brief propofol anaesthesia. *Can. J. Anaesth.* 1995; **42:** 114–118.
53. **Roberts FL, Dixon J, Lewis GTR,** *et al.* Induction and maintenance of propofol anaesthesia: a manual infusion scheme. *Anaesthesia* 1988; **43** (Suppl.): 14–17.
54. **Tackley RM, Lewis GTR, Prys-Roberts C,** *et al.* Computer controlled infusion of propofol. *Br. J. Anaesth.* 1989; **62:** 46–53.
55. **Dunnet JM, Prys-Roberts C, Holland DE,** *et al.* Propofol infusion and the suppression of consciousness: dose requirements to induce loss of consciousness and to suppress response to noxious and non-noxious stimuli. *Br. J. Anaesth.* 1994; **72:** 29–34.
56. **Gepts E, Jonckhleer K, Maes V,** *et al.* Disposition kinetics of propofol during alfentanil anaesthesia. *Anaesthesia* 1988; **43** (Suppl.): 8–13.
57. **Hull CJ.** The pharmacokinetics of alfentanil in man. *Br. J. Anaesth.* 1983; **55** (Suppl. 2): 157S–164S.
58. **Hartung J.** Twenty-four of twenty-seven studies show greater incidence of emesis associated with nitrous oxide than with alternative anaesthetics. *Anesth. Analg.* 1996; **83:** 114–116.
59. **Sukhani R, Lurie J, Jabamoni R.** Propofol for ambulatory gynaecologic laparoscopy: does omission of nitrous oxide alter postoperative emetic sequelae and recovery? *Anesth. Analg.* 1994; **78:** 831–835.
60. **Ludbrook GL, Upton RN, Grant,** *et al.* Brain and blood concentrations of propofol after rapid intravenous injection in sheep, and their relationship to cerebral effects. *Anaesth. Intens. Care* 1996; **24:** 445–452.
61. **Hughes MA, Glass PSA, Jacobs JR.** Context-sensitive half-time in multicompartment pharmacokinetic models for intravenous anaesthetic drugs. *Anesthesiology* 1992; **76:** 334–341.

CHAPTER 8

Postoperative nausea and vomiting (PONV)

M. Hitchcock

PONV is common after day surgery[1]. A recent study in a selection of British DSUs found that the incidence of PONV ranged from 30% in the best centres to 68% in others[2].

While common during recovery in the DSU, PONV may only begin after the patient leaves the unit. Carroll *et al.*[3] found that over 35% of patients experienced postdischarge nausea and vomiting and, interestingly, most of these had not suffered from emetic problems while in the DSU. These symptoms were neither mild nor short lived. This study revealed that during the first 5 postoperative days, these patients experienced nausea for an average of 1.7 days and vomiting for 0.7 days[3]. This was suffciently severe that patients in this group were slower to resume their normal activities than those without PONV. Similarly, Watson *et al.*[2] found that 17% of patients complained of nausea and/or vomiting on the first postoperative day and 11% on the second.

> PONV is common and its published incidence has changed little in the past 10 years[1,4]. Day case operations introduced more recently, such as laparoscopic cholecystectomy, are associated with an increased incidence[5]. PONV remains a problem for every clinician working in day surgery.

The importance of PONV

Unpleasantness of nausea and vomiting
Orkin[6] found that of all forms of minor morbidity associated with day surgery, patients were most keen to avoid PONV. In order to do so, they were willing to tolerate a variety of other forms of morbidity or inconvenience, including more pain, longer hospital stays and increased cost. However those working in the field of day surgery may view this form of 'minor' morbidity, to patients it is a most serious and important problem.

Duration of stay and unplanned admission
Green and Jonsson[7] demonstrated that postoperative nausea was the most important factor in determining the length of hospital stay after ambulatory surgery, and PONV has been shown to be one of the main reasons for unplanned overnight admission[7,8]. In addition, unplanned admission may also result from sedation and other side-effects of potent antiemetics such as droperidol[9], although this is not common[10].

Cost
Carroll *et al.*[11] found that personnel, supply and drug costs for the management of PONV in day case surgery averaged $US14.94 per patient. PONV also increased the

running costs of the unit by prolonging recovery room stay; and in units running at near capacity, this was estimated to cost as much as $US415 per patient.

> *PONV increases costs and decreases efficiency in day surgery. More importantly, it is the aspect of postoperative morbidity dreaded most by patients.*

Prevention of PONV

Good day surgery practice focuses on primary prevention of PONV rather than treatment of established morbidity. This entails more than simply administering antiemetics (*Table 8.1*).

Table 8.1. Strategies for the reduction of PONV

Identify high-risk patients and operations
Consider prophylactic antiemesis for these groups
Use general measures to reduce the likelihood of triggering PONV
Choose an anaesthetic technique which minimizes PONV
Treat established PONV using protocols that can be followed by recovery staff without recourse to an anaesthetist

> *Good day surgery organization and treatment is the key to reducing PONV.*

Identify those at increased risk

Surgical factors.
Type of surgery. Patients and surgeons traditionally attribute PONV to the anaesthetic, but there is good evidence that the type of surgery, irrespective of the anaesthetic technique, makes a significant contribution to the incidence and severity of PONV[12]. Certain operations are associated with a high incidence of PONV (*Table 8.2*).

Table 8.2. Operations associated with a high risk of PONV

Adults	Children
Laparoscopy – especially sterilization or cholecystectomy	Bat ear correction
	Strabismus surgery
Dental procedures	Circumcision
Ovum retrieval	Orchidopexy
	Inguinal hernia repair

Duration of surgery and anaesthesia. This may influence the incidence of PONV. Watson *et al.*[2] found that operations lasting longer than 1 hour were associated with a higher incidence of PONV. This may be due to a number of factors, including increased effects of anaesthesia, type of surgery, prolonged fasting and increased pain.

Pain. Certain types of day case surgery are associated with increased postoperative pain. While it is true that some patients may feel nauseous with severe pain, a direct causal relationship between pain and PONV is unproven. While Jakobsson *et al.*[13] found that pain increases the severity of PONV, Parnass *et al.*[14] found the incidence of PONV to be unrelated to the incidence of postoperative pain. Anderson and Krohg[15] found that 90% of in-patients with nausea after abdominal surgery also had accompanying pain, and that in 80% of these patients, pain relief using opioid medication also resulted in relief of nausea. However, a much more common day case scenario is one in which an opioid, usually morphine, administered to relieve postoperative pain, produces nausea in addition to analgesia.

Patient factors (Table 8.3).

Table 8.3. Patient characteristics predisposing to PONV

Age: highest in children and young adults
Gender: females > males
?BMI >30
History of previous PONV
History of motion sickness

Age. Several studies have shown that the incidence of PONV varies with age[16]. PONV is least in infants below 12 months of age (5%), increases to 20% in children under 5 years, remains at between 34 and 40% from 6 to 65 years and declines thereafter.

Sex. Women are recognized to be two to three times more prone to PONV than males, and PONV is likely to be of greater severity[17]. This is only true for females older than 11 years[18]. A possible link between the incidence of PONV and the phase of the menstrual cycle has been found. Honkavaara *et al.*[19] have shown that PONV is more likely during the menstrual period itself. This implies that female patients with other risk factors for PONV should, if possible, be scheduled for elective day case surgery during the phase of the menstrual cycle least associated with PONV, although which time of the cycle is least likely to exacerbate PONV is disputed[20]. Such forethought requires more organization than many busy day surgery units can achieve, but might represent an ideal.

Obesity. Palazzo and Strunin[21] found that patients with a BMI >30 were more likely to suffer from PONV. The reasons for this may include difficulty with face mask ventilation leading to gastric distention. In a later study, in which patients were not ventilated by face mask before intubation, no relationship between BMI and PONV was found[1].

History of PONV and motion sickness. Patients with a history of PONV after previous anaesthetics have been found to have a threefold greater incidence of PONV in the first 24 hours postoperatively than patients without such a history[22]. Many patients only begin to experience emetic symptoms as they begin their journey home following discharge. Several studies have demonstrated an increase in PONV after discharge, especially in patients who have received morphine, due to its vestibular effect[23]. In addition, anti-motion sickness drugs such as hyoscine are more beneficial in patients prone to motion sickness than ondansetron, although ondansetron has a better side-effect profile[24]. Patients should be assured that while some patients will experience PONV despite all measures, everything will be done to try to prevent or reduce it.

> *A history of previous PONV or motion sickness should merit prophylactic antiemetic treatment.*

Antiemetic prophylaxis
For those patients at increased risk of PONV, prophylactic antiemetics may be indicated. Van den Berg[25] suggests that an antiemetic should produce a reduction in the incidence of PONV of 55% to justify its routine prophylactic use. Most groups of antiemetics fall far short of this ideal. The choice of antiemetic medication used in the day surgery setting will depend on its efficacy, cost and side effect profile. $5HT_3$ antagonists (most studies have used ondansetron) and droperidol most closely satisfy these criteria[26,27]. They have generally been given IV, either immediately prior to induction or during surgery.

Droperidol. This has been shown to be equally effective at doses of 2.5, 1.25 and 0.625 mg[28]. It is difficult to give 0.625 mg in the dilutions available in the UK, and 0.5 mg is satisfactory. Lower doses are less likely to cause side-effects, which include drowsiness, restlessness, anxiety and acute dystonia, reported even after doses as low as 0.625 mg[9]. The incidence of restlessness, or akathisia, after droperidol in day surgery may be underestimated[10]. Some consider that the side-effect profile of droperidol, even in low doses, makes it unsuitable for routine prophylaxis.

Ondansetron. This is usually given in a dose of 4 or 8 mg. There would appear to be little evidence that the higher doses are more effective[24]. The $5HT_3$ receptor antagonists, ondansetron, granisetron and tropisetron, have all been shown to be equally effective for the prophylaxis of PONV[29]. They have few side-effects, making them attractive in day surgery, but their cost makes their routine prophylactic use in large numbers of day case patients expensive. These additional costs may be justified: Watcha and Smith[30] showed prophylactic ondansetron to be cost effective, but only for operations with a high incidence of PONV, when the frequency of emesis was greater than 33%.

> *For prophylactic antiemesis, droperidol 0.5 or 0.625 mg IV at induction is the treatment of choice where cost is an issue, but in view of its reported side-effects, it should be limited to at-risk patients. If the expected incidence of PONV for the procedure is greater than 33%, or the patient is at particularly high risk of PONV, the use of ondansetron 4 mg IV is justified.*

General measures
For general measures applicable to all patients, see *Table 8.4*.

Alleviate anxiety. A direct relationship between increased preoperative anxiety and an increased incidence of PONV is not well established. However, there are theoretical reasons why anxious patients may be at an increased risk of PONV, due both to delayed gastric emptying and increased gastric volume from swallowed air[31,32]. Measures to alleviate anxiety are discussed in Chapter 4.

Premedication with anti-acid and prokinetic drugs. The use of ranitidine and metoclopramide may help reduce PONV. While the efficacy of metoclopramide as an antiemetic is questionable, it is a potent prokinetic agent for gastric motility. Ranitidine given preoperatively may also reduce PONV[33], although it is not as effective as droperidol[34]. Metoclopramide 10 mg and ranitidine 150 mg PO 60–90 minutes before surgery have therefore been recommended[35,36]. These drugs should be administered on arrival, to allow sufficient time for them to work.

Table 8.4. General measures to reduce the incidence of PONV

Alleviate anxiety
Premedication with ranitidine and metoclopramide
Keep patients warm
Maintain appropriate fluid balance
Avoid gastric distention. Consider LMA
Avoid unnecessary pharyngeal suction
Limit unnecessary movement

Keep patients warm. Being cold postoperatively is unpleasant, may increase the need for oxygen if associated with shivering, and contributes to an increased incidence of PONV[36].

Maintain appropriate fluid balance. Preoperative fasting guidelines have changed in the past 5 years to allow preoperative fluids up to 2–3 hours preoperatively (see Chapter 3). This may reduce thirst and PONV[37].

Peroperative IV fluids (see Chapter 5) may reduce PONV after longer operations[38]. However, for shorter procedures, it may be simpler and as effective to encourage oral fluids preoperatively.

Intraoperative IV fluids, ideally 4% dextrose, 0.18% saline in volumes of between 15 and 20 ml kg^{-1} should be administered intraoperatively, where the assessed risk of PONV is high, or in operations lasting longer than 20 minutes.

Postoperative oral fluid intake may increase PONV in certain patients. With decreased periods of preoperative fasting and intraoperative fluid replacement, thirst in the immediate postoperative period is reduced in most patients[39]. Postoperative vomiting is often precipitated by the first oral fluids. Patients are a good guide as to when to offer them food and drink postoperatively: they should be allowed to drink or eat when they wish.

Avoid gastric distention. This may result from face mask ventilation, and has been shown to increase the incidence of PONV[1]. Transient apnoea after intravenous agents, particularly if large bolus doses of opioids are used, can be minimized by slow injection and reducing the dose of opioid. Airway maintenance using the LMA may decrease the incidence of PONV through a variety of factors, including less gastric distention, avoiding the need for muscle relaxants and anticholinesterase drugs, and by allowing lighter planes of anaesthesia[40] (Chapter 6).

Avoid unnecessary pharyngeal suction. Pharyngeal suction can precipitate retching and vomiting. Trepanier[41] found that the aspiration of gastric contents via an orogastric tube during surgery increased the incidence of PONV, possibly due to stimulation of pharyngeal reflexes. Where the LMA has been used, removing it without cuff deflation may reduce the need for suction by sweeping out pooled secretions.

Limit unnecessary movement of patients, especially postoperatively and ensure it is gentle, and smooth. Kamath *et al.*[22] found that 66% of patients who cited a cause for their PONV blamed movement, and these patients had a particular susceptibility to motion sickness. Sudden or violent movement has been shown to increase the incidence of PONV, especially in those patients given opioid analgesics[42].

> *General measures to reduce PONV should be routine practice in day surgery for all patients, but particularly for at-risk patients.*

Anaesthetic technique

Induction agents. The choice of induction agent can affect the incidence of PONV. Myles *et al.*[43] found that induction with propofol reduced PONV by 18% compared with thiopentone. Similarly, Boysen *et al.*[44] found that PONV and recovery time were reduced with propofol, compared with both thiopentone and etomidate, in minor gynaecological surgery. Etomidate has a higher incidence of PONV associated with its use than thiopentone[45].

> *Propofol is undoubtedly the induction agent of choice in the avoidance of PONV.*

Maintenance: propofol versus volatiles. Several studies have compared a propofol-based TIVA technique with propofol induction and volatile maintenance. Most have found a decreased incidence of PONV associated with a TIVA technique[46]. Maintenance of anaesthesia with an infusion of propofol has also been shown to be associated with a low incidence of PONV when compared with the newer volatile anaesthetics, sevoflurane[47] and desflurane[48]. Ericksson and Korttila[49] recommend the use of prophylactic ondansetron when using desflurane, but even this combination is associated with a greater incidence of PONV than TIVA. Propofol has been shown to be more effective than ondansetron in preventing PONV, but only when used for both induction and maintenance of anaesthesia in a TIVA technique[50].

> *TIVA using propofol is the technique of choice to minimize PONV.*

Nitrous oxide. The role played by nitrous oxide in PONV is controversial. Lonie and Harper[51] found that the omission of nitrous oxide from their anaesthetic technique, for patients undergoing day case laparoscopic surgery, resulted in a lower incidence of PONV. However most reports investigating the emetic potential of nitrous oxide used to supplement volatile anaesthetics have failed to demonstrate a convincing causal relationship between nitrous oxide and PONV[52,53] although meta-analysis has concluded that it does contribute to PONV[54].

When propofol is used for induction and maintenance, increased PONV with nitrous oxide is more difficult to demonstrate. Sukhani *et al.*[55] investigated the effect of nitrous oxide on PONV in patients undergoing day case gynaecological laparoscopy anaesthetized with propofol with or without nitrous oxide. They found that nitrous oxide supplementation did not increase the incidence of PONV. Furthermore, the use of nitrous oxide reduced the requirements for propofol and produced a faster immediate recovery. No opioid drugs were used during this study. It has been suggested that nitrous oxide may increase the incidence of PONV only when used in conjunction with longer-acting opioids to supplement propofol anaesthesia, although the study of Sukhani *et al.*[55] does not support this theory. Where the risk of PONV is high, the balance of evidence suggests that nitrous oxide may increase the incidence of PONV[54], but its usefulness in preventing awareness must not be overlooked.

> *There is little evidence that nitrous oxide is a major factor in the incidence of PONV, but it should be omitted where the risk of PONV is high.*

Opioids. Although longer-acting opioids such as morphine undoubtedly increase PONV[23], potent but relatively short-acting opioid drugs, such as alfentanil and fentanyl, may not do so. These short-acting opioids are essential for the successful prevention and treatment of pain following many day surgery procedures.

Forrest *et al.*[56] have shown that the use of fentanyl in a balanced anaesthetic technique, as a substitute for volatile agents, is associated with increased PONV. However, several studies have demonstrated that both fentanyl and alfentanil, when used to supplement anaesthesia, are associated with reduced PONV and earlier ambulation and discharge[57].

> *In day case procedures where opioids are needed to prevent and treat postoperative pain, shorter-acting drugs, such as fentanyl and alfentanil, are the drugs of choice. Longer-lasting analgesia should be provided by the use of local anaesthetics and non-opioid analgesics, such as NSAIDs. Avoid morphine.*

Local anaesthesia. While it is generally accepted that the incidence of PONV following local anaesthesia is very low, controversy surrounds the use of spinal anaesthesia in day surgery[58], which may increase PONV if hypotension results.

> *The use of local anaesthesia, alone or with sedation, is strongly recommended where possible, and where the risk of PONV is high.*

Muscle relaxants and reversal agents. Muscle relaxants themselves are not thought to be implicated in the causation of PONV. However, anticholinesterase drugs, used to reverse their effect, may be pro-emetic[59]. The use of non-depolarizing muscle relaxants such as mivacurium, which do not require reversal, have been shown to be associated with a decreased incidence of PONV, and may be the drugs of choice[60].

Management of established PONV

Scoring severity. DSUs should routinely score PONV. Nausea is subjective and visual analogue scoring systems have been used to measure this[61]. Retching and vomiting can be objectively measured. Antiemetic treatment should be given to any patient with retching, vomiting, moderate or severe nausea (>4 on a visual analogue score), or who requests antiemetic therapy.

Antiemetic treatment. Similar considerations of efficacy, side-effects and cost apply to the antiemetics used to treat PONV which results despite the measures described above. The most effective antiemetics currently available to treat PONV are droperidol and the $5HT_3$ antagonists. The majority of studies have investigated the efficacy of ondansetron[26].

Although several placebo-controlled studies have used ondansetron in doses of 8 mg[62,63], it is an effective antiemetic for the treatment of established PONV in doses as low as 1 and 4 mg[64]. Watcha and Smith[30] concluded that treatment of established symptoms with ondansetron was cost effective even when the incidence of PONV was low, and that droperidol was a cost-effective alternative when the incidence of PONV was only 10%.

> *For established PONV, ondansetron 4 mg IV should be the first-line therapy. If prophylactic ondansetron has already been given, droperidol 0.5 or 0.625 mg IV should be used.*

An example of a PONV management protocol is shown in *Figure 8.1.*

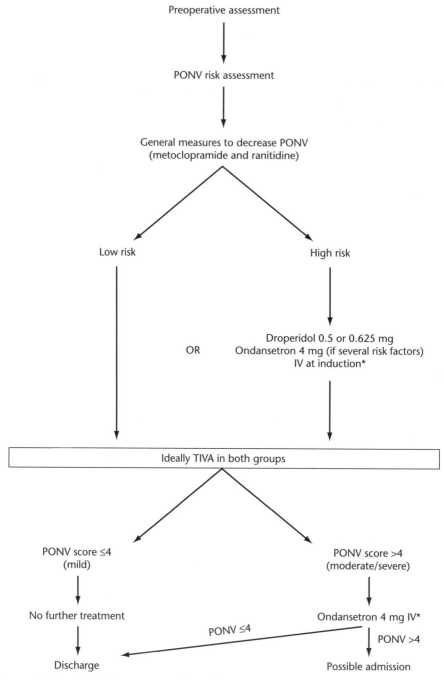

Figure 8.1. Postoperative nausea and vomiting treatment protocol.
*If ondansetron is used for prophylaxis, use droperidol for treatment of PONV scores >4.

In addition....
Ephedrine. It is well known that hypotension can cause nausea and vomiting. Ephedrine is a useful drug to prevent and treat PONV, even where BP is within normal limits: 0.5 mg kg^{-1} IM has been shown to be as effective as droperidol[65].

Ephedrine 3–6 mg IV is especially useful in patients with increased postural hypotension postoperatively, typically young females with low/normal preoperative blood pressure.

The efficacy of ephedrine may be due to correction of relative hypovolaemia produced by prolonged preoperative starvation. If so, more widespread use of pre- and intraoperative hydration may decrease the need for this drug.

Steroids. Dexamethasone has been shown to decrease the incidence of swelling, nausea and vomiting following dental surgery[66]. In addition it has been found to exert a synergistic effect on other antiemetics, such as granisetron, in gynaecological surgery[67]. Dexamethasone, in an IV dose of 8 mg for an adult patient, should be considered for antiemetic prophylaxis, especially in oral surgery.

Metoclopramide. Fifty percent of the studies reviewed by Rowbotham revealed that metoclopramide was no more effective than placebo in the prevention of PONV[68]. Furthermore, IV metoclopramide is not free from side-effects, the most important of which are extrapyramidal reactions. On current evidence there is nothing to recommend the use of IV metoclopramide as an antiemetic in day case anaesthesia. Its prokinetic effect when given as an oral premedication may be of value in emptying the stomach.

Alternative antiemetic therapy. Many other additional methods have been used to prevent and treat PONV, e.g. ginger root, acupuncture, hypnosis and transdermal scopolamine patches. While some success is claimed for all of these measures, none is consistently better than the antiemetics described[69-71]. DSUs may choose to have a number of supplementary measures available.

Conclusions

PONV is very common following day surgery. It has a significant effect on the patients' perceptions of the quality of their care, and on day unit efficiency in terms of throughput and costs. Patients must be assessed preoperatively for risk factors for PONV.

Simple measures may help to decrease the incidence of PONV in those at low risk, but for patients at higher risk, prophylactic antiemetic therapy is indicated. Droperidol is the drug of choice in this situation, given IV in a low dose at induction. For patients with several risk factors for PONV, the use of ondansetron would be justified. If established symptoms develop, first-line therapy should be with ondansetron, unless already used, in which case droperidol should be used.

However, the most effective strategy in reducing PONV may be the avoidance of volatile anaesthetic agents, and the use of propofol for induction and maintenance of anaesthesia[50]. Rescue antiemetics may then be used only if needed.

> *Successful management of PONV should be focused on prevention. This requires the use of techniques with a low incidence of PONV for all patients, the detection of those most at risk, in whom additional measures can be employed, and the use of antiemetic protocols to prevent and treat PONV where indicated.*

References

1. **Watcha MF, White PF.** Postoperative nausea and vomiting. Its aetiology, treatment and prevention. *Anesthesiology* 1992; **77**: 162–184.
2. **Watson BJ, Hitchcock M, Swailes R, et al.** Nausea and vomiting after day surgery under general anaesthesia. A multicentre survey of symptoms after discharge. *Ambulatory Surg.* 1997; in press.
3. **Carroll NV, Miederhoff P, Cox FM, et al.** Postoperative nausea and vomiting after discharge from outpatient surgery centres. *Anesth. Analg.* 1995; **80**: 903–909.
4. **Cohen MM, Duncan PG, DeBoer DP, et al.** The postoperative interview: assessing risk factors for nausea and vomiting. *Anesth. Analg.* 1994; **78**: 7–16.
5. **Madsen MR, Jensen KEJ.** Postoperative pain and nausea after laparoscopic cholecystectomy. *Surg. Laparosc. Endosc.* 1992; **2**: 303–305.
6. **Orkin F.** What do patients really want? Preferences for immediate postoperative recovery. *Anesth. Analg.* 1992; **74**: S225.
7. **Green G, Jonsson L.** Nausea: the most important factor in determining length of hospital stay after ambulatory anaesthesia. A comparative study of isoflurane and/or propofol techniques. *Acta Anaesthesiol. Scand.* 1993; **37**: 742–746.
8. **Gold BS, Kitz DS, Lecky JH, et al.** Unanticipated admission to the hospital following ambulatory surgery. *J. Am. Med. Assoc.* 1989; **262**: 3008–3010.
9. **Melnick B, Sawyer R, Karambelkar D, et al.** Delayed side-effects of droperidol after ambulatory general anaesthesia. *Anesth. Analg.* 1989; **69**: 748–751.
10. **Davis PJ, McGowan FX Jr, Landsman I.** Effect of antiemetic therapy on recovery and hospital discharge time. A double-blind assessment of ondansetron, droperidol, and placebo in paediatric patients undergoing ambulatory surgery. *Anesthesiology* 1995; **83**: 956–960.
11. **Carroll NV, Miederhoff PA, Cox FM, et al.** Costs incurred by outpatient surgical centres in managing postoperative nausea and vomiting. *J. Clin. Anesth.* 1994; **6**: 364–369.
12. **Lerman J.** Surgical and patient factors involved in postoperative nausea and vomiting *Br. J. Anaesth.* 1992; **69** (Suppl. 1): 24S–32S.
13. **Jakobsson J, Davidson S, Andreen M, et al.** Opioid supplementation to propofol anaesthesia for outpatient abortion: a comparison between alfentanil, fentanyl and placebo. *Acta Anaesthesiol. Scand.* 1991; **35**: 767–770.
14. **Parnass SM, McCarthy RJ, Ivankovich AD.** The role of pain as a cause of postoperative nausea/vomiting after outpatient anaesthesia. *Anesth. Analg.* 1992; **74**: S233.
15. **Anderson R , Krohg K.** Pain as a major cause of postoperative nausea. *Can. Anaesth. Soc. J.* 1976; **23**: 366–369.
16. **Cohen MM, Cameron CB, Duncan PG.** Paediatric anaesthetic morbidity and mortality in the perioperative period. *Anesth. Analg.* 1990; **70**: 160–167.
17. **Zelcer J, Wells DG.** Anaesthetic related recovery room complications. *Anaesth. Intens. Care* 1987; **15**: 168–174.
18. **Rowley MP, Brown TCK.** Postoperative vomiting in children. *Anaesth. Intens. Care* 1982; **10**: 309–313.
19. **Honkavaara P, Lehtinen AM, Hovorka J, et al.** Nausea and vomiting after gynaecological laparoscopy depends upon the phase of the menstrual cycle. *Can. J. Anaesth.* 1991; **38**: 876–879.
20. **Beattie WS, Lindblad T, Buckley DN, et al.** The incidence of postoperative nausea and vomiting in women undergoing laparoscopy is influenced by the day of the menstrual cycle. *Can. J. Anaesth.* 1991; **38**: 298–302.
21. **Palazzo MGA, Strunin L.** Anaesthesia and emesis. I: aetiology. *Can. J. Anaesth.* 1984; **31**: 178–187.
22. **Kamath B, Curran J, Hawkey C, et al.** Anaesthesia, movement, and emesis. *Br. J. Anaesth.* 1990; **64**: 728–730.
23. **Weinstein MS, Nicholson SC, Schreiner MS.** A single dose of morphine sulphate increases the incidence of vomiting after outpatient inguinal surgery in children. *Anesthesiology* 1994; **81**: 572–577.
24. **Honkavaara P.** Effect of ondansetron on. nausea and vomiting after middle ear surgery during general anaesthesia. *Br. J. Anaesth.* 1996; **76**: 316–318.
25. **Van den Berg AA.** The prophylactic antiemetic efficacy of prochlorperazine and ondansetron in nasal septal surgery: a randomised double-blind comparison. *Aust. Soc. Anaesth.* 1996; **24**: 538–545.

26. **Russell D, Kenny GNC.** 5HT$_3$ antagonists in postoperative nausea and vomiting. *Br. J. Anaesth.* 1992; **69** (Suppl. 1): 63S–68S.

27. **Gan TJ, Collis R, Hetreed M.** Double-blind comparison of ondansetron, droperidol and saline in the prevention of postoperative nausea and vomiting. *Br. J. Anaesth.* 1994; **72**: 544–547.

28. **Tang J. Watcha MF, White PF.** A comparison of cost efficacy of ondansetron and droperidol as prophylactic therapy for elective outpatient gynaecologic procedures. *Anesth. Analg.* 1996; **83**: 304–313.

29. **Naguib M, Bakry AKE, Khoshim MHB,** *et al.* Prophylactic antiemetic therapy with ondansetron, tropisetron, granisetron and metoclopramide in patients undergoing laparoscopic cholecystectomy: a randomised, double-blind comparison with placebo. *Can. J. Anaesth.* 1996; **43**: 226–231.

30. **Watcha MF, Smith I.** Cost-effectiveness analysis of antiemetic therapy for ambulatory surgery. *J. Clin. Anaesth.* 1994; **6**: 370–377.

31. **Jenkins LC, Lahay D.** Central mechanisms of vomiting related to catecholamine responses: anaesthetic implications. *Can. Anaesth. Soc. J.* 1971; **18**: 434–441.

32. **Ong BY, Palahnuik RJ, Cumming M.** Gastric volume and pH in out-patients. *Can. Anaesth. Soc. J.* 1978; **25**: 36–39.

33. **Kraynack BJ, Bates MK.** Antiemetic action of ranitidine in out-patient laparoscopy under propofol–isoflurane anaesthesia. *Anesthesiology* 1990; **73**: A14.

34. **Cozanitis D, Asantila R, Eklund P,** *et al.* A comparison of ranitidine, droperidol or placebo in the prevention of nausea and vomiting after hysterectomy. *Can. J. Anaesth.* 1996; **43**: 106–109.

35. **Miller JR, Anderson WG.** Silent regurgitation in day case gynaecological patients. *Anaesthesia* 1988; **43**: 321–323.

36. **Kallar SK.** New modalities in postoperative nausea and vomiting. *J. Clin. Anaesth.* 1992; **4** (Suppl. 1): 16S–19S.

37. **Gilbert SS, Easy WR, Fitch WW.** The effect of preoperative oral fluid on morbidity following anaesthesia for minor surgery. *Anaesthesia* 1995; **50**: 79–81.

38. **Yogendran S, Asokumar B, Cheng DCH,** *et al.* A prospective randomised double-blinded study of the effect of intravenous fluid therapy on adverse outcomes in outpatient surgery. *Anesth. Analg.* 1995; **80**: 682–686.

39. **Strunin L.** How long should patients fast before surgery? Time for new guidelines. *Br. J. Anaesth.* 1993; **70**: 1–3.

40. **Luff AJ, Morris RJ, Wainwright AC.** Day case management in adjustable suture squint surgery. *Eye* 1993; **7**: 694–696.

41. **Trepanier CA.** Perioperative gastric aspiration increases postoperative nausea and vomiting in outpatients. *Can. J. Anaesth.* 1993; **40**: 325–328.

42. **Muir JJ, Warner MA, Offord KP,** *et al.* Role of nitrous oxide and other factors in postoperative nausea and vomiting: a randomised and blinded study. *Anaesthesiology* 1987; **66**: 513–518.

43. **Myles PS, Hendrata M, Bennett AM.** Postoperative nausea and vomiting. Propofol or thiopentone: does choice of induction agent affect outcome? *Anaesth. Intens. Care* 1996; **24**: 355–359.

44. **Boysen K, Sanchez R, Krintel J,** *et al.* Induction and recovery characteristics of propofol, thiopentone, and etomidate. *Acta Anaesthesiol. Scand.* 1989; **33**: 689–692.

45. **Korttila K, Tammisto T, Aromaa U.** Comparison of etomidate in combination with fentanyl of diazepam, with thiopentone as an induction agent for general anaesthesia. *Br. J. Anaesth.* 1979; **51**: 1151–1157.

46. **Raftery S, Sherry E.** Total intravenous anaesthesia with propofol and alfentanil protects against postoperative nausea and vomiting. *Can. J. Anaesth.* 1992; **39**: 37–40.

47. **Huang S, Wong CH, Yang JC,** *et al.* Comparison of emergence and recovery times between sevoflurane and propofol as maintenance in adult outpatient surgery. *Anesthesiology* 1994; **81**: A6.

48. **Rapp SE, Conahan TJ, Pavlin DJ,** *et al.* Comparison of desflurane with propofol in outpatients undergoing peripheral orthopaedic surgery. *Anesth. Analg.* 1992; **75**: 572–579.

49. **Eriksson H, Korttila K.** Recovery profile after desflurane with or without ondansetron compared with propofol in patients undergoing outpatient gynaecological laparoscopy. *Anesth. Analg.* 1996; **82**: 533–538.

50. **Gan TJ, Ginsberg B, Grant AP,** *et al.* Double-blind, randomised comparison of ondansetron and intraoperative propofol to prevent postoperative nausea and vomiting. *Anesthesiology* 1996; **85**: 1036–1042.

51. **Lonie DS, Harper NJN.** Nitrous oxide anaesthesia and vomiting: the effect of nitrous oxide anaesthesia on the incidence of vomiting following gynaecological laparoscopy. *Anaesthesia* 1986; **41:** 703–707.

52. **Hovorka J, Korttila K, Erkola O.** Nitrous oxide does not increase nausea and vomiting following gynaecological laparoscopy. *Can. Anaesth. Soc. J.* 1989; **36:** 145–148.

53. **Sengupta P, Plantevin OM.** Nitrous oxide and day case laparoscopy: effect on nausea, vomiting, and return to normal activity. *Br. J. Anaesth.* 1988; **60:** 570–573.

54. **Tramer M, Moore A, McQuay H.** Omitting nitrous oxide in general anaesthesia: meta-analysis of intraoperative awareness and postoperative emesis in randomised controlled trials. *Br. J. Anaesth.* 1996; **76:** 186–193.

55. **Sukhani R, Lurie J. Jabamoni R.** Propofol for ambulatory gynaecologic laparoscopy: does omission of nitrous oxide alter postoperative emetic sequelae and recovery? *Anesth. Analg.* 1994; **78:** 831–835.

56. **Forrest JB, Cahalan MK, Rehder K.** Multicentre study of general anaesthesia. *Anesthesiology* 1990; **72:** 262–268.

57. **Millar JM, Jewkes CF.** Recovery and morbidity after day case anaesthesia. A comparison of propofol with thiopentone–enflurane anaesthesia with and without alfentanil. *Anaesthesia* 1988; **43:** 738–743.

58. **Rabey PG, Smith G.** Anaesthetic factors contributing to postoperative nausea and vomiting. *Br. J. Anaesth.* 1992; **69** (Suppl. 1): 40S–45S.

59. **King MJ, Milazkiewicz R, Carli F.** Influence of neostigmine on postoperative nausea and vomiting. *Br. J. Anaesth.* 1988; **61:** 403–406.

60. **Ding Y, Fredman B, White PF.** Use of mivacurium during laparoscopic surgery: effect of reversal drugs on postoperative recovery. *Anesth. Analg.* 1994; **78:** 450–454.

61. **Hitchcock M, Ogg TW.** Quality assurance in day case anaesthesia. *Ambulatory Surg.* 1994; **2:** 193–204.

62. **Bodner M, White PF.** Antiemetic efficacy of ondansetron after outpatient laparoscopy. *Anesth. Analg.* 1991; **73:** 250–254.

63. **Larijani GE, Gratz I, Afshar M, et al.** Treatment of postoperative nausea and vomiting with ondansetron: a randomised, double-blind comparison with placebo. *Anesth. Analg.* 1991; **73:** 246–249.

64. **Scuderi P, Wetchler BV, Sung YF, et al.** Treatment of postoperative nausea and vomiting after outpatient surgery with the 5HT3 antagonist ondansetron. *Anesthesiology* 1993; **78:** 15–20.

65. **Rothenberg DM, Parnass SM, Litwack K, et al.** Efficacy of ephedrine in the prevention of postoperative nausea and vomiting. *Anesth. Analg.* 1991; **72:** 58–61.

66. **Baxendale BR, Vater M, Lavery KM.** Dexamethasone reduces pain and swelling following extraction of third molar teeth. *Anaesthesia* 1993; **48:** 961–964.

67. **Fujii Y, Tanaka H, Toyooka H.** Granisetron–dexamethasone combination reduces postoperative nausea and vomiting. *Can. J. Anaesth.* 1995; **42:** 387–390.

68. **Rowbotham DJ.** Current management of postoperative nausea and vomiting. *Br. J. Anaesth.* 1992; **69** (Suppl. 1): 46S–59S.

69. **Phillips S, Ruggier R, Hutchinson SE.** Zingiber Officinale (Ginger) – an antiemetic for day case surgery. *Anaesthesia* 1993; **48:** 715–717.

70. **Ghaly RG, Fitzpatrick KTJ, Dundee JW.** Antiemetic studies with traditional Chinese acupuncture. *Anaesthesia* 1987; **42:** 1108–1110.

71. **Arfeen Z, Owen H, Plummer JL, et al.** A double-blind randomised trial of ginger for the prevention of postoperative nausea and vomiting. *Anaesth. Intens. Care* 1995; **23:** 449–459.

CHAPTER 9

Pain management in the adult day surgery patient

G.E. Rudkin

The selection of suitable day surgery procedures depends primarily on adequate pain management. This is increasingly important as we are presented with patients with more 'complex' procedures. Acute pain management in day surgery requires a planned, balanced approach, incorporating combinations of analgesic methods, and the assessment and institution of a pain management plan. This allows nursing staff to implement therapy efficiently, resulting in improved patient comfort and avoiding complications associated with inadequate pain control. See *Table 9.1* for aims of pain management.

Table 9.1. Aims of pain management

To improve patient comfort
To reduce side-effects which delay discharge and increase morbidity
To allow early return to normal function and activity
To control pain safely at home
To provide cost-effective pain management

What is the result of inadequately controlled pain?

Pain prolongs the patient's time to discharge from the recovery room or the DSU, so that extra nursing staff or extended nursing hours are needed, resulting in a cost-inefficient system[1]. Excessive and uncontrolled pain is also a cause of nausea and vomiting, further extending the patient's stay in the recovery room[2].

Uncontrolled pain is one of the major causes of unplanned admission following day surgery[3]. This is inconvenient to patients and carers, and is a costly exercise[4].

Pain adversely affects surgical recovery. Restlessness from inadequate pain control may result in haematoma formation and infection[5]. The patient's ability to mobilize is directly related to the amount of postoperative pain. Inadequate pain control may limit early mobilization, which may be crucial to early return of function[5].

Uncontrolled pain may prolong the patient's return to normal activity[6]. It is also distressing to the patient and sleep disturbances are frequently reported.

Uncontrolled pain after discharge will increase the burden on GPs and community health services[7]. It is poor publicity for the DSU in particular and day surgery in general.

Uncontrolled pain following patient discharge adversely affects attitudes relating to day surgery for the individual patient, the public and the general practitioner.

What does the choice of pain management depend on?

Day surgery analgesia must allow the patient to be discharged safely and without delay. Additionally, after the patient has been discharged, he must not require close medical or nursing supervision, either for the administration of analgesia or for safety reasons. This means that many in-patient methods of pain control, such as morphine by injection or as patient-controlled analgesia (PCA), epidural infusions and long-lasting central neural blockade, currently have no place in day surgery.

Suitable drugs are chosen on the basis of their availability, freedom from side-effects, convenience of administration and safety. Patient preference and cost may be issues, although analgesic methods used in day surgery are often inexpensive.

Analgesia needs to be tailored to the severity of the pain associated with the procedure. Laparoscopy, hernia repair and arthroscopy have all been associated with severe pain, but are amenable to specific methods of pain control[8–10].

The knowledge and expertise of the DSU staff, anaesthetists, surgeons and nurses, gleaned from clinical experience and, more importantly, from well-conducted outcome studies of local pain management, are possibly the most important factors in ensuring that pain control is effective.

Measurement of pain

The severity of postoperative pain must be adequately assessed in order that day surgery staff can institute a prompt and effective pain management plan for the patient. The best scoring system is one of 'self-reporting' by the patient (*Figure 9.1*)[7].

Alternatively, an observer-reporting system (reported by the nurse) can be used in situations where there are communication difficulties. The great advantage of a patient pain assessment system is that it is a measurement of changes in pain rating and effectiveness of the pain management. Particularly during the first stage of recovery, day surgery staff should assess and reassess patients' pain levels frequently, increasing the frequency of assessment if pain is poorly controlled.

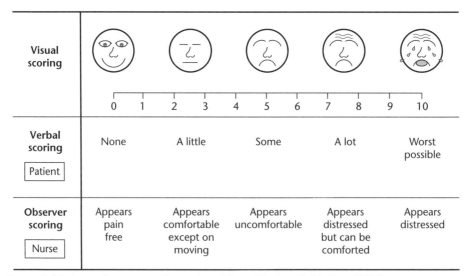

Visual scoring					
	0 1 2 3 4 5 6 7 8 9 10				
Verbal scoring / Patient	None	A little	Some	A lot	Worst possible
Observer scoring / Nurse	Appears pain free	Appears comfortable except on moving	Appears uncomfortable	Appears distressed but can be comforted	Appears distressed

Figure 9.1 Pain scoring system. Reproduced from **Hitchcock M, Ogg TW.** Day surgery analgesia. *J. One Day Surg.* 1993; **3**: 20–21 with permission from Newton Mann.

When should we assess pain management: at rest or during activity?

Good postoperative analgesia should allow patients to mobilize more comfortably. Differences between analgesic methods may only be evident when pain is assessed during activity, e.g. walking or coughing rather than at rest[11], hence it is mandatory to assess efficacy of analgesia during activity and at rest[12].

A practical scheme for pain assessment in the day patient is to assess pain at rest in first-stage recovery, and at rest *and* during activity in second-stage recovery, at discharge and after discharge.

Strategies to manage pain in day surgery

A useful day surgery pain management plan is given in *Figure 9.2*. This emphasizes the importance of a predetermined strategy to deal with pain through all the stages of day surgery: preoperative, intraoperative, in first- and second-stage recovery, and home after discharge.

Pain management should be discussed with the patient, either at assessment or on admission to the DSU. Honest discussion and explanations are essential (*Table 9.2*). Patient preferences should be respected; for instance with regard to the use of suppositories or central neural blockade.

Frequent monitoring of pain scores (at rest and during activity) and assessment of the adequacy of pharmacological and non-pharmacological interventions and their side-effects is essential. A pain management plan allows rescue analgesia to be given and side-effects treated quickly so that patient discharge is not delayed.

The following are key issues in pain management.

Table 9.2. Preoperative patient preparation for optimal pain management

Discuss with patients their previous experiences and expectations of pain
Be honest about the anticipated intensity and duration of postoperative pain
Explain that not **all** postoperative pain will be eliminated
Discuss pain assessment and the management plan
Explain the importance of factual reports of pain, avoiding stoicism and exaggeration
Discuss potential side-effects of analgesics
Discuss management of side-effects, e.g. modified diet for codeine-related constipation
Enable patients to feel confident that their pain be controlled
Discuss realistic expectations for return to work or sporting activities
Provide printed information in layman's terms concerning postoperative pain and return-to-work
   expectations for specific day surgery procedures

Preoperative patient preparation

Much of the distress of postoperative pain is linked to anxiety and patients' fear of the unknown[13]. It has been shown that postoperative pain can be reduced by proper preoperative preparation and education[13].

Clinicians can identify patients preoperatively who are more likely to experience postoperative pain, such as those who express high levels of anxiety or pain expectations[6,14]. Patients undergoing specific surgical procedures such as gynaecological laparoscopy and hernia repair are also more likely to experience more severe pain than those undergoing lens extraction[15].

Multimodal analgesia
There have been many different approaches to pain management in day surgery. More recently, a balanced or 'multimodal' method has been found to be most successful[16]. This is the combination of two or more analgesics or analgesic methods, chosen to improve analgesia and minimize side-effects[17] (*Figure 9.2*).

For mild pain, simple analgesics such as paracetamol may be sufficient. Patients with mild to moderate pain in day surgery benefit from combinations of NSAIDs and opioids (most commonly codeine analgesics)[18,19], in addition to regional or local anaesthesia[20].

How to choose the analgesia
Aim at a balanced or multimodal analgesic plan. Start with a combination of NSAID, short-acting opioid plus local or regional analgesia where appropriate. The patient response to drugs varies, so rescue analgesia for postoperative pain beyond acceptable levels may be needed.

Allow time for maximum effect to be reached before increasing the dose. Be wary of potential side-effects which may appear as the dose is increased. The drug effect should be achieved with the smallest effective dose to reduce side-effects.

If side-effects occur, treat specific side-effects, document them, and choose an alternative drug if pain is still not adequately relieved.

Pre-emptive analgesia
The concept of pre-emptive analgesia has been developed as the hypothesis of 'preventing pain'. Experimental studies have demonstrated that pre-injury neuronal block or opioid administration reduces pain[21]. However, results so far have not confirmed that this treatment has a major impact on postoperative pain management[22]. Recent work also suggests that pre-emptive NSAIDs are of no clinical benefit[23], confirming previous studies undertaken in patients undergoing minor oral surgical procedures[24–26]. In the future, effective pre-emptive analgesia may be more readily achieved with neuronal block.

However, pre-emptive analgesia is a good model for the management of acute pain in that prevention is better than treatment. There is clinical evidence that patients who wake up comfortably tend to remain so, and those that wake up in pain are difficult to get comfortable. Established pain that is severe is difficult to control.

In the context of day surgery where operations tend to be short, the analgesia should be working maximally when the patient wakes from anaesthesia, so preoperative or early analgesia may allow time to effect rather than being pre-emptive. This may be particularly true of NSAIDs, which take some time to reach maximum effect, depending on the route of administration.

Local and regional anaesthesia
Local anaesthetics may be infiltrated at the wound site or at a distance from the surgical site as in regional techniques. Good local anaesthesia will inhibit the peripheral nociceptive response to pain, which has been shown to be very beneficial[27]. The widespread use of local anaesthetic solutions, both alone and in conjunction with other analgesia, can result in excellent pain relief for the day patient. Early pain, which is often refractory to analgesics, can be prevented or treated by local application of anaesthetics. The requirements for opioid analgesics in the perioperative period can therefore be reduced.

The place of spinal and epidural anaesthesia is more controversial in day surgery, but regional and local anaesthesia offer day patients substantial benefits, both from a pre-

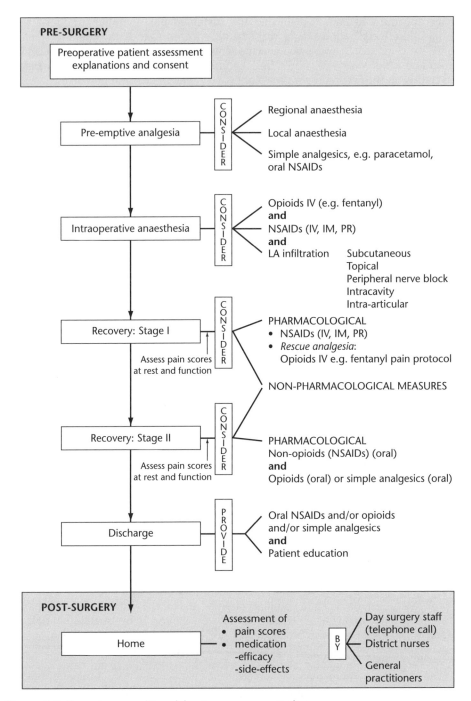

Figure 9.2. Day surgery multimodal pain management plan.
LA, local anaesthetic.

emptive approach to pain control and the sustained postoperative analgesia with minimal side-effects[28]. However, it must be recognized that extra time and space is required to administer these blocks. Also, patients should be warned that the effects will wear off and other analgesia should be taken before this happens, particularly before going to bed on the first postoperative night.

The choice of local anaesthetic agent is important. Agents such as bupivacaine should be chosen for their long-lasting effect. All surgeons should be encouraged to use bupivacaine whether it be for local anaesthetic procedures alone or as an adjunct in a balanced pain management plan where general anaesthesia is used.

Local anaesthesia can be administered by the following methods.

- Wound infiltration by subcutaneous infiltration[29,30]: single dose or by continuous infusion by means of an indwelling catheter left *in situ*[31,32].
- Topical application: EMLA® cream and lignocaine aerosol or gel[33].
- Peripheral nerve blocks, e.g. ilioinguinal, iliohypogastric, which prolong postoperative pain relief and reduce the requirements for oral analgesia[9].
- Intracavity instillation, e.g. laparoscopy[34,35].
- Intra-articular: instillation of local anaesthetics into joints after knee arthroscopy has been shown to reduce opioid requirements and to allow patients to ambulate sooner[36].
- Intravenous regional anaesthesia for upper and lower limb procedures.
- Plexus blocks, such as brachial plexus.
- Central neural blocks (spinal, epidural).

> *Local anaesthesia should be used in as many day patients as possible; alone, with sedation or with general anaesthesia. It maintains the best balance between effectiveness and side-effects for postoperative analgesia. If it can be used, use it.*

This is discussed in detail in Chapter 10 and relevant aspects in Chapter 14.

Pharmacological agents

Opioids

Opioids are naturally occurring or synthetic drugs with morphine-like actions. All opioids, however short-acting they are, are limited by their postoperative sequelae: PONV, sedation and respiratory depression[37]. Opioids such as morphine and pethidine are considered to have a length of action too long for day surgery, with potent emetic effects.

Investigators who have reviewed the use of morphine in day surgery have noted that the incidence of nausea and vomiting increases significantly in the first 24 hours after surgery[38]. Moreover, nausea and vomiting often occurs for the first time after discharge, because morphine can act as an emetic stimulus on the trip home resulting in delayed vomiting[39]. Discharge may also be delayed or prevented by PONV and sedation.

> *Always consider more suitable alternatives before giving morphine to day cases.*

Commonly used intravenous opioids in the day surgery setting are fentanyl and alfentanil.

Fentanyl. This is used most frequently as an intraoperative analgesic, as its length of action will last into the initial period of recovery. It has a fast onset of action and its half-life is 3–4 hours; this hangover effect into the recovery period may be useful. It is also considered the opioid of choice in the immediate recovery period for patients with moderate to severe pain. Trained nursing staff can administer fentanyl according to a pain protocol (*Figure 9.3*)[40]. Sedation scores must also be monitored during the administration of the fentanyl pain protocol.

When fentanyl is given intravenously for a pain score ≥5 according to the pain protocol, supplementary oral or rectal analgesia should also be given. This allows the oral or rectal analgesic to take effect as the short-acting opioid is wearing off.

Patient-controlled analgesia (PCA) has been used in day surgery with fentanyl as the popular opioid choice. It has little advantage over a fentanyl pain protocol where patient request is also considered in the decision to give intravenous fentanyl (*Figure 9.3*). One of the practical problems associated with PCA is when to cease it and commence oral analgesia. Clinical experience with this method has shown that patients are often reluctant to relinquish their control device, thus prolonging recovery room times (unpublished data).

Alfentanil. This is most commonly used in combination with propofol as a TIVA technique in day surgery, with the advantages of a rapid recovery and minimal side-effects such as nausea and vomiting[41]. Alfentanil differs from fentanyl, as its onset of action is three times more rapid than that of fentanyl[42], its duration of action one-third shorter[42] and it is four times less potent than fentanyl[43].

PONV may be associated with the use of fentanyl or alfentanil, potentially delaying discharge. However, problems are minimal because of their short duration of action[44].

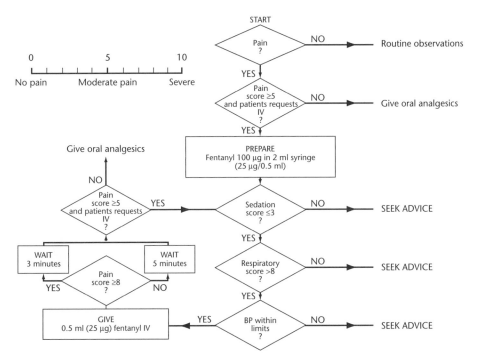

Figure 9.3. Fentanyl pain protocol. Reproduced from **Rudkin G**. Patient choice in sedation anaesthesia and recovery room analgesia. *Ambulatory Surg.* 1994; **2**: 75–80 (Figure 3) with permission from Elsevier Science - NL.

Remifentanil. This is a new ultra-short-acting opioid, suitable for infusion techniques, having rapid onset and offset of its effects[45]. However, reported disadvantages intraoperatively are a lowered arterial oxygen saturation and higher end-tidal CO_2 in spontaneously breathing patients[46]. Due to its short-lasting analgesic effect after cessation of the infusion, the anaesthetist must provide an immediate alternative analgesic, which may limit its usefulness in day surgery.

Oxycodone. This is a potent synthetic opioid, structurally related to morphine, but with better oral bioavailability. It is a very effective analgesic for moderate to severe pain and can be given alone or in combination with paracetamol. Dosage can be titrated to the patient's needs until sedation occurs.

Codeine. This is one of the most commonly used oral opioids following day surgery, given for mild-to-moderate pain. Preparations are generally given in combination with paracetamol. Codeine has an additive analgesic effect with paracetamol for moderate to strong postoperative pain[47]. Paracetamol 500 mg plus codeine phosphate 30 mg is effective in 97% of day case oral surgery patients[48]. However, constipation is a frequent and often distressing adverse effect, therefore patient explanation is important and prophylactic strategies should be considered.

Dextropropoxyphene. This is structurally related to methadone, but is less potent and has more dysphoric adverse effects. It is often used in combination with paracetamol.

Tramadol. This is a centrally acting analgesic which can be used for acute pain postoperatively. It has low affinity for opioid receptors and also has a non-opioid mechanism of action, inhibiting both noradrenaline and 5-hydroxytryptamine neuronal uptake. Its analgesic potency is only 5–10 times less than that of morphine[49] and is equal to that of pethidine[50]. Tramadol has advantages over other opioids in the postoperative setting as it does not cause significant respiratory depression. However, its major drawback is the incidence of nausea and vomiting which has been reported to be as high as 30–35%[50,51]. Further clinical studies are required to determine the role of tramadol in day surgery acute pain management.

Paracetamol
Paracetamol has analgesic and antipyretic properties, but little anti-inflammatory activity. It is well-absorbed orally and almost entirely metabolized by the liver, with a half-life of about 4 hours. It has few adverse effects in normal dosage (up to 4 g in 24 hours). It is a cheap, safe and effective agent when combined with other drugs in a balanced analgesic approach, where it has been shown to have a 15–25% morphine-sparing effect[52]. However, on its own it is usually insufficient.

NSAIDs (non-steroidal anti-inflammatory drugs)
These drugs are now the basis of most day surgery analgesic regimes. As well as providing effective analgesia, their anti-inflammatory effects may help reduce local oedema. In the early postoperative period NSAIDs should not be used alone in the management of severe pain, but be combined with opioids. Present literature suggests that there is no great benefit in administering NSAIDs before surgery, apart from allowing time for them to be effective. Their place in day surgery is part of a multimodal analgesic plan in combination with local and regional anaesthesia and opioids[20]. Their morphine-sparing effects are well recognized and this improves pain relief and

minimizes the use of more potent drugs and their accompanying side-effects. Overall their benefits greatly outweigh their risks.

When should you avoid NSAIDs? A concise history and examination of the patient is important before NSAIDs are prescribed to day patients, as contraindications must be respected. Side-effects of NSAIDs appear minimal in low-risk patients but there is concern with patients who have active gastroduodenal ulceration, renal or heart failure or a bleeding tendency[19]. All asthmatics should be questioned as to whether they have taken aspirin or other NSAIDs and whether symptoms of bronchospasm developed. Only 5% of asthmatics will react to NSAIDs in this way, so it is worth asking if they have taken aspirin or ibuprofen as these drugs are freely available 'over the counter'. If the patient has taken these drugs without wheezing, then it is safe to use NSAIDs for day surgery. See *Table 9.3* for a list of patients who are at high risk of developing side-effects from NSAIDs.

Table 9.3. Patients at high risk of developing side-effects from NSAIDs

Age over 60 years	Aspirin-induced or other severe asthma
Pre-existing	Concurrent use of
peptic ulcer disease	other NSAIDs
renal dysfunction	diuretics
congestive cardiac failure	other nephrotoxic agents
bleeding or anticoagulant disorder	anticoagulants
liver dysfunction	Children less than 16 years of age
Dehydration	Pregnant and lactating women
Hypersensitivity to NSAIDs	

Ranitidine and omeprazole have been used for prophylactic purposes against the development of gastrointestinal side-effects in patients taking NSAIDs[53], with misoprostol shown recently to be most effective[54].

What about the patient who has been on chronic NSAID therapy prior to surgery? These patients should cease their medication at least 24–48 hours prior to surgery, or in enough time to allow elimination of the drug[55], to decrease the risk of bleeding complications. NSAIDs with long half-lives need to be stopped at least 4–5 half-lives prior to surgery to allow elimination of the drug. The general recommendation is to stop aspirin therapy 5–10 days prior to surgery[56,57]. This drug is then restarted after surgery. These patients should not be given an additional NSAID for pain control, but may be treated with local or regional anaesthetics or opioids.

Which NSAID is the best? There is no scientific documentation asserting the superiority of any individual NSAID. However, relative potencies in terms of anti-inflammatory, analgesic and antipyretic qualities may vary between different agents. Ketorolac possesses potent analgesic properties, but minor anti-inflammatory properties compared with other NSAIDs. More recently ketorolac dosage regimes have been under review in some countries. Ketorolac has been implicated as the causative agent for renal failure in healthy patients[58]. Many countries have now accepted a revised dose schedule (*Table 9.4*) which is considered safe for clinical practice provided there are no contraindications to its use.

It is important that drugs are administered according to recommended dosage schedules. Recent published work has shown that tenoxicam administered intravenously at the commencement of anaesthesia at the recommended dose (20 mg) is an

Table 9.4. Revised dose schedule for ketorolac

Dose	Age <65 years	Age >65 years or <50 kg weight
Initial dose	10 mg	10 mg
Subsequent dose	10 mg 4–6 hourly prn	10 mg 4–6 hourly prn
Maximum daily dose	90 mg	60 mg

prn, whenever necessary.

ineffective analgesic for laparoscopy[59]. It is suggested that higher doses are required for efficacy. However, the incidence of side-effects increases with higher dose levels.

Piroxicam, another oxicam NSAID, is often administered sublingually as 'Feldene melts', but there is little evidence supporting its efficacy in day surgery, and again larger doses than recommended may be needed for efficacy[60].

Choice of preparation will depend on the availability, desired route of administration (oral, rectal, IV), duration of effect and cost. Some NSAIDs are better for elderly patients, for example, because of their shorter half-life or lesser effects on renal function (*Table 9.5*).

A major advantage of NSAIDs is that they can easily be combined with opioids and the toxicities do not overlap. The toxicity of these drugs is lower when they are used for shorter periods – such as in the day surgery setting – than compared with chronic use.

NSAIDs have significant opioid dose-sparing effects and can be used for pain in the immediate postoperative period, reducing the opioid side-effects. When pain cannot be adequately controlled despite increasing the opioid dose, it is important to reassess the patient and be aware that there may be an underlying surgical cause for the patient's continuing pain.

Routes of drug administration

Intravenous

This route is most commonly used when a bolus dose is administered intra- or postoperatively. Some of the newer NSAIDs (ketorolac, diclofenac and tenoxicam) can be administered intravenously.

Table 9.5. Commonly used NSAIDs in day surgery

Name	Dose (mg)	Dosing interval (hours)	Daily max. (mg)	Onset (hours)	Duration (hours)	$T_{1/2}$ (hours)
Short half-life						
Ibuprofen	200–400	4–6	1200	0.5	4–6	2±0.5
Ketoprofen[a]	50–100	6–8	200	0.5–2	6–8	1.8±0.3
Diclofenac[a]	25–75	8–12	150	1–3	12	1.1±0.2
Indomethacin	25–50	6–8	200	0.5	4–6	2.4±0.4
Ketorolac[a]						
oral	10	4–6	40	1	6	5.3±1.2
IM	10	4–6	90	0.5–1	6	5.3±1.2
IV	10	4–6	90	0.05	6	5.3±1.2
Long half-life						
Tenoxicam[a]	10– 20	24	20	1	24	72±26
Naproxen	500 then 250	6–12	1000	1	6–8	14±1

[a]Available for intravenous administration in some countries.

Intramuscular

Intramuscular opioids cause pain and trauma and may prevent patients from requesting more pain relief. Diclofenac administered intramuscularly has resulted in the formation of sterile abscesses, with patients suffering severe pain. There is no place for IM injections in day surgery if there are other alternative routes of analgesic administration.

Oral

The oral route is convenient and inexpensive and is the mainstay of day surgery analgesia. Oral medication can be offered to patients as soon as they are able to tolerate fluids. If the patient cannot tolerate oral medication, alternative routes such as rectal administration can be used.

Rectal

This administration is an alternative mode of delivery. However, it must be recognized that there is a lag time for absorption into the circulation compared with the intravenous route. NSAIDs given by the rectal route are absorbed no faster than tablets and many patients find suppositories unacceptable[61]. In a published report of patient opinions on rectal administration of analgesics, 98% patients felt that the use of rectally administered drugs should always be discussed with the patient beforehand[61]. Discussion and patient consent is important, as has recently been emphasized in a reported case where failure to consider this resulted in a charge of serious professional misconduct[62].

Other routes

Other routes such as intra-articular, transdermal, transmucosal and transnasal, are becoming increasingly popular, and further research will determine their place in the management plan of day patient pain relief.

When should analgesia be given?

For severe pain, IV opioids (preferably fentanyl) should be administered as soon as practical according to a pain protocol (see *Figure 9.3*). For moderate or mild pain, simple oral analgesics are usually sufficient, given regularly. Regular frequent assessment of pain is important.

Withholding analgesia or encouraging patients to 'wait longer' increases discomfort. A relatively small dose of an analgesic given early in the development of pain is usually more effective than a larger dose given when the pain has become more severe.

Recently, a PCA technique using intranasal fentanyl has been reported[63]. The high patient satisfaction for this technique and its potential for use in the home setting opens up exciting new possibilities in pain control. However, further research is required to determine its suitability and safety.

What non-pharmacological means can supplement the pain management plan?

Elevation

Oedema is a significant cause of pain immediately after surgery. Proper elevation of the affected part, e.g. upper or lower limb, can greatly reduce this pain. Elevation must be at an appropriate height, e.g. heart level for upper limbs[64]. Patients with elevated systolic blood pressure require higher elevation.

Ice
This helps reduce oedema, reduce muscle spasm and alter the patient's pain threshold[65]. Ho *et al.* have shown that application of ice to a knee for 25 minutes produces a maximal response in the ability to reduce blood flow and bone metabolites, but for more than 30 minutes can result in a temporary loss of nerve function[66].

Bandages
These applied too tightly can increase postoperative pain and local oedema, and impede the patient's ability to mobilize and early return to function.

Other therapies
Relaxation and distraction therapies may reduce pain and anxiety in the postoperative period. These methods take only a few minutes to teach and are worthwhile for anxious patients. TENS (transcutaneous electric nerve stimulation) has been shown to be useful in allowing an increased range of function in patients postoperatively, reducing their pain scores and requirements for analgesia[67]. Other modalities, such as acupuncture, hypnotherapy and aromatherapy, have some place. However, they are no substitute in the management of moderate to severe pain in the early postoperative period.

Pain management in difficult patient groups

The elderly
Elderly patients can develop oversedation disproportionate to the amount of opioid administered. All major organ system functions are decreased in the elderly, so reduce dosages appropriately and be aware of the agitated or restless patient. Pain assessment may be difficult as these patients may have problems such as dementia, deafness and visual disturbances. NSAIDs can be used safely in this patient group. However, extra vigilance is required for side-effects which may develop, such as gastric irritation and renal toxicity.

Cognitively impaired, emotionally disturbed and non-English speaking
Patients in these groups may require extra explanation, attention and time with interpreters or specialized health care workers. Patients in long-term care may benefit from being accompanied by their usual carer. The cost-effectiveness of managing these patient groups in a day surgery setting must also be considered.

Patients who have severe anxiety states associated with postoperative pain may benefit from anti-anxiety drugs such as the benzodiazepines or antipsychotic drugs in addition to their analgesic management.

Chronic pain
Patients who have been receiving opioid analgesics prior to surgery may require higher starting and maintenance doses postoperatively.

Patient discharge

The clinician should review the patient prior to discharge, assess the efficacy of pain relief and provide specific drugs and discharge instructions. Pain scores should be included in discharge criteria.

The patient should be instructed that as the local anaesthetic agent begins to wear off, prescribed analgesia should be commenced. Before going to bed, oral analgesia should be taken so that the patient does not wake up in severe pain.

Dispensing appropriate analgesia with clear instructions for the patient is crucial. Prepacked analgesics for anticipated mild, moderate or severe pain, with clear directions has the potential for improving patient comfort at home (*Table 9.6*). However, a recently conducted audit at The Churchill Hospital, Oxford, UK showed that day patients with severe pain at home do not always take their analgesia as prescribed in adequate doses

Table 9.6(a). Anticipated postoperative pain by surgery type

Mild	Moderate	Severe
Minor gynaecological surgery Toenail surgery Removal of breast lumps Removal of lumps and bumps	Knee arthroscopy Varicose vein surgery	Open hernia repair Laparoscopic cholecystectomy Laparoscopic hernia repair Haemorrhoidectomy Laparoscopic tubal ligation

Table 9.6(b). Suggested take home analgesia for day surgery patients by pain severity[a]

Mild	Moderate	Severe
Oral NSAIDs 8 hourly diclofenac/ibuprofen or 4–6 hourly ketorolac		
Plus these drugs (mg) Codeine phosphate 8 + paracetamol 500[b] • 2 tablets 6–8 hourly	Dihydrocodeine 10 + paracetamol 500[b] • 2 tablets 6–8 hourly	Codeine phosphate 30 + paracetamol 500[b] • 1–2 tablets 4 hourly • maximum 8 in 24 hours
Or these alternative drugs (mg) Dihydrocodeine 10 + paracetamol 500[b] • 2 tablets 6–8 hourly	Dextropropoxyphene 32.5 + paracetamol 325[b] • 2 tablets 6–8 hourly	Oxycodone 5 mg (oral) • 1–2 tablets 4 hourly • maximum 8 in 24 hours
Or these alternative drugs (mg) Dextropropoxyphene 32.5 + paracetamol 32.5[b] • 2 tablets 6–8 hourly	Codeine phosphate 30 + paracetamol 500[b] • 2 tablets 6–8 hourly	

[a]Preoperatively all patients must be questioned as to any contraindications to NSAIDs.
[b]See *Table 9.6(c)*.

Table 9.6(c). Generic names for proprietary drugs

Generic name (mg)	Proprietary name: UK	Proprietary name: Australia
Codeine phosphate 8 + paracetamol 500	Co-codamol®	Panadeine®
Dihydrocodeine 10 + paracetamol 500	Co-dydramol®	Not available
Dextropropoxyphene 32.5 + paracetamol 325	Co-proxamol® or Distalgesic®	Digesic® or Capadex®
Codeine phosphate 30 + paracetamol 500	Tylex® or Co-codamol 30/500® or Solpadol®	Panadeine Forte®

and may even mix in their own analgesics containing additional paracetamol. Clear instructions are therefore mandatory (see *Table 16.6*).

In order to provide satisfactory care for patients in the postdischarge period, some form of continued assessment and management of pain therapy is mandatory. More attention should be paid to patients' pain, discomfort and other troublesome outcomes following day surgery from the patient's perspective[68].

A follow-up telephone call the next morning provides feedback on whether analgesic regimes are satisfactory and reassures the patient. General practitioners, district nurses and day surgery staff can all play a vital role in this important link in high-quality patient care in day surgery.

Successful treatment of pain in day surgery requires a flexible approach that is tailored to the individual patient.

Three issues must be addressed to ensure optimal pain management in day surgery.

- Assessment of pain both during rest and function.
- The implementation of a pain management plan emphasizing preoperative patient education and combination therapy.
- Outcome studies especially in the postdischarge period, reflecting quality patient care and cost.

Postoperative sequelae, such as nausea and vomiting, patient mobility and a return to normal activities, should also be considered in relevant outcome studies. Improved drugs with minimal emetic sequelae and new drug delivery techniques may improve day surgery patient outcome for the future.

> *Analgesic strategies using local anaesthesia, short-acting IV opioids, NSAIDs and paracetamol combinations as part of a pain management plan provide effective analgesia, improved recovery and faster discharge. After discharge, patient follow-up is essential to monitor the effectiveness of pain management.*

References

1. **Hitchcock M, Ogg TW**. Quality assurance in day case anaesthesia. *Ambulatory Surg.* 1994; **2:** 193–204.
2. **Anderson R, Krohg K**. Pain as a major cause of post operative nausea and vomiting. *Can. Anaesth. Soc. J.* 1976; **23:** 366–369.
3. **Gold BS, Kitz DS, Lecky JH, et al.** Unanticipated admission to the hospital following ambulatory surgery. *J. Am. Med. Assoc.* 1989; **69:** 1009–1012.
4. **Meridy HW**. Criteria for selection of ambulatory surgical patients and guidelines for anaesthetic management: a retrospective study of 1553 cases. *Anesth. Analg.* 1982; **61:** 921–926.
5. **Burt A**. Physiotherapy following joint replacements in the hand. *Physiotherapy* 1986; **72:** 445–448.
6. **Payne FB, Ghia JN, Levin KJ, et al.** The relationship of preoperative and intraoperative factors on the incidence of pain following ambulatory surgery. *Ambulatory Surg.* 1995; **3:** 127–130.
7. **Hitchcock M, Ogg TW**. Day surgery analgesia. *J. One Day Surg.* 1993; **3:** 20–21.
8. **Fraser RA, Hotz SB, Hurtig JB, et al.** The prevalence and impact of pain after day-care tubal ligation surgery. *Pain* 1989; **39:** 189–201.
9. **Ding Y, White PF.** Post-herniorrhaphy pain in outpatients after preincision ilioinguinal–hypogastric nerve block during monitored anaesthesia care. *Can. J. Anaesth.* 1995; **42:** 12–15.
10. **Kinnard P, Truchon R, St-Pierre A, et al.** Interscalene block for pain relief after shoulder surgery. *Clin. Orthopaed. Rel. Res.* 1994; **304:** 22–24.
11. **Dahl JB, Rosenberg J, Hansen BL, et al.** Differential analgesic effects of low dose epidural morphine and morphine–bupivacaine at rest and during mobilisation after major abdominal surgery. *Anesth. Analg.* 1992; **74:** 362–365.

12. **Kehlet H**. Postoperative pain relief – what is the issue? (Editorial) *Br. J. Anaesth.*1994; **72**: 375–378.
13. **Hekmat N, Burke M, Howell S**. Preventative pain management in the postoperative hand surgery patient. *Orthopaed. Nursing* 1994; **13**: 3.
14. **Wallace LM**. Surgical patients' expectations of pain and discomfort: does accuracy of expectation minimise post-surgical pain and distress? *Pain* 1985; **22**: 363–373.
15. **Osborne GA, Rudkin GE**. Outcome after day-care surgery in a major teaching hospital. *Anaesth. Intens. Care* 1993; **21**: 822–827.
16. **Michaloliakou C, Chung C, Sharma S**. Preoperative multimodal analgesia facilitates recovery after ambulatory laparoscopic cholecystectomy. *Anesth. Analg.* 1996; **82**: 44–51.
17. **Kapur PA**. Preoperative multimodal analgesia facilitates recovery after ambulatory laparoscopic cholecystectomy. *Anesth. Analg.* 1996; **82**: 44–51.
18. **Kehlet H, Dahl JB**. The value of multi-modal or balanced analgesia in postoperative pain relief. *Anesth. Analg.* 1993; **77**: 1048–1056.
19. **Kehlet H, Mather LE (Eds)**. The value of non-steroidal anti-inflammatory drugs in postoperative pain. *Drugs* 1992 **44** (Suppl. 5): 1–63.
20. **Dahl JB, Møiniche S, Kehlet H**. Wound infiltration with local anaesthetics for postoperative pain relief – a review. *Acta Anaesthesiol. Scand.* 1994; **38**: 7–14.
21. **Coderre TJ, Katz J, Vaccarino AL, et al**. Contribution of central neuroplasticity to pathological pain: review of clinical and experimental evidence. *Pain* 1993; **52**: 259–285.
22. **Dahl JB, Kehlet H**. The value of pre-emptive analgesia in the treatment of postoperative pain. *Br. J. Anaesth.* 1993; **70**: 434–439.
23. **Rogers JE, Fleming BG, Macintosh KD, et al**. Effect of timing of ketorolac administration on patient-controlled opioid use. *Br. J. Anaesth.* 1995; **75**: 15–18.
24. **Flath RK, Hick ML, Dionne RA, Pelleu GB**. Pain suppression after pulpectomy with preoperative flurbiprofen. *J. Endodontics* 1987; **13**: 339–347.
25. **Sisk AL, Mosley RO, Martin RP**. Comparison of preoperative and postoperative diflunisal for suppression of postoperative pain. *J. Oral Maxillofac. Surg.*1989; **47**: 464–468.
26. **Sisk AL, Grover BJ**. A comparison of preoperative and postoperative naproxen sodium for suppression of postoperative pain. *J. Oral Maxillofac. Surg.* 1990; **48**: 674–678.
27. **Flanagan JF, Edkin B, Spindler K**. 3 in 1 femoral nerve block following ACL reconstruction allows predictably earlier discharge and significant cost savings. *Anesthesiology* 1994; **81**: A950.
28. **Brown AR, Weiss R, Greenberg CP, et al**. Interscalene block for shoulder arthroscopy: a comparison with general anesthesia. *J. Arthro. Relat. Surg.* 1993; **9**: 295–300.
29. **Owens H, Galloway DJ, Mitchell KG**. Analgesia by wound infiltration after surgical excision of benign breast lumps. *Ann. R. Coll. Surg. Engl.* 1985; **67**: 114–115.
30. **Moss G, Regal ME, Lichtig L**. Reproducing postoperative pain, narcotics, and length of hospitalization. *Surgery* 1986; **99**: 206–210.
31. **Levack ID, Holmes JD, Robertson GS**. Abdominal wound perfusion for the relief of postoperative pain. *Br. J. Anaesth.* 1986; **58**: 615–619.
32. **Gibbs R, Purushotam A, Auld C, et al**. Continuous wound perfusion with bupivacaine for postoperative wound pain. *Br. J. Surg.* 1988; **75**: 923–924.
33. **Sinclair R, Cassuto J, Hostrom S, et al**. Topical anesthesia with lidocaine aerosol in the control of postoperative pain. *Anesthesiology* 1988; **68**: 895–901.
34. **Ræder JC, Børdahl PE, Nordentoft J, et al**. Outpatient laparoscopic sterilization: is local anaesthesia better? *Ambulatory. Surg.* 1993; **1**: 158–161.
35. **Goulding ST, Hovell BC**. Laparoscopic inguinal hernia repair: quality of recovery following the use of intraperitoneal bupivacaine. *Ambulatory Surg.* 1995; **3**: 75–77.
36. **Smith I, Van Hemelrijk J, White PF, et al**. Effects of local anesthesia on recovery after outpatient arthroscopy. *Anaesth. Analg.* 1991; **73**: 536–539.
37. **Campbell WI**. Analgesic side effects and minor surgery: which analgesic for minor day-care surgery? *Br. J. Anaesth.* 1990; **64**: 617.
38. **Weistein MS, Nicolson SC, Schreiner MS**. A single dose of morphine sulfate increases the incidence of vomiting after outpatient inguinal surgery in children. *Anesthesiology* 1994; **81**: 572–577.
39. **Munro HM, Riegger LQ, Reynolds PI, et al**. Comparison of the analgesic and emetic properties of ketorolac and morphine for outpatient strabismus surgery. *Br. J. Anaesth.* 1994; **72**: 624–628.

40. **Rudkin GE.** Patient choice in sedation anaesthesia and recovery room analgesia. *Ambulatory Surg.* 1994; **2**: 75–80.

41. **Raftery S, Sherry E.** Total intravenous anaesthesia with propofol and alfentanil protects against postoperative nausea and vomiting. *Can. J. Anaesth.* 1992; **39**: 37–40.

42. **Dollery C (Ed.).** (1991) *Therapeutic Drugs,* Vol. 1. Churchill Livingstone, Edinburgh.

43. **Janssen P.** (1984) The development of new synthetic narcotics. In: *Opioids in Anaesthesia* (Ed. FG Estafanous). Butterworth-Heinemann, Boston, MA. p. 37.

44. **Cardosa M, Rudkin GE, Osborne GA.** Outcome after day-case knee arthroscopy in a major teaching hospital. *Arthroscopy* 1994; **10**: 624–629.

45. **Bürkle H, Dunbar S, Van Aken H.** Rementanil: a novel, short-acting, μ-opioid. *Anesth. Analg.* 1996; **83**: 646–651.

46. **Smith I, Avramov M, White PF.** Remifentanil versus propofol for monitored anesthesia care-effects on ventilation. *Anesthesiology* 1995; **83**: A4.

47. **Bjune K, Stubhaug A, Dodgson MS,** *et al.* Additive analgesic effect of codeine and paracetamol can be detected in strong, but not moderate, pain after Caesarean section. Baseline pain-intensity is a determinant of assay-sensitivity in a postoperative analgesic trial. *Acta Anaesthesiol. Scand.* 1996; **40**: 399–407.

48. **Chye EPY, Young IG, Osborne GA.** Outcomes after same-day oral surgery: a review of 1180 cases at a major teaching hospital. *J. Oral Maxillofac. Surg.* 1993; **51**: 846–849.

49. **Hennies HH, Friderichs E, Schneider J.** Receptor binding, analgesic and antitussive potency of tramadol and other selected opioids. *Arzneimittelforschung* 1988; **38**: 877–880.

50. **Eggers KA, Power I.** Tramadol. *Br. J. Anaesth.* 1995; **74**: 247–249.

51. **Rodriguez MJ, De la Torre MR, Perez-Iraola P,** *et al.* Comparative study of tramadol versus NSAIDs as intravenous continuous infusion for managing postoperative pain. *Curr. Ther. Res.* 1993; **54**: 375–383.

52. **Jesperson TW, Christensen KS, Kjersgaard-Anderson P,** *et al.* Treatment of post-operative pain with morphine compared with morphine and paracetamol. A double-blind clinically controlled investigation with placebo. *Ugeskr. Lager* 1989; **151**: 1615–1618.

53. **Wilde MI, McTavish D.** Omeprazole . An update of its pharmacology and therapeutic use in acid-related disorders. *Drugs* 1994; **48**: 91–132.

54. **Shah K, Price AB, Talbot IC,** *et al.* Effect of longterm misoprostol coadministration with non-steroidal anti-inflammatory drugs: a histological study. *Gut* 1995; **37**: 195–198.

55. **Connelly CS, Panush RS.** Should nonsteroidal anti-inflammatory drugs be stopped before elective surgery? *Arch. Intern Med.* 1991; **151**: 1963–1966.

56. **McEvoy GK (Ed.).** (1996) *AHFS Drug Information 96.* American Society of Health System Pharmacists, Bethesda, pp. 1368, 1571, 2267.

57. **Guarnieri KM, Mckeon BP.** (1994) Drug metabolism reactions and interaction in the surgical patient: prevention of medication-induced morbidity. In: *Perioperative Medicine: the Medical Care of the Surgical Patient,* 2nd Edn (Eds DR Goldman, FH Brown, DM Guarnieri). McGraw Hill, New York. pp. 479–490.

58. **Smith K, Halliwell RMT, Lawrence S,** *et al.* Acute renal failure associated with intramuscular ketorolac. *Anaesth. Intens. Care* 1993; **21**: 700–703.

59. **Windsor A, McDonald P, Mumtaz T,** *et al.* The analgesic efficacy of tenoxicam versus placebo in day case laparoscopy: a randomised parallel double blind study. *Anaesthesia* 1996; **51**: 1066–1069.

60. **Lysak SZ, Anderson PT, Carithers RA,** *et al.* Postoperative effects of fentanyl, ketorolac and piroxicam as analgesics for outpatient laparoscopic procedures. *Obstet. Gynaecol.* 1994; **83**: 270–275.

61. **Vyvyan HAL, Hanafiah Z.** Patients' attitudes to rectal drug administration. *Anaesthesia* 1995; **50**: 983–985.

62. **Mitchell J.** A fundamental problem of consent. *Br. Med. J.* 1995; **310**: 43–48 .

63. **Striebel HW, Oelmann T, Spies C,** *et al.* Patient-controlled intranasal analgesia: a method for noninvasive postoperative pain management. *Anesth. Analg.* 1996; **83**: 547–551.

64. **Tegtmeier R.** How high should the hand be elevated after hand surgery? *Orthop. Rev.* 1981; **5**: 117–120.

65. **Cohn BT, Draeger RI, Jackson DW.** The effects of cold therapy in the postoperative management of pain in patients undergoing anterior cruciate ligament reconstruction. *Am. J. Sports Med.* 1989; **17**: 344–349.
66. **Ho SS, Illgen RL, Meyer RW,** *et al.* Comparison of various icing times in decreasing bone metabolism and blood flow in the knee. *Am. J. Sports Med.* 1995; **23**: 74–76.
67. **Brown RE.** (1992) Transcutaneous electrical nerve stimulation for acute and postoperative pain. In: *Acute Pain: Mechanisms and Management* (Eds RS Sinatra, AH Hord, B Ginsberg, *et al.*). Mosby, St Louis, MO. pp. 379–389.
68. **Cohen MM, Duncan PG, DeBoer DP.** Assessing discomfort after anaesthesia: should you ask the patient or read the record? *Qual. Health Care* 1994; **3**: 137–141.

CHAPTER 10

Local and regional anaesthesia in the adult day surgery patient

G.E. Rudkin

Local anaesthesia can be defined as the temporary loss of sensation from local anaesthetic applied directly to the wound site. It is often performed by the surgeon for minor procedures. In regional anaesthesia, nerves are blocked at a distance from the surgical site. This is mostly performed by the anaesthetist for more complex procedures, and includes peripheral nerve blocks, plexus blockade and central neural blockade (spinal, epidural).

Day surgery performed under local or regional anaesthesia is becoming increasingly popular. This is due to the development of minimally invasive surgical techniques, improved sedation and recognition that postoperative problems such as drowsiness, nausea and vomiting and uncontrolled pain can be minimized. Local or regional anaesthesia can be used alone, in combination with sedation anaesthesia or, most commonly, as part of a multimodal analgesia plan with general anaesthesia[1] (see *Figure 9.2*). A range of local/regional anaesthetic techniques can be used in day surgery (*Table 10.1*).

Table 10.1. Local and regional anaesthetic techniques in day surgery

Topical anaesthesia
Infiltration techniques
Instillation into joints and body cavities
Intravenous regional blocks (Bier's block)
Peripheral nerve blocks, e.g. ilioinguinal block
Plexus blockade, e.g. brachial plexus block
Central neural blockade
    spinal
    epidural/caudal

Day surgery performed under local anaesthesia is often the simplest, safest and cheapest. Dexter and Tinker have shown that the major determinant of postanaesthesia cost is overnight admission[2]. Procedures performed under local anaesthesia minimize postoperative problems such as pain and nausea and vomiting, which are the major causative factors of patient admission. The cost of local anaesthetic drugs is a very small part of the economics of day surgery.

Many procedures which have previously been performed on an in-patient basis under general anaesthesia are now performed on a day basis under local/regional anaesthesia alone or combined with sedation techniques. Examples of procedures performed in this way are breast reduction[3], lens extraction[4], septoplasty[5], prostatectomy[6,7], tonsillectomy[8] and thyroidectomy[9]. Cases managed in this way incur fewer expenses, and techniques have been shown to be safe and acceptable to patients and medical personnel. In properly equipped centres and for selected procedures, local/regional anaesthesia provides the means for 'office-based' surgery (conducted in surgeons' private operating facilities) rather than 'hospital day surgery management', which is an additional cost-effective option[10].

> *It is important to monitor safety, cost effectiveness and patient acceptability for newly adopted local anaesthetic techniques for cases previously performed under general anaesthesia.*

Is regional anaesthesia preferable to general anaesthesia?

A controversial issue in day surgery is whether regional anaesthesia offers significant benefits over general anaesthesia for the day patient. Literature presents conflicting reports; however, its real place will vary from one institution to another[11,12]. This will depend upon the physical layout of the facility for ease of block insertion, surgeon and patient acceptance of the technique, and the expertise of the anaesthetist. It is essential that each facility audit its own complication rates, recovery room times and patient opinions to determine the relevance of regional or general anaesthesia.

There are benefits for patients, surgeons and the day surgery facility when local or regional anaesthesia is used. Advantages and disadvantages are summarized in *Tables 10.2 and 10.3.*

Table 10.2. Advantages of local/regional anaesthesia

Patient advantages
Avoidance of general anaesthetic with its related complications
Minimal incidence of nausea and vomiting
Improved postoperative pain relief
Shortened recovery room time
Communication with staff during surgery
Observation of the procedure
Earlier mobilization

Surgeon advantages
Accurate assessment of function before wound is closed
Discussion of operative findings and treatment options at surgery

Facility advantages
Option of direct transfer to second-stage recovery
Shortened patient recovery room time
Reduced postoperative nursing requirements
Fewer hospital admissions
Overall reduction in facility costs

Advantages

In an outcome study of 6000 day cases, anaesthesia-related complications were more frequent with general anaesthesia than with local anaesthesia and sedation or regional anaesthesia[13]. The incidence of PONV can be minimized by using regional techniques alone or using local/regional anaesthesia in combination with general anaesthesia[14]. Opioid requirements are fewer, and investigators have consistently shown that patients have less postoperative pain[14–16].

The application of local anaesthesia before the surgical stimulus may have a pre-emptive analgesic effect[15,17]. It has been suggested that with general anaesthesia, pain treatment started before surgery is more effective in the reduction of postoperative pain than treatment given at recovery[18]. Clinically, there is less postoperative pain when the blockade of noxious stimuli is complete and extended into the initial postoperative period[19]. Although there have been conflicting reports in the literature as to whether pre-emptive analgesia can be proven or not, there are clinical advantages for patients who wake up comfortably, as they tend to remain comfortable. In the authors' experience, patients who wake with significant pain are difficult to settle and require more analgesia.

It is preferable for the surgeon to discuss local and regional advantages at the patient's initial surgical consultation. Patients should be given the choice of being awake during their surgery[20,21]. If awake, they may be able to to view their surgery on a video screen – for instance during knee arthroscopy. The surgeon can then discuss operative findings, treatment options and postoperative care with the patient during surgery. Some surgeons find patient co-operation useful during surgery for testing functional repair before wound closure, as in hernia repair or trigger finger release.

Local or regional anaesthesia can shorten recovery room times, and first-stage recovery can often be bypassed (see *Figure 16.2*)[14,22]. Earlier mobilization is also possible; and for surgery such as knee arthroscopy under local anaesthesia, the opportunity for immediate physiotherapy has been shown to be an advantage[23]. Nursing requirements are reduced, providing inherent cost advantages[24]. Fewer unanticipated hospital admissions occur with local or regional techniques, which also assists facilities in reducing overall costs[25].

Table 10.3. Disadvantages of local/regional anaesthesia

Additional time requirements
   discussion with patient
   block insertion
   onset time
   gentle tissue handling
   incomplete block necessitating supplementation or conversion to general anaesthetic
Potential nerve damage
Surgeon and patient co-operation required
Prolonged regional block may result in urinary retention and delayed discharge

Disadvantages

The additional time needed to persuade some patients of the benefits of regional anaesthesia can be a problem, e.g. when cultural differences dictate that patients be asleep during surgery. In this instance, sedation (with amnesic drugs) and regional anaesthesia can be combined, leaving the patient with no memory of the surgical event – a preferred option over general anaesthesia. A practical issue is the extra time taken to perform the block, which is of relevance to the single-handed anaesthetist. Onset time must be considered, and on occasions the block may require supplementation, causing further delays in operating schedules.

> *Local and regional anaesthesia offer significant benefits to the day surgery patient. Its place , either as part of a general anaesthetic technique or used alone, will depend on the facility, patient, surgeon and skills of the anaesthetist.*

Patient issues

Careful patient assessment is as important for patients undergoing local or regional techniques, as for general anaesthesia. The final decision can be made with the anaesthetist on the day of surgery. However, a planned work-up is necessary (*Table 10.4*).

The anaesthetist must be confident of performing the block (to inspire trust in the patient), and come to an agreement with the patient for sedation or conversion to general anaesthesia if necessary.

Table 10.4. Key factors in planned approach for local/regional anaesthesia

Prior to day of surgery
Surgeon states benefits at initial patient consultation
Assessment nurse
assesses patient
discusses benefits of local/regional approach
provides printed information
plays instructional videos on relevant block (if available)
refers to anaesthetist for special consultation if necessary
Day of surgery
Anaesthetist discusses and agrees to perform local/regional anaesthesia

In discussing aspects of local/regional anaesthesia, special emphasis should be placed on the following:

- patient's previous experience with local/regional anaesthesia;
- relative or absolute contraindications to use of local or regional anaesthesia (*Table 10.5*);
- advantages of local/regional anaesthetic techniques and anaesthetic alternatives;
- explanation of block administration: needle insertion, expectation of motor and sensory blockade and block duration;
- complications and side-effects and known incidence of these;
- discussion of combined use of sedative agents, emphasizing amnesic, sedative and control aspects;
- examination of appropriate anatomy, e.g. spine;
- expectation of the recovery time and postoperative analgesic requirements, contrasting differences between local/regional anaesthesia and general anaesthesia.

Patients appreciate hearing-aids, dentures and wigs being left in place. A relaxing atmosphere with their choice of music and use of personalized tapes is recommended. Staff should provide a supportive pillow for comfort, warmth and an interpreter if required. A screen to prevent the patient seeing the operation may be needed. Avoid inappropriate chatter in the operating theatre – patients hate staff chatting over them as

Table 10.5. Relative or absolute contraindications to use of local/regional anaesthesia

History of bleeding problem
Allergies to local anaesthetic
Neurological deficit in area of planned blockade
Infection at site of block
Patient unwilling or uncooperative

if they do not exist. It is surprising how little sedation patients require if the atmosphere is conducive and the surgeon handles the tissues gently.

Technical issues

Performing the block
The anaesthetist must have a good understanding of the relevant anatomy and have gained a degree of expertise in performing the block. Anticipate the length of time for insertion and onset time and move straight into theatre following the block – valuable time is often gained at this stage.

If the block fails, the surgeon may be able to supplement with additional local anaesthetic and the anaesthetist must be on stand-by to convert to general anaesthesia immediately.

Tourniquet
A bloodless field, with the aid of a tourniquet, will assist the surgeon identify structures, aid accurate dissection and reduce surgical time. However, a tourniquet should always be used carefully. The pneumatic tourniquet is less likely to cause permanent paralysis of the limb than an elastic or rubber bandage. It must be judiciously applied as its use can result in prolonged oedema, stiffness and temporary weakness or paralysis. Misapplication can also result in paraesthesia – a complication that can be confused with neural damage from a nerve block[26]. Tourniquet nerve damage is mostly a consequence of mechanical pressure; muscle damage results from ischaemia[27].

When applying a tourniquet:

- elevate the limb before application (4 minutes optimal time)[27];
- respect safe tourniquet time (not greater than 2 hours);
- the width of the cuff should be approximately the diameter of the upper or lower limb;
- apply soft padding beneath the tourniquet;
- select appropriate pressures; range 250–300 mmHg or 20–100 mmHg above systolic pressure.

Most patients can tolerate a cuff pressure of 250 mmHg for 10–15 minutes, and this tolerance can be extended in the following ways.

- Using a forearm or lower leg tourniquet rather than an arm or thigh tourniquet, as patient tolerance is significantly greater[28].
- Intraoperative sedation using a propofol infusion and/or an amnesic agent.
- 'Ring' the upper arm at the proximal edge of the tourniquet with local anaesthetic to block the superficial sensory nerves. This can be performed conveniently with a spinal needle, placing the local anaesthetic subcutaneously.

- Exsanguinate the entire limb, e.g. fingertips to axilla, with an Esmarch bandage, then apply the tourniquet on top of the exsanguination wrap. Pain-free ischaemia can then be extended to 60–75 minutes[29].

> *Sensible application of the tourniquet is important. The anaesthetist can implement a number of strategies to extend patient tolerance for greater than 15 minutes.*
>
> *The patient must understand the benefits and potential side-effects of local/regional anaesthesia, and be co-operative and accepting of the block.*
>
> *The surgeon should sow the seeds for successful local/regional anaesthesia at the initial patient consultation. At surgery, gentle tissue handling and a relaxing ambience are advantageous.*
>
> *The anaesthetist should be skilled in performing the local/regional anaesthetic technique and have a knowledge of appropriate dosage of local anaesthesia.*

Local anaesthetic agents and toxicity

Long-acting local anaesthetic agents will provide the patient with prolonged postoperative analgesia. Short-acting local anaesthetic drugs may be appropriate for plexus blockade if mobilization and early return to function is considered necessary. Patients may have a perception of increased pain when the local anaesthetic wears off. It is therefore necessary to encourage patients to take oral analgesics when the local anaesthetic begins to wear off rather than wait for total return of sensation when pain is unremitting.

Seizures occur when the local anaesthetic exceeds a certain minimum blood level. Signs and symptoms in the unsedated patient are a dysphoric feeling, ringing in the ears, and a metallic taste in the mouth followed by circumoral numbness. Dizziness may occur, together with slurring of speech. As the local anaesthetic blood levels rise, fine twitching of the small muscles of the face, especially the eyelids, and hand, become apparent. With some agents, particularly lignocaine, the patient may feel drowsy. These are the prodroma to a generalized convulsion. However, most convulsions are short lived.

Preventing seizures is the objective. Take care not to inject directly into a blood vessel by aspirating when injecting. A few milligrams of lignocaine in the vertebral artery will cause a convulsion. If injecting into vascular tissues such as the face, neck and penis, there is a greater likelihood of higher blood levels. Less vascular areas such as the foot and inguinal region will give more leeway for increased dosage[30]. When considering the use of high doses of local anaesthetic, close to the presumed toxic limits, intravenous midazolam is advisable. Benzodiazepines have proven to be highly specific and effective in seizure management – with a role in preventing and treating convulsions[31].

If seizures occur, oxygenate and hyperventilate the patient, administer intravenous fluids and intravenous midazolam.

Cardiac changes can be observed with bupivacaine well before seizures are noticed. The more recently introduced local anaesthetic agent, ropivacaine, has many of the properties of bupivacaine with less motor blockade and less cardiotoxicity. It may have advantages for local infiltration because of a greater vasoconstrictive effect, which may prolong its action[32].

The addition of adrenaline (1/200000) to the local anaesthetic agent will not only assist haemostasis but will also reduce absorption, prolonging anaesthesia. This is contra-indicated in procedures on the penis and digits. It is particularly useful for shorter-acting agents such as lignocaine. However, longer-acting agents such as bupivacaine outlast the duration of the vasoconstriction and blood levels are little affected. *Table 10.6* offers manufacturers' suggested dose ranges. The anaesthetist must choose doses appropriately: doses recommended may be too high for the elderly and too low for the healthy. Studies have supported almost double the dose range for local anaesthetic administered in the inguinal area[30].

Table 10.6. Suggested local anaesthetic doses

Drug	Dose range (mg kg^{-1})	Adult dose (mg)
Procaine	14	1000
Prilocaine	10	600
Lignocaine	7[a]	500[a]
Mepivacaine	7[a]	500[a]
Bupivacaine	1–2	150
Ropivacaine	1–2	150–200

[a]With adrenaline.

> *The anaesthetist must select suitable doses of local anaesthetic agent with length of action appropriate for the day surgical procedure.*

Sedation and monitoring

Monitoring of the patient is essential with regional anaesthesia so that early desaturation, ventilatory changes or arrhythmias can be detected. Prior to regional blockade, the anaesthetist should check the anaesthetic machine and availability of anaesthetic drugs in case patient resuscitation or conversion to general anaesthesia is necessary.

The anaesthetist may choose to use local/regional anaesthesia in combination with sedation techniques for patient comfort and surgeon convenience (Chapter 11). Sedation should be commenced prior to the administration of the initial local anaesthetic injection, with care taken to avoid oversedation. Analgesics are generally not necessary but if they are used the anaesthetist must provide vigilant monitoring, as the combination of sedative and opioid can cause significant respiratory depression[33]. Sedation should not be given as a cover-up for an incomplete or inadequate block. Amnesic agents should be administered discretely, as their use may limit patients' recall of surgery and postoperative instructions.

> *Sedative agents can be combined with local and regional anaesthesia for patient comfort and surgeon convenience. The patient should be alert postoperatively so that recovery room stays are minimized.*

Local/regional anaesthesia combined with general anaesthesia

General anaesthesia may be a preferred patient or surgeon option. If so, local/regional anaesthesia can be used as an adjunctive measure. There are advantages to blocks being performed before induction of general anaesthesia because of their pre-emptive effect and the safety margin in having the patient awake when injecting local anaesthetic near a nerve. Time management is essential so that undue delays do not occur. Simple local anaesthetic infiltration can easily be performed during the operative procedure, with the added advantage of lessening the requirements of general anaesthesia. Additional long-acting local anaesthetic can be instilled into appropriate surgical sites before the patient wakes. The limits are only in the imagination!

Commonly used blocks in day surgery

Topical local anaesthesia
The use of topical local anaesthetic agents such as EMLA® cream have been successful for day case myringoplasty[34]. Topical application of lignocaine gel has also been shown to be effective for up to 6 hours post-circumcision[35]. It is useful to provide the gel for patients at discharge for application when regional anaesthesia wears off.

Local/regional anaesthesia for the eye (see Section 14.6)
Local/regional anaesthesia offers significant advantages to patients undergoing ophthalmic surgery – often elderly with significant medical problems[4]. This technique provides for an efficient system, with considerable time saving as the block can be performed while the previous patient is being transferred to second-stage recovery. It also allows for a rapid recovery with minimal disruption to patients' mental function.

Peribulbar (periconal) anaesthesia. This is commonly performed by the anaesthetist or surgeon. It is an easy technique which provides good operating conditions, avoiding the serious complications of retrobulbar blocks. At least 30 minutes should be allowed for block onset. Up to 10 ml of local anaesthetic is placed outside the muscle cone, with the needle tip no further back than the equator of the eye. There are many variations of the peribulbar technique but with the transconjunctival approach patients experience minimal pain. A pressure device is required to ensure spread of local anaesthetic and to decrease intraocular pressure.

Retrobulbar (intraconal) anaesthesia. Although still widely practised, this is less popular than the peribulbar technique because of the serious but fortunately rare local complications: retrobulbar haemorrhage, globe perforation and optic nerve damage. Block onset is more rapid than peribulbar anaesthesia, with a lower incidence of chemosis. A small volume of local anesthetic (2 ml) is deposited within the extraocular muscle cone. A facial nerve block is used in conjunction with this block to prevent contraction of the orbicularis oculi.

Topical anaesthesia. Amethocaine used as a topical local anaesthetic is gaining popularity for cataract surgery. Advantages are its fast onset of action and avoidance of risks associated with needle use. Disadvantages include suboptimal operating conditions with patient eye movement; and some patients experience discomfort during surgery. Maximum dose is 5 mg (15 drops of 0.5%). It is important not to exceed safe clinical doses as serious, even fatal, reactions occur with overdosing.

Instillation into joints and body cavities
The instillation of local anaesthetic into joints is safe but there have been conflicting reports as to the benefits of this technique[36,37]. Smith *et al.* have shown intra-articular local anaesthesia to reduce analgesic requirements and facilitate early mobilization

following arthroscopic knee surgery[38]. Local anaesthetic has also been successfully instilled into cavities following laparoscopy (Chapter 13).

Intravenous regional anaesthesia (IVRA) (Bier's block)

IVRA is a simple, reliable and suitable technique for upper and lower limb surgery. It may be less reliable in the lower than upper limb[39] and a larger volume of local anaesthetic must be used, which is an additive risk if cuff failure occurs. IVRA is suitable for most superficial surgical procedures, allowing for early mobilization and return to function. However, there are time limitations due to tourniquet use.

Guidelines for safety and improvement of IVRA.

- Appropriate monitoring and resuscitative facilities must be available.
- Use of an Esmarch bandage to exsanguinate the limb.
- A reliable tourniquet is mandatory.
- Use of a double tourniquet to reduce tourniquet pain. This is difficult in patients with obese or short upper arms. In this situation, a single tourniquet is preferable as it ensures that the tourniquet occludes the deep arterial branches which may not be compressed if the tourniquet is placed too distally or if it slides distally during manipulation of the arm.
- Local anaesthetic agents most commonly used are plain lignocaine (0.5%) or prilocaine (0.5%) approximately 50 ml for the arm and 100 ml for the lower limb.
- Alkalinization of the local anaesthetic (1 ml 8.4% sodium bicarbonate to each 10 ml of lignocaine). This will reduce pain on injection and improve the quality of the block[40].
- The addition of 60 mg ketorolac to 0.5% lignocaine has been shown to improve analgesia by controlling tourniquet pain and diminishing postoperative pain[41].
- The patient must be provided with alternative analgesia as soon as possible following deflation of the tourniquet, as there is no residual anaesthesia. NSAIDs are a good choice and are best started before the commencement of the procedure so that they are acting at the end of the procedure.

Brachial plexus blockade

For day surgery the axillary and the interscalene approaches are commonly used. The supraclavicular approach is not advisable because of the risk of pneumothorax. An axillary block is appropriate for elbow, lower arm, hand or finger surgery. The success rate has been shown to be similar using paraesthesia, transarterial fixation or nerve stimulation techniques[42].

The drawbacks of brachial plexus blockade are the time necessary to achieve surgical anaesthesia, failure rate and the potential for postoperative paraesthesia from nerve damage. However, by scheduling the patient first on the operating list and with a skilled anaesthetist, this block can provide prolonged analgesia with minimal recovery problems. An interscalene block can be quickly performed and is most useful for shoulder surgery. It is used as an adjunct to general anaesthesia in a balanced analgesia plan or as a single technique for surgical anaesthesia. D'Alessio has demonstrated shorter turnover times with an interscalene block than a general anaesthetic technique[43]. Lignocaine will provide a fast onset of action and will enable the anaesthetist to assess the success of the block in a short period of time. Early mobilization can also be achieved, which may be an advantage for selected shoulder surgery. If bupivacaine is used, the patient can expect up to 24 hours of analgesia, but both patients and staff must be advised of these expectations.

Wrist block

Wrist block is easily performed by blocking the three terminal nerves at the wrist: median, ulnar and superficial branch of the radial nerve. It is suitable for short procedures on the wrist or hand. Patient comfort from tourniquet use will limit the application of this block. The advantages of a wrist block are control of muscle movement and postoperative control of the upper limb.

Digital nerve blocks

These are appropriate for finger surgery. However, adrenaline should be avoided in the local anaesthetic solution.

Lateral femoral cutaneous nerve block

This is a simple block to perform which is suitable for skin graft excision from the upper thigh.

Ankle block

Ankle block is a good choice for foot surgery, with a high success rate achieved for the block. Approximately 30 minutes should be allowed to perform the block. Patients appreciate a short-acting sedative agent at block insertion as blocking the deep peroneal nerve in the deep planes below the fascia is painful. An infusion of a short-acting opioid such as remifentanil may be a suitable alternative at block insertion. (Chapter 9). Use of a mid-calf tourniquet will assist patient comfort in the awake patient.

Perivascular 3 in 1 nerve block

This block (femoral, obturator and lateral femoral cutaneous nerve) was used by Flanagan for patients undergoing anterior cruciate ligament reconstruction. The reported technique was safe and had a high success rate, allowing patients to be discharged within 24 hours with significant cost savings[44].

Penile blocks

Dorsal nerve blocks or ring blocks are simple and satisfactory blocks for the paediatric group undergoing circumcision or hypospadias repair. Local anaesthesia without adrenaline should be used. Vater and Wandless have shown that a dorsal nerve block had specific advantages over caudal analgesia in boys undergoing circumcision. Micturition occurred earlier, boys were able to stand sooner and there was a lower incidence of vomiting[45].

Block of ilioinguinal, iliohypogastric and genitofemoral nerves

Infiltration of the operative site with local anaesthetic is the least invasive and safest of all techniques for hernia repair. However, reliability and success for the technique is necessary. Sparks *et al.* have described a short bevel needle technique, facilitating correct needle placement, which has a high success rate and high patient and surgeon satisfaction for the block[46]. Patient advantages for an infiltration technique when bupivacaine is used, compared with a control group, are decreased recovery room pain and postdischarge oral analgesic requirements[47]. Care should be taken to infiltrate local anaesthetic in the subfascial rather than the subcutaneous layer after herniorrhaphy, as studies have demonstrated a better analgesic effect with this technique[48]. Day surgery staff should be aware of the transient femoral nerve blockade which can follow 'blind' ilioinguinal field block[49]. The use of a short bevel blunt needle which accurately identifies fascial planes may minimize this risk of large volumes of local anaesthetic tracking down to the femoral nerve.

> *Patients should be able to lift their leg on the side of the hernia repair before they are mobilized following an inguinal field block.*

Central neural blockade: spinal and epidural

Spinal and epidural anaesthesia are viable alternatives to general anaesthesia in day surgery, with some investigators demonstrating advantages of fewer side-effects and earlier discharge times[50]. However, this remains a controversial issue as some clinicians are concerned about delayed patient recovery. Selection of short-acting local anaesthetic drugs is therefore appropriate. Lignocaine is the most common spinal drug for day patients. A 2% solution can be used as an isobaric preparation. The amount required to block below the inguinal ligament is 3–4 ml, and 4–5 ml above the inguinal ligament. The 5% solution is less popular because of reports of radicular irritation presenting as pain in the back radiating to the legs[51]. The duration of lignocaine spinal anaesthesia is variable.

Epidural lignocaine will provide 60–90 minutes of anaesthesia, with possible discharge 5–6 hours after the block. Spinal has distinct advantages over epidural anaesthesia with less time required to achieve an adequate block, lower incidence of incomplete sensory and motor block and pain during surgery[52].

There are potential problems with the use of central neural blockade in day surgery.

- Time to insert the block, which may affect efficiency.
- Incomplete block or return of sensation part way through surgery.
- Delayed ambulation, necessitating prolonged time in first-stage recovery.
- Patients must have complete return of sensation prior to discharge. Therefore additional analgesics are required in the late recovery period.
- Urinary retention.
- Post-dural puncture headache. Recently, the incidence of this problem in day patients has been shown to be reduced to 1% by selecting an older group of patients and the use of 25- or 26- gauge, non-cutting, pencil-point spinal needles[53,54].

Caudal anaesthesia. This is used for anorectal surgery, but the following disadvantages limit its use in the adult patient.

- Pain on insertion.
- Landmarks are difficult to feel.
- Varying anatomy.
- Higher failure rate than spinal or epidural anaesthesia.
- Delay in re-establishing micturition.

Perianal infiltration of local anaesthetic with a balanced analgesia plan offers a suitable alternative.

> *The choice of neural blockade will depend on the surgical procedure, patient and surgeon factors, anaesthetic skill for the administration of the block and nursing expertise.*

Patient discharge, instructions and follow-up

Patients receiving local and regional anaesthesia should meet standard discharge criteria before being discharged from the day surgery facility (Chapter 16). However, special attention must be paid before discharging patients following either spinal or epidural blockade. In addition to meeting standard discharge criteria, they need to be able to void and plantar flex the foot with proprioception of the big toe[55]. Voiding is an extra check that there is no residual blockade[56]. Full recovery of motor and sensory functions is required before discharge. Once sensation has returned, residual sympathetic blockade and orthostatic hypotension are rarely a problem, and patients may ambulate. Elderly males who may have prostatic enlargement are at risk of urinary retention, so fluid restriction in the perioperative period is appropriate.

For patients who have had brachial plexus anaesthesia, discharge before full sensation returns is safe and practical. However, very clear verbal and written instructions must be given. For patient safety, the anaesthetized arm should be placed in a sling, with clear instructions about protection strategies (*Table 10.7*). Instructions for patients following foot surgery are given in *Table 10.8*.

> *Patients must meet standard discharge criteria following day surgery local or regional anaesthesia. In addition, patients who have undergone central neural blockade should have full return of motor and sensory function and void before discharge. Patient instructions relating to limb protection are important to those who have residual numbness following limb anaesthesia.*

Table 10.7. Patient instructions following an arm block

You have had a nerve block anaesthetic. During the time the block is effective the area remains numb. Your armpit may be sore for a day or two after your anaesthetic. This will improve with time
While the arm is numb
    you will be unable to feel discomfort and you could injure, burn or hurt yourself
    avoid bumping the numb area
    elevate your hand above your heart
    wear a sling to protect your arm
    resume normal activities after the numbness has worn off
Commence a full range of exercises every hour. Light use of fingers is encouraged (eating, combing hair, etc.). Heavy lifting should be restricted
If you have any questions, concerns or problems relating to your nerve block anaesthetic, please do not hesitate to contact your anaesthetist or the Day Surgery Unit (telephone number)

Strategies to overcome problems with local/regional anaesthesia in day surgery

- When designing a facility, plan for a 'block room' adjacent to theatre so as not to encroach on recovery space or theatre availability[43].
- Surgeons should inform all patients of local/regional benefits at the initial patient visit.

Table 10.8. Instructions to patients following foot surgery

For your comfort and to aid healing following surgery you should (delete as necessary)
  not walk on your affected foot, but use crutches or a walker
  or
  walk on your affected foot as you find comfortable
Elevate your foot as soon as possible following surgery. Elevation should be above your heart level
  with your hip and knee flexed. A pillow should be placed under your calf for support. Use a foot
  cradle made from a large cardboard box or pillows to keep bed covers off your foot
If you do not have full feeling back in your foot following surgery, make sure that it is protected
  from injury
Exercise your legs regularly by alternately flexing your hips, knees, and ankles. This will stimulate
  your circulation
Ice may be applied to your foot on specific instruction from your doctor
Keep the bandage clean and dry. Do not remove the dressing or inspect the wound. Some
  bleeding through the dressing may occur. This can be expected. If there is progressive bleeding
  after 24 hours, contact your doctor
If you have any questions, concerns or problems relating to your nerve block anaesthetic, please
  do not hesitate to contact your anaesthetist or the Day Surgery Unit (telephone number)

- An assessment nurse can provide patients with more detailed information on local/regional blocks prior to the day of surgery and identify the anaesthetist who will be performing the block.
- The anaesthetist should discuss risks of general anaesthesia and advantages of the local/regional technique with the patient preoperatively.
- In plexus anaesthesia or central neural blockade, where time is required for block insertion and onset time, schedule patients first on the operating list.
- For fast onset of action, lignocaine is an appropriate local anaesthetic choice; however, supplementation with a longer-acting agent such as bupivacaine will prolong postoperative analgesia.
- To speed the onset of the block and decrease discomfort at the time of infiltration, add bicarbonate (8.4% solution) just before injection[57,58]. It is recommended that 1 ml of bicarbonate for each 10 ml of lignocaine is used. Onset time can further be improved by warming the local anaesthetic to body temperature before use[59].
- The anaesthetist must learn relevant anatomy and practise the block for greater success.
- A nerve stimulator will determine the proximity of the needle to the nerve and may be useful in the sedated or uncooperative patient; however, this has not been shown to improve success rates for brachial plexus blocks[60].
- Use short bevel needles to minimize the incidence of nerve damage[61].
- Minimize delays by assuming the block will be successful. Move the patient to the operating table, instruct the surgical team to scrub and drape the relevant area.
- Avoid using sedative agents with long half-lives or combination agents that cause postoperative drowsiness.
- If a 'fair' block results which is unsuitable for surgical anaesthesia, the surgeon should supplement the surgical site with long-acting local anaesthesia. This also assists prolonged postoperative analgesia .
- Encourage patients to take oral analgesics such as NSAIDs *before* the block wears off.
- Follow patients postoperatively to ascertain patient satisfaction and morbidity for the block.

> *With appropriate patient selection and sedation, local and regional techniques can be used for day surgery patients. Skilful application of peripheral neural blockade broadens the anaesthetist's range of options in providing quality and cost-effective day surgery care.*

References

1. **Bridenbaugh LD, Soderstrom RM.** Lumbar epidural block anesthesia for outpatient laparoscopy. *J. Reprod. Med.* 1979; **23**: 85–86.
2. **Dexter F, Tinker JH.** Analysis of strategies to decrease postanesthesia care unit costs. *Anesthesiology* 1995; **82**: 94–101.
3. **Zukowski ML, Ash K, Klink B, et al.** Breast reduction under intravenous sedation: a review of 50 cases. *Plast. Reconstruct. Surg.* 1996; **97**: 952–956.
4. **Berry CB, Murphy PM.** Regional anaesthesia for cataract surgery. *Br. J. Hosp. Med.* 1993; **49**: 689, 692–701.
5. **Srinivasan V, Arasaratnam RB, Jankelowitz GA.** Day-case septal surgery under general anaesthesia and local anaesthesia with sedation. *J. Laryngol. Otol.* 1995; **109**: 614–617.
6. **Leach Ge, Sirls L, Ganabathi K, et al.** Outpatient visual laser-assisted prostatectomy under local anesthesia. *Urology* 1994; **43**: 149–153.
7. **Hugosson J, Bergdahl S, Norlen L, et al.** Outpatient transurethral incision of the prostate under local anesthesia: operative results, patient security and cost effectiveness. *Scand. J. Urol. Nephrol.* 1993; **27**: 381–385.
8. **Krespi YP, Ling EH.** Laser-assisted serial tonsillectomy. *J. Otolaryngol.* 1994; **23**: 325–327.
9. **Hochman M, Fee WE.** Thyroidectomy under local anesthesia. *Arch. Otolaryngol., Head Neck Surg.* 1991; **117**: 405–407.
10. **Van Sickels JE, Tiner BD.** Cost of a genioplasty under deep intravenous sedation in a private office versus general anesthesia in an outpatient surgical center. *J. Oral Maxillofac. Surg.* 1992; **50**: 687–690.
11. **Michaloliakou C, Chung F, Sharma S.** Preoperative multimodal analgesia facilitates recovery after ambulatory laparoscopic cholecystectomy. *Anesth. Analg.* 1996; **82**: 44–51.
12. **Monk TG, Boure B, White PF, et al.** Comparison of intravenous sedative–analgesic techniques for outpatient immersion lithotripsy. *Anesth. Analg.* 1991; **72**: 616–621.
13. **Osborne GA, Rudkin GE.** Outcome after day-care surgery in a major teaching hospital. *Anaesth. Intens. Care* 1993; **21**: 822–827.
14. **Bridenbaugh LD.** Regional anaesthesia for outpatient surgery. *Can. Anaesth. Soc. J.* 1983; **30**: 548.
15. **Tverskoy M, Cozacov C, Ayache M, et al.** Postoperative pain after inguinal herniorraphy with different types of anesthesia. *Anesth. Analg.* 1990; **70**: 29–35.
16. **Parnass SM, McCarthy RJ, Bach B, et al.** A prospective evaluation of epidural versus general anesthesia for outpatient arthroscopy. *Anesthesiology* 1990 **73**: A23.
17. **Jebeles JA, Reilly JS, Gutierrez JF, et al.** The effect of pre-incisional infiltration of tonsils with bupivacaine on the pain following tonsillectomy under general anesthesia. *Pain* 1991; **47**: 305–308.
18. **Ejlersen E, Andersen HB, Eliasen K, et al.** A comparison between pre- and postincisional lidocaine infiltration on postoperative pain. *Anesth. Analg.* 1992; **74**: 495–498.
19. **Kissin I.** Preemptive analgesia. Why its effect is not always obvious. *Anesthesiology* 1996; **84**: 1015–1019.
20. **Rudkin GE.** Patient choice in sedation anaesthesia and recovery room analgesia. *Ambulatory Surg.* 1994; **2**: 75–80.
21. **Tetzlaff JE, Spevak C, Yoon H, et al.** Patient acceptance of interscalene block. *Anesth. Analg.* 1991; **72**: S295.
22. **Rudkin GE, Maddern GJ.** Peri-operative outcome for day-case laparoscopic and open inguinal hernia repair. *Anaesthesia* 1995; **50**: 586–589.
23. **Wallace DA, Carr AJ, Loach AB, et al.** Day case arthroscopy under local anaesthesia. *Ann. R. Coll. Surg. Engl.* 1994; **76**: 330–331.
24. **Allen HW, Mulroy MF, Fundis K, et al.** Regional versus Propofol general anesthesia for outpatient hand surgery. *Anesthesiology* 1983; **79**: A1.

25. **Brown AR, Weiss R, Greenberg C,** *et al.* Interscalene block for shoulder arthroscopy: comparison with general anesthesia. *Athroscopy* 1993; **9**: 295–300.
26. **Crenshaw AH, Milford L.** (1963) The hand. In: *Campbell's Operative Orthopaedics*, Vol. 1, 4th Edn (Eds AH Crenshaw and L Milford). CV Mosby, St Louis, MO. pp. 140–141.
27. **Green DP.** (1988) General principles: the tourniquet. In: *Operative Hand Surgery*, Vol. 11, 2nd Edn (Ed. DP Green). Churchill Livingstone, Edinburgh. pp. 7–26.
28. **Hutchinson DT, McClinton MA.** Upper extremity tourniquet tolerance. *J. Hand Surg.* 1993; **18A**: 206–210.
29. **Dushoff IM.** Hand surgery under wrist block and local infiltration anesthesia, using an upper arm tourniquet (letter). *Plast. Reconstruct. Surg.* 1973; **51**: 685.
30. **Karatassas A, Morris RG, Slavotinek AH.** The relationship between regional blood flow and absorption of lignocaine. *Aust. N.Z. J. Surg.* 1993; **63**: 766–771.
31. **de Jong RH.** (1994) *Local Anesthetics.* CV Mosby, St Louis, MO. p. 299.
32. **Johansson B, Glise H, Halleräck B,** *et al.* Preoperative local infiltration with ropivacaine for postoperative pain relief after cholecystectomy. *Anesth. Analg.* 1994; **78**: 210–214.
33. **Bailey PL, Pace NL, Ashburn MA,** *et al.* Frequent hypoxemia and apnea after sedation with Midazolam and Fentanyl. *Anesthesiology* 1990; **73**: 826–830.
34. **Kaddour HS.** Myringoplasty under local anaesthesia: day case surgery. *Clin. Otolaryngol.* 1992; **17**: 567–568.
35. **Tritrakarn T, Pirayavaraporn S.** Postoperative pain relief for circumcision in children: comparison among morphine, nerve block, and topical analgesia. *Anesthesiology* 1985; **62**: 519–522.
36. **Milligan KA, Mowbray MJ, Mulrooney L,** *et al.* Intra-articular bupivacaine for pain relief after arthroscopic surgery of the knee joint in daycase patients. *Anaesthesia* 1988; **43**: 563–564.
37. **Henderson RC, Campion ER, DeMasi RA,** *et al.* Postarthroscopy analgesia with bupivacaine. *Am. J. Sports Med.* 1990; **18**: 614–617.
38. **Smith I, Van Hemelrijck J, White PF,** *et al.* Effects of local anesthesia on recovery after outpatient arthroscopy. *Anesth. Analg.* 1991; **73**: 536–539.
39. **Kim DD, Shuman C, Sadr B.** Intravenous regional anesthesia for outpatient foot and ankle surgery: a prospective study. *Orthopedics* 1993; **16**: 1109–1113.
40. **Armstrong P, Watters J, Whitfield A.** Alkalinisation of prilocaine for intravenous regional anaesthesia. Suitability for clinical use. *Anaesthesia* 1990; **45**: 935–937.
41. **Reuben SS, Steinberg RB, Kreitzer JM,** *et al.* Intravenous regional anesthesia using Lidocaine and Ketorolac. *Anesth. Analg.* 1995; **81**: 110–113.
42. **Davis WJ, Lennon RL, Medel DJ.** Brachial plexus anesthesia for outpatient surgical procedures on an upper extremity. *Mayo Clin. Proc.* 1991; **66**: 470–473.
43. **D'Alessio JG, Rosenblum M, Shea KP,** *et al.* A retrospective comparison of interscalene block and general anesthesia for ambulatory surgery shoulder arthroscopy. *Reg. Anesth.* 1995; **20**: 62.
44. **Flanagan JFK, Edkin B, Spindler K.** 3 in 1 femoral nerve block following ACL reconstruction allows predictably earlier discharge and significant cost savings. *Anesthesiology* 1994; **81**: A950.
45. **Vater M, Wandless J.** Caudal or dorsal nerve block? A comparison of two local anaesthetic techniques for postoperative analgesia following day case circumcision. *Acta Anaesthesiol. Scand.* 1985; **29**: 175–179.
46. **Sparks CJ, Rudkin GE, Agiomea K,** *et al.* Inguinal field block for adult inguinal hernia repair using a short-bevel needle. Description and clinical experience in Solomon Islands and an Australian teaching hospital. *Anaesth. Intens. Care* 1995; **23**: 143–148.
47. **Ding Y, White PF.** Post-herniorrhaphy pain in outpatients after pre-incision ilioinguinal–hypogastric nerve block during monitored anaesthesia care. *Can. J. Anaesth.* 1995; **42**: 12–15.
48. **Yndgaard S, Holst P, Bjerre-Jepsen K,** *et al.* Subcutaneously versus subfascially administered Lidocaine in pain treatment after inguinal herniotomy. *Anesth. Analg.* 1994; **79**: 324–327.
49. **Rosario DJ, Skinner PP, Raftery AT.** Transient femoral nerve palsy complicating preoperative ilioinguinal nerve blockade for inguinal herniorrhaphy. *Br. J. Surg.* 1994; **81**: 897.
50. **Parnass SM, McCarthy RJ, Bach BR,** *et al.* Beneficial impact of epidural anesthesia on recovery after outpatient arthroscopy. *Arthroscopy* 1993; **9**: 91–95.
51. **Schneider M, Ettlin T, Kaufmann M,** *et al.* Transient neurologic toxicity after hyperbaric subarachnoid anesthesia with 5% lidocaine. *Anesth. Analg.* 1993; **76**: 1154.

52. **Seeberger MD, Lang ML, Drewe J, *et al*.** Comparison of spinal and epidural anesthesia for patients younger than 50 years of age. *Anesth. Analg.* 1994; **78:** 667–673.

53. **Halpern S, Preston R.** Postdural puncture headache and spinal needle design. *Anesthesiology* 1994; **81:** 1376–1383.

54. **Mulroy MF, Wills RA.** Spinal anesthesia for outpatients: appropriate agents and techniques. *J. Clin. Anesth.* 1995; **7:** 622.

55. **Pflug AE, Aashein GM, Foster C.** Sequence of return of neurological function and criteria for safe ambulation following subarachnoid block. *Can. Anaesth. Soc. J.* 1978; **25:** 133.

56. **Wetchler BV.** (1990) Problem solving in the postanesthesia care unit. In: *Anesthesia for Ambulatory Surgery* (ed. BV Wetchler). JB Lippincott Co., Philadelphia, PA. pp. 375–436.

57. **Capogna G, Celleno D, Laudano D, *et al*.** Alkalinization of local anesthetics: which block, which local anesthetic? *Reg. Anesth.* 1995; **20:** 369.

58. **Hilgier M.** Alkalinization of bupivacaine for brachial plexus block. *Reg. Anesth.* 1985; **8:** 59.

59. **Heath PJ, Brownlie GS, Herrick MJ.** Latency of brachial plexus block. The effect on onset time of warming of local anaesthetic solutions. *Anaesthesia* 1990; **45:** 297–301.

60. **Goldberg ME, Gregg C, Larijani GE, *et al*.** A comparison of three methods of axillary approach to brachial plexus blockage for upper extremity surgery. *Anesthesiology* 1987; **66:** 814.

61. **Moore DC, Mulroy MF, Thompson GE.** Peripheral nerve damage and regional anesthesia. *Br. J. Anaesth.* 1994; **73:** 436.

CHAPTER 11

Sedation

G.E. Rudkin

Sedation anaesthesia is becoming increasingly popular due to improved delivery techniques and newer, short-acting drugs suitable for sedation. Sedation techniques in combination with local or regional anaesthesia, or as an adjunct to common diagnostic and therapeutic procedures, can improve patient care and reduce costs in day surgery compared with general anaesthetic techniques (*Tables 11.1* and *11.2*).

Table 11.1. Sedation ± analgesia for day surgery procedures: advantages to the patient

Reduced patient anxiety
Less pain on the initial injection of local anaesthetic
Reduced deep traction pain during surgery
Greater patient tolerance of long procedures
Avoidance of risks associated with general anaesthesia
Amnesia for the surgical or procedural event
More streamlined recovery room process with faster patient discharge
Fewer postoperative complications compared with general anaesthesia

Table 11.2. Sedation ± analgesia for day surgery procedures: advantages to the surgeon or proceduralist

Optimal operating conditions for surgery can be achieved, with improved patient tolerance[1]
Better control over the course of proceedings[1,2]
Reduced sympathetic response to surgery
Operating times can be reduced with a co-operative patient
More complete examinations can be performed in procedural work[3]

There needs to be a general ambience in the operating theatre which instils calmness in the patient. The surgeon must be trained in performing procedures with patients under sedation anaesthesia. Gentle surgical techniques should be used, with careful tissue handling. However, sedation is not a substitute for inadequate pain control, the basis of which is effective local or regional anaesthesia (*Table 11.3*).

Definitions and end points

The objective is to produce a level of sedation where the patient is relaxed, and calm and rational verbal communication is continuously possible.

Table 11.3. Sedation ± analgesia for day surgery procedures: advantages to the day surgery facility

Patients may be able to move directly to second-stage recovery
Overall patient time in the facility can be reduced
Cost-effective alternative to general anaesthesia[4]
Overall cost to the facility can be reduced

Various terminologies have been used for sedation which have led to confusion (*Table 11.4*). Those administering sedation must identify the specific patient needs for the procedure before choosing analgesic, anxiolytic, sedative and amnesic drugs to use alone or in combination[5].

Administration of sedative drugs results in a continuum from drowsiness to deep sleep and can progress quickly to unconsciousness or general anaesthesia. Once this has happened the sedationist has become an anaesthetist whether or not this was intended, and the same standard of monitoring and expertise as for general anaesthetic care is required (*Figure 11.1* and *Table 11.5*).

> *The drugs and techniques used should provide a margin of safety which is wide enough to render unintended loss of consciousness unlikely.*

Table 11.4. Terminologies used for sedation

Term	Definition	Comment
Conscious sedation	State of depressed level of consciousness where the patient has the ability to maintain an airway and respond appropriately to verbal communication	Term introduced by Bennett 1978[6]; first used by dentists. *Limitation:* does not incorporate monitoring, i.e. safety aspect
Neurolept analgesia	State of depressed consciousness achieved by a combination of drugs consisting of a tranquillizer, opioid and nitrous oxide	Term introduced in 1959 by DeCastro and Mundeleer[7]. Term often used inappropriately
Sedoanalgesia	State of depressed consciousness achieved by combination of analgesia and sedation[4]	More specific term used when analgesics are added to sedation regime
Monitored anaesthesia care (MAC)	Term encompasses both patient monitoring and the administration of sedative medications	Advantage: incorporates monitoring, i.e. safety aspect. *Limitation:* does not include 'extent' of depression of conscious state

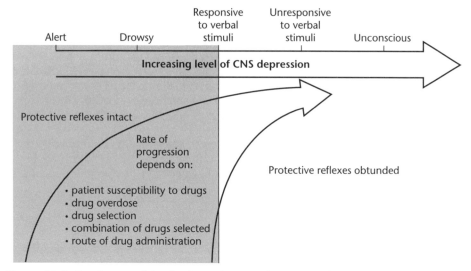

Figure 11.1. Continuum of depth of consciousness between sedation and general anaesthesia.

Table 11.5. Potential pitfalls associated with sedation which may cause patients' protective reflexes to be obtunded

Wide variety of combinations of drugs administered
Difficulty in predicting absorption, distribution and efficacy of drugs
Wide individual patient variation in response to drug
Inexperience of the person administering sedation
Potentially excessive drug used to compensate for inadequate analgesia
Wide variety of procedures performed with differing levels of surgical stimuli
Differing standards of equipment and staffing where procedures are performed[8]

Safety and monitoring

Anaesthetic surveillance

The poor safety profile attributed to sedation anaesthesia is largely due to those without anaesthetic skills administering sedation. This was demonstrated in a large, multicentre study conducted by FASA, where the complication rate was higher for patients undergoing local anaesthesia and sedation (1/106) than for general anaesthesia (1/120) and local anaesthesia (1/268)[9]. If sedation is given by skilled anaesthetists and titrated to maintain safe sedation levels, morbidity should be minimal[10].

Anaesthetists are ideally suited to provide sedation anaesthesia, with their expertise in infiltration techniques, airway management and patient monitoring and their ability to titrate drugs to patient needs. Moreover, induction agents such as propofol, a very suitable sedative agent, should not be administered by non-anaesthetists. It is mandatory that the sedationist has responsibility only for sedation and cardiorespiratory monitoring and is not involved in performing the procedure itself.

A common pitfall in sedation is to induce a confusional state, where the patient is a long way along the sedation continuum line (*Figure 11.1*). If the anaesthetist gives additional sedative drugs this will further contribute to the patient's disorientation. Failure to distinguish between the common causes of agitation may result in inappropriate therapeutic decisions[11]. The anaesthetist must have experience in sedation techniques to recognize this 'risky' state. Failure to do so will compromise patient care. In the American Society of Anesthesiologists' closed claims analysis study, Caplan *et al.* reported that the cause of cardiac arrest in a group of healthy patients undergoing spinal anaesthesia and sedation may have been due to unappreciated respiratory insufficiency secondary to drug-induced central nervous system (CNS) depression[12].

> *It is essential to have an experienced sedationist, preferably an anaesthetist, to monitor and maintain safe levels of sedation. This person should not be involved in the procedure being undertaken, so that full attention is paid to the patient's conscious level.*

Variation in patient needs

Patients vary in their needs for sedation and amnesia. Some patients will be comfortable without sedation, and the role of the anaesthetist will be simply to observe. Others will want complete amnesia. The situation may change during the procedure and the anaesthetist needs to titrate drugs according to the changing surgical stimuli and noise level associated with surgical equipment.

The anaesthetist must also differentiate between pain and anxiety. Pain should be treated by additional local anaesthetic supplemented by a potent, rapid-acting intravenous analgesic such as fentanyl. Anxiety is best treated by an anxiolytic drug such as midazolam.

> *The sedationist must be sensitive to patient requirements and titrate appropriate drugs to reduce anxiety and pain in response to surgical events.*

Monitoring

Level of consciousness. Patients' responses to sedative agents vary considerably. It is therefore important that the same monitoring facilities employed for safe general anaesthesia are applied to sedation anaesthesia. Close contact between the anaesthetist and the patient is essential. Acceptably safe sedation is up to and including sedation level 3, where the patient's eyes are closed but he or she is rousable to command[13] (*Table 11.6*).

Essential monitoring. This is continuous measurement of oxygen saturation[14] during the procedure and until the patient meets the discharge criteria in the recovery area[15]. A review of 2000 anaesthetic incidents showed that pulse oximetry detected more

Table 11.6. Sedation scale

1. Fully awake
2. Drowsy
3. Eyes closed but rousable to command
4. Eyes closed but rousable to mild physical stimulation
5. Eyes closed and unrousable to mild physical stimulation

incidents than any other monitor. In an incident-monitoring review, Webb *et al.* considered that the proper use of pulse oximetry would have alerted the anaesthetists in over 80% of incidents, had the incidents remained undetected by other means[16]. However oxygen desaturation is a late indicator of hypoventilation.

Hypoventilation may be detected earlier with a capnometer to measure end-tidal Pco_2 which is a clinically accurate estimate of $Paco_2$. The expired gas can be sampled through a nasal cannula or a Hudson mask (*Figure 11.2*). The set-up can be simple and inexpensive[17].

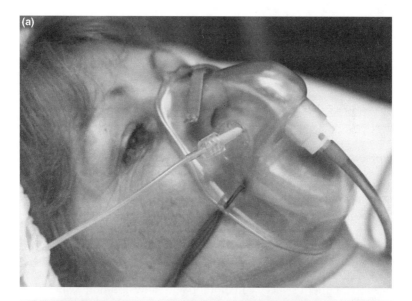

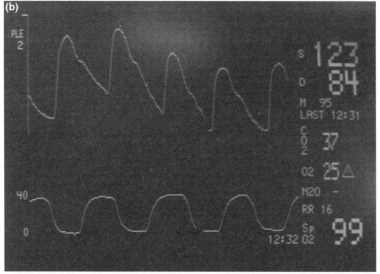

Figure 11.2. End-tidal CO_2 monitoring in the sedated patient. (a) Simple set up for expired gas sample through a Hudson mask; (b) capnograph tracing from expired gas.

There are limitations with this form of monitoring with respect to reliability and accuracy. Spurious readings, large arterial to end-tidal carbon dioxide gradients, mouth breathing, obstruction to catheters and dilution by supplemental oxygen are commonly cited problems that cause reductions in measurement accuracy[18]. However, with further improvements in equipment and clinical experience in capnography during sedation monitoring, these problems are likely to be overcome[19]. In the past, some centres have used pre-cordial stethoscopes for breath-by-breath monitoring, but these have been largely replaced by capnometry.

Capnography immediately identifies respiratory obstruction and rising end-tidal P_{CO_2} levels. In high-risk patients it gives early warning of respiratory decompensation.

Monitoring of BP and ECG is useful in general, and essential for patients with a history of ischaemic heart disease or arrhythmias.

Emergency equipment must always be available, as well as trained staff who are able to cope with potentially lethal complications.

> *Monitoring of conscious level and oxygen saturation is mandatory and capnometry is highly recommended, both during the procedure and in the recovery room.*

Oxygen supplementation

Oxygen may be given via oxygen mask or nasal cannula. Dislodgement of a nasal cannula can be prevented by secure taping. A guide to the oxygen flow rate required to achieve adequate inspired oxygen concentrations (FIO_2) where normal ventilatory pattern is assumed[20] is given in *Table 11.7*. For abnormal ventilatory patterns, the larger the tidal volume or the faster the respiratory rate, the lower the FIO_2.

For surgical procedures performed around the nose, oxygen tubing can be put into the patient's mouth which is tolerated particularly well. There is concern that increased oxygen concentration in patients undergoing head and neck procedures, where surgical drapes cover the patient's face, can potentially allow ignition[21]. In this instance, particularly in patients undergoing lens extraction under local anaesthesia, the administration of air/O_2 mix, with close observation of pulse oximetry, is appropriate. A flow rate of at least 10 l minute^{-1} should be used to prevent accumulation of CO_2.

Table 11.7. Flow rate guidelines for estimating inspired oxygen concentrations (FIO_2)

100% O_2 flow rate (litres minute^{-1})	FIO_2
Nasal cannula	
1	0.24
2	0.28
3	0.32
4	0.36
5	0.40
6	0.44
Oxygen mask	
4–5	0.30
5–6	0.40
6–7	0.50
7–8	0.60

SEDATION ANAESTHETIC RECORD

Operation .... Surgeon ....
Patient's name .... Age .... Weight .... kg
Allergies .... ASA status .... Medications ....

Questionnaire evaluated –   Yes/No   Special requirements for sedation:
Patient fasted –   Yes/No   Awake –   Yes/No
Carer available –   Yes/No   Drowsy –   Yes/No
                                     Amnesia –   Yes/No

DRUGS

1 ....
2 ....
3 ....
4 ....
5 ....
6 ....
7 ....

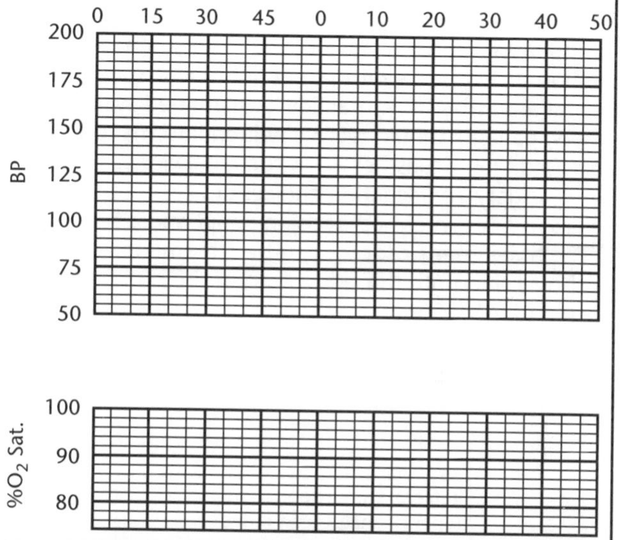

IV ACCESS

Site

Gauge

COMMENTS

Uneventful – Yes/No

MONITORING

BP, ECG, %O_2 Sat., Pulse, etCO_2

ANAESTHETIST
SIGNATURE:

....

Procedure time   Recovery

0   15   30   45   0   10   20   30   40   50

BP: 200 175 150 125 100 75 50

%O_2 Sat.: 100 90 80

DISCHARGE CRITERIA   **COMMENTS**

1. Vital signs stable ....

2. Postanaesthesia
   recovery score 10 ....

3. Able to ambulate ....

4. Alert & orientated ....

5. Responsible adult
   present ....

6. Patient given discharge
   instruction sheet ....

7. Discharge time ....

SIGNATURE:

....

Figure 11.3. Sedation anaesthetic record.

Drapes should be displaced from the patient's face, to allow air flow and allay any feeling of claustrophobia.

Standards
When sedation is used, it is imperative that trained personnel and appropriate facilities are provided, as well as emergency equipment and drugs for full resuscitation of the patient in the event of an untoward reaction. Each facility must comply with national standards laid down by governing health bodies, to ensure safe standards for the administration of sedative drugs[22–24].

The anaesthetic record for sedation anaesthesia is a communication record to all staff concerned in the day surgery facility, a guidance for future administration of sedation anaesthesia, and a medico-legal document. An example of a sedation record is given in *Figure 11.3*.

Assessment

Comprehensive preoperative patient assessment is as important for patients undergoing sedation anaesthesia with regional or local anaesthesia, as it is for those undergoing general anaesthesia. A practical streamlined system is outlined in *Figure 11.4*. Before surgery, patients should receive written information relating to safety aspects of general versus sedation anaesthesia. Instructional videos both on information pertaining to the day of surgery and sedation choices are also useful. This information allows the patient to make a more informed decision about anaesthetic options.

The assessment process can be streamlined by the use of a health questionnaire which will orientate those involved in the patient assessment to the patient's general health and behavioural state.

A fully informed patient who has received a thorough preoperative explanation will have less preoperative anxiety on the day of surgery, and better rapport between patient, surgeon and anaesthetist. This will also assist the informed consent process.

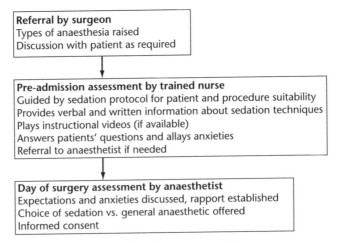

Figure 11.4. Flow chart for streamlined patient assessment.

Patient sedation choices

The anaesthetist must consider the patient's needs[25] and choice[26] of sedation. Discussion with patients about their expectations has been shown to improve patient satisfaction[27]. The preoperative assessment allows appropriate sedation drugs and techniques to be tailored to the patient's needs (*Table 11.8*) and patients can be reassured about any concerns that they may have. The needs of every patient must be assessed individually. The anaesthetist should explain to the patient that every effort will be made to meet their requests but that in some cases this cannot be guaranteed.

> *Preoperatively, the anaesthetist should discuss sedation issues with the patient. These relate to the patient's perceived needs for drowsiness, amnesia, control and specific concerns that he or she may have.*

Table 11.8. Suggested questions for patient choice in sedation anaesthesia

Patient question	On entering the operating theatre	During local anaesthetic administration	During surgery
Do you wish to be awake?			
Do you wish to be drowsy?			
Do you wish to have no memory of events? (amnesia)			

Patient question	YES	NO
Do you want to control your own sedation?		
Do you want the anaesthetist to control your sedation?		
Do you have any particular concerns or fears relating to your sedation anaesthesia?		
(a) lack of personal control		
(b) fear of going to sleep		
(c) fear of pain		
(d) fear of the unknown		
(e) fear of seeing the operating room		
(f) fear of witnessing surgery		
(g) fear of overhearing conversation related to the surgery		

Difficult patient groups

Particular care should be taken when administering sedation anaesthesia in the following cases.

Sedation outside the operating theatre
Sedation outside the operating theatre, such as in the magnetic resonance imaging (MRI) suite, requires careful patient selection, vigilant monitoring and adherence to

safety guidelines. There may be minimal staff assistance, and observation of the patient may be difficult. It is imperative that trained staff assistance is available and that substandard levels of monitoring are not accepted.

The elderly patient
Hypotension and respiratory depression readily occur. This can be minimized by slow administration, careful titration and assessing the effect before supplementing the dose of drugs. Close communication and careful monitoring are required.

The uncooperative patient
In uncooperative patients, particularly those who have extreme anxiety, significant psychiatric problems and severe learning disabilities, sedation can be successful, provided a preoperative planned approach, with an agreement of sedation techniques and establishment of rapport, is made.

The sleep apnoeic patient
Obstructive sleep apnoea is a common condition. Davies and Stradling have estimated that 1 in 50 males have some airway obstruction when lying supine[28]. This is made worse when sedative drugs are administered. The anaesthetist must be aware that early airway obstruction can occur before a deeper level of sedation is achieved and vigilant monitoring is required.

Suspected sleep apnoea should be investigated preoperatively with a sleep study and relevant management instituted before day surgery. How do you identify the sleep apnoeic patient preoperatively?

- History of snoring (often reported by partner).
- History of sleep apnoea witnessed by partner.
- Reports of daytime sleepiness.
- A neck circumference greater than 43 cm is suggestive[29].

If the patient has his or her own nasal continuous positive airway pressure mask, this should be brought to day surgery and used perioperatively. These machines are light and portable and require only a mains power supply. Supplementary oxygen may be added to the nasal mask if required.

Intraoperatively, use only short-acting sedative drugs such as propofol. Vigilant monitoring of the patient's conscious level and airway is necessary and the patient roused should snoring occur.

The patient should be returned to the sitting position as soon as practical as this will improve airway patency. Patient discharge is appropriate when routine discharge criteria are met.

Patient preparation

Patients who are scheduled for sedation anaesthesia should be fasted appropriately according to general anaesthetic guidelines (see Chapter 3). This is important from a safety aspect, in case of loss of protective airway reflexes or if general anaesthesia must be administered.

In the day surgery setting, sedative premedication is inappropriate, drugs are better accurately titrated at the time of surgery. Preoperative patient anxiety can be reduced by:

- a full explanation about surgery and sedation anaesthesia before admission;
- minimizing preoperative waiting time ;
- providing a relaxing atmosphere;
- encouraging patients to bring their own music for personal headphones.

Commonly used sedative drugs

Benzodiazepines
These have remained popular for sedation anaesthesia because anxiolysis and amnesia are dose-related and relatively controllable. Diazepam, with its long half-life (24–48 hours), has been largely replaced with midazolam which has a shorter half-life (2–4 hours) and is water soluble, resulting in fewer venous complications such as thrombophlebitis. It has also been shown to be a much better anxiolytic and amnesic drug than diazepam. It has no active metabolites, permitting rapid patient recovery. Careful intravenous titration to the desired clinical effect will minimize side-effects from inadvertent overdosage. However, there is wide variation in patient sensitivity to midazolam[30].

Flumazenil
This is a competitive benzodiazepine antagonist which is useful in midazolam oversedation. It is important to recognize that resedation may occur after flumazenil, which has a half-life of approximately 1 hour compared with 2–4 hours for midazolam, therefore caution is needed to avoid premature discharge[31]. Midazolam and flumazenil have reciprocal dose-dependent effects (*Figure 11.5*); the effect of flumazenil declines while sedative levels of midazolam persist[32]. There are also cost considerations associated with its use: the cost of flumazenil being approximately four times that of midazolam.

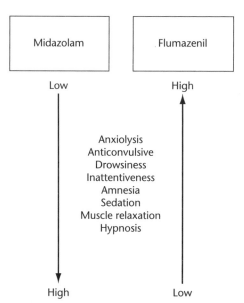

Figure 11.5. Reciprocal dose-dependent effects of midazolam and flumazenil.

Propofol
Used in subanaesthetic doses, this has now become popular as a sedative agent. It has a rapid redistribution, a short elimination half-life and very rapid patient recovery, with less postoperative drowsiness in the early phases of patient recovery compared with midazolam and diazepam[33]. Propofol is suited to continuous infusion techniques due to its favourable pharmacodynamic–kinetic profile. Greater accuracy in drug titration can be achieved, with a reduced incidence of oversedation.

Propofol and midazolam have similar sedative effects, both immediately after bolus doses and following 1 hour of continuous infusion of the drug. However, midazolam has a more profound amnesic effect than propofol[34]. Reduced doses of propofol are required when combined with midazolam[35].

Propofol–midozolam
This combination is synergistic when used in the commonly accepted dose range. Using this combination for hypnosis, a 44% reduction in the ED_{50} of each agent was found. The combination may prove useful for sedation, induction and maintenance of anaesthesia[36]. Co-induction – the concurrent administration of two or more drugs for the induction of anaesthesia[37] – has the advantages of decreased interpatient variability, decreased toxicity and earlier recovery. Midazolam will also assist amnesia, and respiratory depression can be avoided[38]. However, these clinical advantages have yet to be demonstrated for sedation anaesthesia.

Ketamine
A phencyclidine derivative, this can be a useful addition to the anaesthetist's armamentarium for its analgesic qualities, particularly in the event of an incomplete local anaesthetic block. However, it can produce dissociative anaesthesia with restlessness, dreaming and postoperative confusion, which can be most disturbing to the patient.

Opioids
In addition to sedative drugs for anxiolysis and amnesia, supplemental analgesic opioid agents are useful at the initial injection of local anaesthetic, and can help prevent deep traction pain. However, opioids have increased side-effects, with a higher incidence of nausea and vomiting, respiratory depression and hypotension. Sedative techniques that are more frequently associated with episodes of severe hypotension are more frequently associated with adverse outcomes[39].

Bailey *et al.* showed that in healthy volunteers, fentanyl administered together with low doses of midazolam resulted in clinically significant ventilatory depression with hypoxaemia[40]. Therefore, care must be exercised when fentanyl and midazolam are used in combination. In future, remifentanil, a new opioid analgesic, may find its place in clinical practice because of its short elimination half-life (8–10 minutes) and minimal risk of prolonged recovery, although respiratory depression and chest wall rigidity may limit its use in sedation[41].

Techniques

Routes of administration
A wide variety of routes may be used to administer sedation anaesthesia.

The oral and rectal routes. These routes are limited by slow onset of action. There is also considerable individual variation when drugs are administered by these routes.

Inhalation sedation. This may be used and is popular in dentistry. However, pollution of the atmosphere and the unacceptable smell to patients make this route of administration a less acceptable alternative.

Oral transmucosal. Used for drug delivery, such as 'fentanyl lollipops', this route has been reported to be a pleasant and effective way of producing preoperative sedation in children. Close monitoring is required as respiratory depression can occur[42].

Nasal. This route has also been used, particularly for paediatric patients, where drugs such as midazolam have been used in doses of 0.2 mg kg^{-1} [43].

Intravenous. This remains the most preferable route of administration, as the drug can be more easily titrated. Bolus and infusion techniques may be used.

Infusion techniques

Continuous intravenous (IV) infusions of sedative drugs provide stable intraoperative sedation while minimizing cardiorespiratory depression[44]. Midazolam infusion produces good intraoperative sedation and amnesia during regional anaesthesia. However, residual amnesia persists well into the postoperative period and return of cognitive function is delayed. Propofol infusion is an excellent alternative with its rapid patient recovery[38].

Propofol infusion rates range between 0.3–4 mg kg^{-1} hour^{-1}. Mackenzie showed that premedicated patients undergoing sedation for spinal anaesthesia required differing propofol infusion rates depending on patient age[13]. No loading dose was given and the dose ranged between 3.0 mg kg^{-1} hour^{-1} for patients over 65 years and 4.1 mg kg^{-1} hour^{-1} for younger patients[13]. In another study, where young, unpremedicated patients underwent extraction of wisdom teeth, a loading dose of 20 mg propofol, 0.7 µg kg^{-1} fentanyl and a propofol infusion of 3.6 mg kg^{-1} hour^{-1} resulted in sedation levels no deeper than eyes closed but rousable to command.

Target controlled infusions (TCI) using propofol have been used for maintenance of anaesthesia (Chapter 7). More recently, target-controlled propofol infusions have been used in patients as an adjunct to regional anaesthesia. During 88% of the total infusion time the desired sedation level was achieved[45]. However, further research is required so that guidelines, advantages and pitfalls of the technique can be more clearly defined for clinical anaesthetists.

Patient-controlled sedation (PCS) techniques

Optimum patient sedation levels may be difficult to achieve due to individual patient response to drugs, differing patient requests and varying surgical stimulation such as peritoneal traction. A PCS technique is a new intraoperative sedation technique where patients have control of their own sedation. Loading dose, bolus dose and lockout interval are programmed into a patient-demand pump by the anaesthetist (see *Figure 11.6*). Published reports to date have shown PCS to be a safe technique with high patient satisfaction[46–49].

Propofol[46–49], alfentanil[50] and midazolam[51] have been used with PCS. Propofol, although not approved for this indication, has been shown to be the drug of choice, with high patient satisfaction and improved postoperative recovery.

The safety and effectiveness of PCS is influenced by the sedative drug used and the settings of the patient-demand variables. In a crossover study with patients presenting for staged wisdom teeth extraction, investigators reported a patient preference for

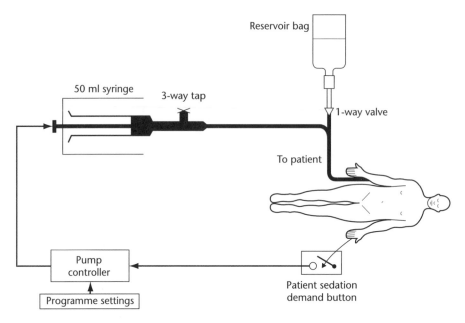

Figure 11.6. Set-up for patient-controlled sedation. Reproduced from **Rudkin G.** Sedation anaesthesia and recovery room analgesia. *Ambulatory Surg.* 1994; **2**: 78 (Figure 2) with permission from Elsevier Science - NL.

patient-controlled propofol rather than propofol by continuous infusion. Approximately half the patients had a strong to moderate preference for PCS, with 15% preferring the infusion technique[52] (*Figure 11.7*).

Other techniques

In addition to pharmacological means of allaying anxiety, patient calmness and comfort can be achieved by non-pharmacological means such as:

- keeping the patient warm;
- a soft mattress and a supportive pillow under the knees;
- talking to the patient;
- music, via personal headphones;
- reduced noise level in the operating theatre;
- hand-holding.

Recovery and discharge

Recovery facilities and discharge criteria are the same as for general anaesthesia, but patients may satisfy these criteria faster with sedation techniques. If patients are alert and have stable vital signs it is appropriate that they be transferred from the operating or procedure room directly to the second-stage recovery room. There are potentially significant cost advantages with this approach, with reduction in recovery room stay and less nursing care (Chapter 16).

Discharge of the sedated patient should be authorized by the practitioner who administered the drugs, or another qualified person using the DSU's discharge criteria.

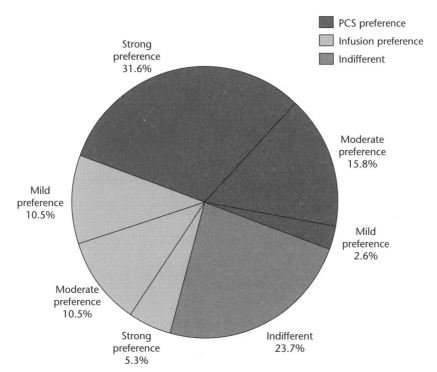

Figure 11.7. Patient preferences for patient-controlled sedation (PCS) or infusion with propofol (*n* = 38). Expressed as a percentage.

The patient must be transferred into the care of a responsible adult to whom written and verbal instructions should be given. This is important as although the patient may appear alert, amnesic drugs such as midazolam may prevent patients from remembering instructions at discharge. Written instructions should also include the prohibition of driving and the operation of machinery until the day following the administration of sedative drugs.

It is important that the anaesthetist select appropriate drugs and routes of administration for sedation anaesthesia so that patient discharge is not delayed. Sedation techniques will remain a cost-effective alternative for surgery compared with general anaesthesia, providing there is quality patient care with minimal postoperative problems. More cost–outcome studies are required for sedation techniques[53].

> *Sedation anaesthesia in conjunction with local, regional anaesthesia or for procedural techniques offers the patient, surgeon and the facility significant advantages. The anaesthetist's ability to provide satisfactory sedation requires sensitivity, experience, expertise in behavioural management, vigilance and an understanding of the pharmacokinetics and dynamics of the drugs involved.*

References

1. **Hiew CY, Hart GK, Thomson KR**, *et al*. Analgesia and sedation in interventional radiological procedures. *Austral. Radiol.* 1995; **39**: 128–134.

2. **Cormio L, Bloem F, Laduc R, et al.** Pain sensation in transurethral microwave thermotherapy for benign prostatic hyperplasia: the rationale for prophylactic sedation. *Eur. Urol.* 1994; **25**: 36–39.

3. **Rodney WM, Dabov G, Orientale E, et al.** Sedation association with a more complete colonoscopy. *J. Fam. Pract.* 1993; **36**: 394–400.

4. **Birch BRP, Anson KM, Miller RA.** Sedoanalgesia in urology: a safe, cost-effective alternative to general analgesia. A review of 1020 cases. *Br. J. Urol.* 1990; **66**: 342–350.

5. **Smith I.** Monitored anesthesia care: how much sedation, how much analgesia? *J. Clin. Anesth.* 1996; **8**: 76S–80S.

6. **Bennett CR.** (1978) The spectrum of pain control. In: *Conscious Sedation in Dental Practice*, 2nd Edn. Mosby, St Louis, MO. pp. 10–23.

7. **DeCastro J, Mundeleer P.** Anesthesie sans barbituriques; la neurolept analgesie (R 1406, R 1625, hydergine, procain). *Anesth. Analg. Paris* 1959; **16**: 1022.

8. **McDermott VG, Chapman ME, Gillespie I.** Sedation and patient monitoring in vascular and interventional radiology. *Br. J. Radiol.* 1993; **66**: 667–671.

9. **Federated Ambulatory Surgery Association** (1986) *FASA Special Study.* FASA, Alexandria, VA.

10. **Chye EP, Young IG, Osborne GA, et al.** Outcomes after same-day oral surgery: a review of 1,180 cases at a major teaching hospital. *J. Oral Maxillofac. Surg.* 1993; **51**: 846–849.

11. **Wansbrough SR, White PF.** Sedation scales: measures of calmness or somnolence? *Anesth. Analg.* 1993; **76**: 219–221.

12. **Caplan RA, Ward RJ, Posner K, et al.** Unexpected cardiac arrest during spinal anesthesia: a closed claims analysis of predisposing factors. *Anesthesiology* 1988; **8**: 5–11.

13. **Mackenzie N, Grant IS.** Propofol for intravenous sedation. *Anaesthesia* 1987; **42**: 3–6.

14. **Association of Anesthetists of Great Britain and Ireland.** (1994) *Recommendations for Standards of Monitoring during Anaesthesia and Recovery*, revised edn. AAGBI, London.

15. **Charlton JE.** Monitoring and supplemental oxygen during endoscopy: one death per 2000 procedures demands action. *Br. Med. J.* 1995; **310**: 886–887.

16. **Webb RK, Van der Walt J, Runciman WB, et al.** Which monitor? An analysis of 2000 incident reports. *Anaesth. Intens. Care* 1993; **21**: 529–542.

17. **Lee G, Shankleton E, Bodlander FMS.** Correspondence: monitoring respiration in sedated patients. *Anaesth. Intens. Care* 1994; **22**: 497

18. **Lenz G, Heipertz W, Epple E.** Capnometry for continuous post-operative monitoring of nonintubated, spontaneously breathing patients. *J. Clin. Monit.* 1991; **7**: 245–248.

19. **Wright SW.** Conscious sedation in the emergency department: the value of capnography and pulse oximetry. *Ann. Emerg. Med.* 1992; **21**: 551–555.

20. **Shapiro BA, Kacmarek RM, Cane RD, et al.** (1991) *Clinical Application of Respiratory Care*, 4th Edn. Mosby-Year Book, Chicago, IL.

21. **Reyes RJ, Smith AA, Mascaro JR, et al.** Supplemental oxygen: ensuring its safe delivery during facial surgery. *Plast Reconstr. Surg.* 1995; **95**: 924–928.

22. **Faculty of Anaesthetists, RACS** (1991) *Sedation for Diagnostic and Minor Surgical Procedures.* P9 Faculty of Anaesthetists, Royal Australasian College of Surgeons, Melbourne.

23. **Association of Anaesthetists of Great Britain and Ireland.** (1994) *Recommendations for Standards of Monitoring During Anaesthesia and Recovery*, revised Edn. AAGBI, London.

24. **American Society of Anesthesiologists.** (1994) Standards for basic intraoperative monitoring. In: *ASA Directory of Members.* ASA, Park Ridge, IL. p. 735.

25. **Solomon SA, Kajla VK, Banerjee AK.** Can the elderly tolerate endoscopy without sedation? *J. R. Coll. Phys. Lond.* 1994; **28**: 407–410.

26. **Rudkin GE.** Patient choice in sedation anaesthesia and recovery room analgesia. *Ambulatory Surg.* 1994; **2**: 75–80.

27. **Schutz SM, Lee JG, Schmitt CM, et al.** Clues to patient dissatisfaction with conscious sedation for colonoscopy. *Am. J. Gastroenterol.* 1994; **89**: 1476–1479.

28. **Davies RJ, Stradling JR.** Acute effects of obstructive sleep apnoea. *Br. J. Anaesth.* 1993; **71**: 725–729.

29. **Davies RJ, Ali NJ, Stradling JR.** Neck circumference and other clinical features in the diagnosis of the obstructive sleep apnoea syndrome. *Thorax* 1992; **47**: 101–105.

30. **Richards A, Griffiths M, Scully C.** Wide variation in patient response to midazolam sedation for outpatient oral surgery. *Oral Surg. Oral Med. Oral Pathol.* 1993; **76**: 408–411.

31. **Philip BK, Simpson TH, Hauch MA,** *et al.* Flumazenil reverses sedation after midazolam-induced general anesthesia in ambulatory surgery patients. *Anesth. Analg.* 1990; **71:** 371–376.

32. **Ghouri AF, Ruiz MA, White PF.** Effect of flumazenil on recovery after midazolam and propofol sedation. *Anesthesiology* 1994; **81:** 333–339.

33. **Valtonen M, Salonen M, Forssell H,** *et al.* Propofol infusion for sedation in outpatient oral surgery. *Anaesthesia* 1989; **44:** 730–734.

34. **Polster MR, Gray PA, O'Sullivan G,** *et al.* Comparison of the sedative and amnesic effects of midazolam and propofol. *Br. J. Anaesth.* 1993; **70:** 612–616.

35. **De Lucia JA, White PF.** Effect of midazolam on induction and recovery characteristics of propofol. *Anesth. Analg.* 1992; **74:** S63.

36. **Short TG, Chui PT.** Propofol and midazolam act synergistically in combination. *Br. J. Anaesth.* 1991; **67:** 539–545.

37. **Vinik HR.** Co-induction: a practical application of anesthetic drug interaction. *Curr. Opin. Anesthesiol.* 1993; **6** (Suppl. 1): S9–S13.

38. **White PF, Negus JB.** Sedative infusions during local and regional anesthesia: a comparison of midazolam and propofol. *J. Clin. Anesth.* 1991; **3:** 32–39.

39. **Daneshmend TK, Bell GD, Logan RFA.** Sedation for upper gastrointestinal endoscopy: results of a nationwide survey. *Gut* 1991; **32:** 12–15.

40. **Bailey PL, Pace NL, Ashburn MA,** *et al.* Frequent hypoxemia and apnea after sedation with midazolam and fentanyl. *Anesthesiology* 1990; **3:** 826–830.

41. **Westmoreland CL, Hoke JF, Sebel PS,** *et al.* Pharmacokinetics of remifentanil and its major metabolite in patients undergoing elective inpatient surgery. *Anesthesiology* 1993; **79:** 893–903.

42. **Streisand JB, Stanley TH, Hague B,** *et al.* Oral transmucosal fentanyl citrate premedication in children. *Anesth. Analg.* 1989; **69:** 28–34.

43. **Fukuta O, Braham RL, Yanase H,** *et al.* The sedative effects of intranasal midazolam administration in the dental treatment of patients with mental disabilities. *J. Clin. Pediatr. Dent.* 1994; **18:** 259–265.

44. **Urquhart ML, White PF.** Comparison of sedative infusions during regional anesthesia – methohexital, etomidate, and midazolam. *Anesth. Analg.* 1989; **68:** 249–254.

45. **Skipsey IG, Colvin JR, Mackenzie N,** *et al.* Sedation with propofol during surgery under local blockade. Assessment of a target-controlled infusion system. *Anaesthesia* 1993; **48:** 210–213.

46. **Rudkin GE, Osborne GA, Curtis NJ.** Intraoperative patient-controlled sedation. *Anaesthesia* 1991; **46:** 90–92.

47. **Osborne GA, Rudkin GE, Curtis NJ,** *et al.* Intraoperative patient-controlled sedation: comparison of patient-controlled propofol with anaesthetist-delivered midazolam and fentanyl. *Anaesthesia* 1991; **46:** 553–556.

48. **Rudkin GE, Osborne GA, Finn BP,** *et al.* Intraoperative patient-controlled sedation: comparison of patient-controlled propofol with patient-controlled midazolam. *Anaesthesia* 1992; **47:** 376–381.

49. **Grattidge P.** Patient-controlled sedation using propofol in day surgery. *Anaesthesia* 1992; **47:** 683–685.

50. **Zelcer J, White PF, Chester S,** *et al.* Intraoperative patient-controlled analgesia: an alternative to physician administration during outpatient monitored anaesthesia care. *Anesth. Analg.* 1992; **75:** 41–44.

51. **Rodrigo C, Chow KC.** A comparison of 1- and 3-minute lockout periods during patient-controlled sedation with midazolam. *J. Oral Maxillofac. Surg.* 1995; **53:** 406–411.

52. **Osborne GA, Rudkin GE, Jarvis IG,** *et al.* Intra-operative patient-controlled sedation and patient attitude to control: a crossover comparison of patient preference for patient-controlled propofol and propofol by continuous infusion. *Anaesthesia* 1994; **49:** 287–292.

53. **Dexter F.** Application of cost-utility and quality-adjusted life years analyses to monitored anesthesia care for sedation only. *J. Clin. Anesth.* 1996; **8:** 286–288.

CHAPTER 12

Practical paediatric day case anaesthesia and analgesia

N.S. Morton

Principles and standards

The multidisciplinary report *Just for the Day*[1] set out 12 quality standards for care of paediatric day cases (*Table 12.1*). These apply whether children are managed in a specialist paediatric unit or in an adult unit which has been adapted for children.

Table 12.1. Twelve quality standards for paediatric day care[1]

1. Integrate the admission plan to include pre-admission, day of admission and post-admission care with planned transfer of care to primary care and/or community services
2. Prepare the child and parents before and during the day of admission
3. Give specific written information to parents
4. Admit the child to an area designated for day cases and do not mix with acutely ill in-patients
5. Do not admit or treat children alongside adults
6. Specifically designated day case staff should care for the child
7. Trained paediatric staff should be used
8. Organize care so that every child is likely to be discharged within the day
9. Ensure that the building, equipment and furnishings comply with paediatric safety standards
10. Ensure that the environment is child friendly
11. Complete essential documents before each child goes home to ensure after care and follow-up are seamless
12. Establish paediatric nursing support for the child at home

Reproduced from **Thornes R.** (1991) *Just for the Day* with permission from Action for Sick Children.

The important principles which can be drawn from these standards are that children should be managed by staff trained in their care, in appropriate child-friendly and child-safe facilities with free parental access to the conscious child.

Preschool paediatric patients gain particular benefit from well-planned and well-conducted day care because separation from parents is reduced. For older children and parents the disruption to schooling and work is minimized.

Patient selection[2,3]

The range of procedures which can be carried out on a day stay basis in children is quite broad (*Table 12.2*) but where there is a significant risk of postoperative haemorrhage (e.g. adenotonsillectomy), the likelihood of prolonged postoperative pain requiring complex pain control (e.g. many orthopaedic procedures) or operations involving

Table 12.2. Range of paediatric day case procedures

Surgical	Medical
General, e.g. herniotomy, hydrocele	Venesection
Urological, e.g. circumcision	Intrathecal injection
ENT, e.g. myringotomy	Radiotherapy
Dental, e.g. extractions	Change of urinary catheter
Ophthalmology, e.g. squint correction	Interventional radiology/cardiology
Orthopaedics, e.g. change of plaster cast	Blood sampling
Plastic surgery, e.g. prominent ear surgery	Bone marrow sampling
	Lumbar puncture
	Needle aspiration cytology
Diagnostic	Metabolic/endocrine tests
Endoscopy ± biopsies	CT, MRI and other scans
Examinations under anaesthesia	
Evoked response audiometry	
Measurement of intraocular pressure	
Biopsy: skin, bone, muscle, lymph node	
Arthroscopy, arthrograms	

opening of a body cavity, in-patient care is required. Even when a given procedure is technically feasible as a day case, there may be other reasons for excluding this option related to the age, maturity, medical condition, anaesthetic risk factors or social circumstances of the child (*Table 12.3*).

Surgeons, paediatricians and anaesthetists may vary in their views about the suitability of individual procedures or patients. Some feel that bilateral procedures, orchidopexy, hypospadias correction, strabismus correction or prominent ear correction are too difficult to manage as day cases but many units have developed techniques to successfully manage all of these.

Adenoidectomy and adenotonsillectomy
Attitudes are changing with regard to the management of adenoidectomy and adenotonsillectomy. More units in Europe and the UK are moving towards North American-style same-day care for adenoidectomy with a postoperative observation period of 4–12 hours and short overnight stay for paediatric tonsillectomy ± adenoidectomy. The risks and benefits of this approach must be weighed for each individual child. Cases should be carefully selected according to the exclusion criteria in *Table 12.3*, and factors such as the experience of the surgeon, pain control, nausea and vomiting, bleeding, postextubation airway problems and re-establishment of oral fluid and dietary intake must be carefully dealt with to ensure success. Good follow-up after discharge and rapid access to help at home are particularly important for this patient group and the call-out rate to the general practitioner may be high[2,3] (K. Mackenzie and J.T. Wilson, personal communication). Same-day paediatric tonsillectomy or adenotonsillectomy is not currently recommended in the UK.

Lower age limit
The lower age limit for day case surgery depends on the facilities available, the experience of staff and the workload. The healthy full-term neonate can safely undergo brief day case surgery provided none of the other exclusion criteria applies and there is access to in-patient neonatal care if required. The preterm or ex-preterm neonate should not be considered for day care before 60 weeks postconceptual age because of the risk

Table 12.3. Exclusion criteria for paediatric day case anaesthesia

---

Anaesthetic and surgical factors
Prolonged surgery and anaesthesia (>1 hour)
Junior unsupervised staff
The occasional paediatric or neonatal case: surgeon and anaesthetist must be suitably trained and carrying out such cases regularly
Opening of body cavity
Significant risk of haemorrhage or body fluid loss requiring replacement
Prolonged postoperative pain (that cannot be adequately controlled with oral analgesics)
Difficult airway
Sleep apnoea
Malignant hyperthermia

Age
Preterm or ex-preterm baby of <60 weeks postconceptual age
Full-term neonate where no in-patient neonatal care available

Medical factors
Poorly controlled systemic disease (e.g. epilepsy, asthma, cardiac disease)
Uninvestigated heart murmur
Metabolic disorders
Diabetes mellitus
Haemoglobinopathy
Active infection (especially of respiratory tract, pertussis, respiratory syncytial virus, measles)

Social factors
Parent unwilling or unable to care for child at home
The very anxious parent or child
Single-parent family with many siblings and no help
Poor housing conditions
No telephone
Inadequate personal transport (not public transport)
Long distance from hospital (>1 hour travelling time)
Sibling of victim of sudden infant death syndrome (SIDS)

---

of perioperative apnoea and, even beyond that age, other complications or sequelae of prematurity may preclude day case management.

Infection
The child with an infection should have surgery postponed for at least 2 weeks after symptoms have resolved and, if there is evidence of lower respiratory tract involvement, this delay should be extended to 4 weeks. If the child has measles, pertussis or respiratory syncytial virus (RSV) infection, a delay of 6 weeks is recommended as respiratory tract irritability is so troublesome[4]. Beware the child with features such as purulent crusting around the nose, pyrexia, lethargy, productive cough and chest signs[5]. Chronic, non-purulent nasal discharge and non-productive cough are very common in children and there is no benefit in postponing their procedure provided they are otherwise suitable for day care.

ASA status
Most paediatric day cases will be normal healthy children (ASA 1) with a specific, often congenital problem requiring investigation or treatment. Those with mild systemic

disease (ASA 2) and well-controlled more severe disease (ASA 3) can also be managed as day cases, and this includes those with stable asthma, epilepsy and simple corrected congenital heart defects. Antibiotic prophylaxis is required for those where prosthetic material or pericardial patches have been used. The child with a heart murmur should not proceed to day surgery until further investigation has been carried out to determine its cause, and paediatric cardiological advice should be sought. Clinical examination, ultrasound and ECG will elucidate the cause in most cases and those infants under age 1 year merit particular caution[6].

> *The criteria for the selection of paediatric patients and operations for day surgery are becoming more relaxed, but prematurity, current infection and operations with associated haemorrhage still need a cautious approach.*

Preparation of child and parents

Preparation for day care (*Table 12.4*) begins at the initial out-patient clinic visit. A clear verbal explanation to parents and the child about what is to happen should be backed up by written information in the form of general instructions about day surgery and specific details about where to go, what time to arrive, what to expect for this particular surgical procedure and clear guidance about preoperative fasting.

Table 12.4. Paediatric preparation for day surgery

Verbal and written information about day surgery and the procedure
Specific instructions – arrival, fasting, etc.
'Saturday Club' or introductory session – visit to the DSU
Videos, toys, games, play therapy, etc.
Physical examination and investigation in a few selected cases
Telephone contact the day before surgery

A pre-admission programme is very useful for teaching the child and parents about the DSU's facilities, staff and ways of working[1]. A visit to the unit at an arranged 'Saturday Club' or special introductory session can be used to great effect in allaying fears and anxieties. Toys, games, computer games, colouring books, videos and play therapy can all be employed, depending on the child's age and maturity. Visits to the anaesthetic induction room and recovery area are very helpful, and the types of anaesthesia, pain relief and postoperative care can be discussed with the parents and child. Badges and certificates of 'bravery' or achievement are useful in young children.

Pre-admission clinics where physical examination, preoperative screening checks and blood tests are carried out can be useful in reducing cancellation of cases, but the vast majority of paediatric day cases do not need preoperative investigations or tests. Telephone contact on the day before surgery is useful and gives an opportunity to re-emphasize preoperative instructions, to confirm attendance and to rule out last minute reasons for postponement such as infections, travel difficulties or family problems. A reserve list can be held to replace these last-minute cancellations so that the operating session is used efficiently.

Fasting

The 643 fasting rules (*Table 12.5*) are easy to teach, although difficult to achieve in practice[7,8].

Table 12.5. Fasting rules

6 hours for solids, milk or milky drinks
4 hours for breast-fed infants
3 hours for clear fluids, including fruit juices, fizzy drinks, water, tea and coffee without milk

This scheme strikes a validated safe balance between prolonged fasting with the attendant risks of dehydration and hypoglycaemia and the risks of regurgitation and aspiration of gastric contents. Clear written instructions to parents with specific times may be helpful, with a statement about encouraging clear fluid intake until a specified time. Those children listed for surgery in the morning should have different timed instructions from those whose surgery is to be in the afternoon. Examples are given in *Table 12.6*. The time of last intake of solids, milk or clear fluids should be noted on admission and if the child has been fasted for an excessively long time, and especially if he or she weighs <15 kg, consideration should be given to placing him or her further down the operating list and giving a clear fluid drink under controlled circumstances on arrival. It must be stressed to parents that prolonged starvation can be harmful and children presenting for surgery in the afternoon should not be starved from the previous evening[9].

> *Children should be psychologically prepared for day surgery before admission. Clear instructions and information, particularly about fasting, are essential.*

Table 12.6. Examples of written fasting instructions

(a) For morning operating list starting at 09.00 a.m.
_____ must have no food, milk or milky drinks after 03.00 a.m. A drink of juice or water should be encouraged up to 06.00 a.m. After that time, no food or drink should be taken
If your child is breast-fed the last feed should be at 05.00 a.m.
You should understand that for safety reasons the surgery will be postponed or cancelled if you do not follow these instructions

(b) For afternoon operating list starting at 13.30 p.m.
_____ must have no food, milk or milky drinks after 07.30 a.m. A drink of juice or water should be encouraged up to 10.30 a.m. After that time, no food or drink should be taken
If your child is breast-fed the last feed should be at 09.30 a.m.
You <u>should not</u> starve your child from the night before their operation as this can cause dehydration and a low blood sugar level
You should understand that for safety reasons the surgery will be postponed or cancelled if you do not follow these instructions

On the day

The time of arrival in the day unit will depend on the time of surgery and although staggered admission times are possible to minimize waiting time, it is usually easier to organize a set arrival time.

Parental involvement and premedication. Sedative premedication is unnecessary in the majority of paediatric day cases if children and parents are well prepared and particularly where there are good preoperative play facilities and child-friendly rooms for induction of anaesthesia. Parental involvement in the induction of anaesthesia can be very helpful, particularly for the preschool age group[10,11]. Parents should not be forced to be present if they do not wish as there is evidence that many parents find this experience very stressful[12–14] and excessively anxious parents may transmit this anxiety to their child[15]. Intravenous induction is thought to be less psychologically disturbing to children than inhalational induction[16,17] and many units in Europe use intravenous induction of anaesthesia as a routine, unless venous access is obviously going to be very difficult or where a child or parent has specifically requested an inhalational technique. The routine use of topical local anaesthesia of the skin with EMLA® cream[18] or amethocaine gel[19] allows painless venous access after 60 and 40 minutes, respectively.

Sedative premedication can be very helpful for selected cases where the child is very anxious, where the child has previously had a traumatic experience with the induction of anaesthesia, where the child has a needle phobia or for the inconsolable child. Oral midazolam, 0.5 mg kg^{-1} is very effective when given 20–30 minutes prior to induction[20–22]. The standard formulation of midazolam is very acidic and tastes very bitter so must be disguised by a sweet liquid either by preparation of a syrup in the pharmacy or by adding the midazolam to a small volume (1–2 ml kg^{-1}) of cola, lemonade, or other sweet drink or by mixing with paracetamol syrup. This presupposes that the child will co-operate in drinking this solution. The same limitation applies to oral ketamine (up to 10 mg kg^{-1}). Other options, such as intranasal midazolam, rectal induction or intramuscular ketamine, are not very satisfactory as they involve a degree of restraint of the child to administer them, which many find unacceptable for elective day case work. For the individual inconsolable child where the surgery is deemed to be essential (e.g. a dental abscess), then with parental consent a degree of restraint to administer an intramuscular premedicant may be justifiable and ketamine 5–10 mg kg^{-1} or midazolam 0.1 mg kg^{-1} can be used.

It is important that the child is carefully monitored after these premedicants as they act very quickly and can produce quite profound sedation. The available evidence suggests that oral midazolam does not delay discharge[20–22].

Recently, fentanyl in the form of a lollipop has been described as a suitable paediatric premedicant[23,24] but many units try to avoid opioids in day cases.

> *Sedative premedication will only be needed for selected cases. Oral midazolam (0.5 mg kg^{-1}) is probably the most suitable. Children must be supervised after premedication.*

Anaesthetic technique

The least invasive technique which is effective should be used. Minor sequelae of anaesthesia[25–27] become magnified in the day surgery setting and many can be avoided by the choice of a suitable anaesthetic technique.

Induction
Intravenous induction. This type of induction with propofol, 4 mg kg^{-1} with added lignocaine, 0.2 mg kg^{-1}, is very effective and results in a slightly earlier recovery in older paediatric day cases than thiopentone induction[28]. Propofol has a product licence down to age 3 years, and has been used in children of lower ages for both induction and

maintenance. The well-known clear-headed recovery and low incidence of PONV are particularly useful in children. Where the laryngeal mask is to be used, insertion is facilitated by the use of propofol[29].

Inhalational induction. There has been a resurgence of interest in inhalational induction with the introduction of sevoflurane into clinical practice and a substantial body of evidence now attests to its efficacy and advantages over halothane, with the main drawback being cost[30–34]. The use of the Humphrey ADE circuit and inspired agent monitoring allows use of very low flows for spontaneous respiration techniques in children, with resultant economy of volatile agent consumption.

Maintenance

The laryngeal mask airway (LMA) has transformed the maintenance of anaesthesia for paediatric day cases[35] and endotracheal intubation and muscle relaxants should only be needed in an emergency or for specific procedures such as upper gastrointestinal endoscopy. Head and neck procedures such as strabismus correction, tongue tie release, correction of prominent ears and dental conservation or extraction can all be performed using the reinforced or conventional LMA with a spontaneous respiration technique[36].

Recovery after maintenance with sevoflurane and desflurane is more rapid and can be associated with restlessness and agitation but this will be minimized if good local or regional analgesia is also used[30,34]. For certain procedures a total intravenous technique such as propofol infusion[29,37,38] can be beneficial, for example, in minimizing emesis after strabismus correction.

Analgesia

Good pain control is critical to the success of paediatric day case surgery. Local analgesia should be used as a component of the anaesthetic technique in all paediatric day cases unless there is a specific reason not to, as it is so effective and safe[2].

Topical and local infiltration. Topical amethocaine or oxybuprocaine for strabismus correction, topical lignocaine gel after circumcision, and wound instillation or wound infiltration with bupivacaine are all simple and highly effective[39,40]. Topical diclofenac drops are also effective analgesics for strabismus surgery[36] and do not carry the risk of inadvertent trauma to the anaesthetized cornea.

Peripheral nerve blocks. These are also highly effective. Single injection techniques are preferred[39,40] and the most useful are penile block, ilioinguinal/iliohypogastric block and great auricular nerve block.

Caudal epidural block. This is also widely applicable in paediatric day surgery and motor block is seldom troublesome if bupivacaine 0.25% is used[36]. Recently, prolongation of analgesia from caudal bupivacaine single injection techniques has been sought by addition of opioids, alpha-2-adrenoceptor agonists and NMDA-antagonists[41], and clonidine or ketamine look particularly promising for paediatric day surgery, although clonidine can produce sedation and hypotension at higher dosage. Clonidine (1 μg kg^{-1}) added to caudal bupivacaine is associated with a doubling of the duration of effective analgesia while ketamine (0.5 mg kg^{-1}) quadruples the analgesia[41]. Preservative-free forms of these drugs must be used.

The NSAIDs should also be routinely used unless specifically contraindicated and several child-friendly formulations are available, for example, ibuprofen syrup

(10 mg kg^{-1}), diclofenac suppositories (1 mg kg^{-1}), and piroxicam melts (0.5 mg kg^{-1}) and these can be given after induction or as a component of the premedication. Ketorolac is available as an intravenous formulation and is widely used at a dose of 0.5 mg kg^{-1}.

The lower age limit for NSAIDs is 1 year or 10 kg, because renal maturation occurs during the first year of life. This corresponds to a diclofenac 12.5 mg suppository every 8 hours (just over 3 mg kg^{-1} day^{-1}). Some centres use 6 months and 6 kg, and give half a diclofenac 12.5 mg suppository. Diclofenac does not have a product licence for paediatric postoperative analgesia, but its widespread use by paediatric anaesthetists, supported by a large body of evidence in the literature, means that it is an acceptable choice provided the contraindications to its use are carefully observed. A locally agreed protocol is the most satisfactory way of dealing with this problem.

Aspirin is associated with Reye's syndrome, but other NSAIDs are not: ibuprofen, for instance, is widely used in large dosages in children with juvenile arthritis without causing Reye's syndrome.

Paracetamol is also ubiquitous and can be given as a premedicant loading dose of 20 mg kg^{-1} or as a suppository after induction of anaesthesia. It is important to realize that the absorption of paracetamol suppositories is slow and poor, so a higher loading dose of around 30–40 mg kg^{-1} must be given to achieve therapeutic plasma concentrations within 90 minutes[39].

> *Good pain control is critical to the success of paediatric day surgery. Local anaesthesia must be used wherever possible, backed up with NSAIDs and/or paracetamol.*

Postoperative care, follow-up and minimizing morbidity

Recovery parameters and discharge criteria

Recovery milestones in children (*Table 12.7*) must be adjusted for the child's age, developmental stage, medical status, surgical procedure and social circumstances[2,3]. The vital signs and conscious level should be normal for the child's age and preoperative level. There should be no respiratory distress or stridor, especially in those children who have been intubated. Swallowing, cough and gag reflexes should be fully regained. Endotracheal intubation *per se* should not contraindicate discharge home in infants, but the reasons for intubation may, for example, severe laryngospasm, unexpected airway problem, traumatic intubation, etc. Children under the age of 5 years are at particular risk of post extubation stridor if the wrong size of tube is used, and care must be taken to ensure that after intubation an audible leak is present with a maximum inflation pressure

Table 12.7. Discharge criteria

Vital signs and conscious level normal for child's age and preoperative state
No respiratory distress or stridor
Swallowing, gag and cough reflexes fully regained
No serious intraoperative anaesthetic problems
Normal movement and ambulation, particularly in older children
PONV absent or mild
Pain well controlled
No bleeding or surgical complications

of 30 cm H_2O. A child who does develop postextubation stridor may require admission to a high dependency or intensive care area for observation and treatment, e.g. nebulized budesonide or adrenaline, or oral or parenteral steroids. The child should be able to move normally for his or her age. Motor blockade of the lower limbs after caudal or inguinal block can be troublesome in older children and may delay safe discharge[8].

Reasons for hospital admission

Inevitably some children (around 1%) may require in-patient admission, and parents should be aware of this possibility. Persistently abnormal vital signs or conscious level, any problem with the airway, motor blockade in an older child, persistent nausea and vomiting, bleeding, severe pain, unexpected surgical problems or unexpected intraoperative events (e.g. regurgitation, aspiration, bronchospasm, hypersensitivity reactions, suxamethonium apnoea, malignant hyperpyrexia) may all lead to admission for further care and investigations.

Postoperative nausea and vomiting (PONV)

Strabismus surgery, orchidopexy, gastroscopy, a past history of PONV or motion sickness, endotracheal intubation and opioids are the main risk factors (*Table 12.8*). Morphine, in particular, causes a high incidence of PONV in children, and this may occur for the first time after discharge[42,43].

Table 12.8. Risk factors for PONV in children

History of PONV or motion sickness
Strabismus surgery
Ear procedures
Orchidopexy
Gastroscopy
Endotracheal intubation
Opioids, especially morphine
Volatile anaesthetics
Early mobilization
Early oral fluids

Propofol and the use of laryngeal mask techniques with local analgesia and avoidance of opioids will minimize PONV. For those with a strong past history of PONV, the $5HT_3$ antagonists have the best efficacy and safety profile and do not produce sedation. Ondansetron 0.1 mg kg^{-1} is an effective prophylactic antiemetic[44,45]. Some units feel that too early or vigorous resumption of oral fluid intake increases the incidence of early PONV, and adequately hydrated children need not necessarily have to take a drink as a prerequisite for being discharged home[46,47].

Postoperative instructions

The surgeon and anaesthetist should give clear verbal instructions about pain control, wound care, mobilization and resumption of activities. This will be reinforced by nursing staff and by clear written instructions specific to each surgical procedure. These should explain the surgical procedure, type of incision, type of sutures and dressing. The measures to control postoperative pain, when to resume normal diet, restrictions on activities, when to allow bathing and washing, notes on wound care and what to do if problems arise should all be made clear. This should include a clear telephone contact, either to the family doctor or to the day surgery unit or hospital. Arrangements for follow-up by a district nurse, health visitor or family doctor and for review at the hospital out-patient clinic should be clearly documented. A discharge letter should be issued to the family doctor and either sent immediately or given to the family to deliver to the doctor.

Dressings
Care of the child at home can be facilitated by simplifying dressings and avoiding unnecessary dressings, for example, after circumcision[48]; after correction of prominent ears[49].

Continuing pain control at home
Oral analgesics are the mainstay of continuing pain control at home after day surgery and it is vital to encourage parents to give analgesics pre-emptively and regularly for 24–48 hours, starting before any local anaesthetic block has worn off. Most hospitals dispense take-home medication to cover the analgesic needs for up to 72 hours. Paracetamol, 15–20 mg kg^{-1} orally, 4–6 hourly is well tolerated and readily available in most households. Ibuprofen, 10 mg kg^{-1}, orally, 6 hourly is suitable for moderate pain. An alternative is to combine oral paracetamol and codeine. After circumcision, parents can be taught to apply topical lignocaine gel very successfully, and after strabismus surgery, topical diclofenac drops can be administered by parents.

Transport home
Children must have a responsible adult escort home after day surgery and this journey should be by private car or taxi, not public transport, and preferably with separate driver and carer. Occasionally a single driver/carer may be the only practical approach. Excessively long travelling time is a contraindication to day case surgery.

Home visits/community liaison
A home visit is not required in all cases but it is well established that a trained paediatric nurse visiting selected cases is very reassuring to parents and children and reduces family doctor call-outs[50–53]. The nurse is involved in reinforcing advice to parents, assessing and giving pain relief, wound care, dressing removal, suture removal and audit.

Conclusion

> *Children can gain particular benefits from well-planned and carefully delivered day care, with particular emphasis on pain control using local anaesthesia and simplification of anaesthetic techniques using modern agents.*

References

1. **Thornes R.** (1991) *Just for the Day*. National Association for the Welfare of Children in Hospital (NAWCH) Ltd, London.
2. **Morton NS, Raine PAM.** (1994) *Paediatric Day Case Surgery*. Oxford Medical Publications, Oxford.
3. **Morton NS, Lord D.** (1994) General principles of paediatric day case anaesthesia. In: *Day Case Anaesthesia and Sedation* (Ed. JG Whitwam). Blackwell Scientific Publications, Oxford. p. 303.
4. **McEwan AI, Birch M, Bingham R.** The preoperative management of the child with a heart murmur. *Paediatr. Anaesth.* 1995; **5:** 151–155.

5. **Keneally JP.** Day stay surgery in paediatrics. *Clin. Anesthesiol.* 1985; **3**: 679–696.
6. **Vanderwalt J.** Anaesthesia in children with viral respiratory tract infections. *Paediatr. Anaesth.* 1995; **5**: 257–260.
7. **Phillips S, Daborn AK, Hatch DJ.** Preoperative fasting for paediatric anaesthesia. *Br. J. Anaesth.* 1994; **73**: 529–531.
8. **Stuart JC, Morton NS.** A clinical audit of day case surgery for children. *J. One Day Surg.* 1991; **1**: 15–18.
9. **Miller DC.** Why are children starved? *Br. J. Anaesth.* 1990; **64**: 409–410.
10. **McCormick ASM, Spargo PM.** Parents in the anaesthetic room: a questionnaire survey of departments of anaesthesia. *Paediatr. Anaesth.* 1996; **6**: 183–186.
11. **Kain ZN, Ferris CA, Mayes LC,** *et al.* Parental presence during induction of anaesthesia: practice differences between the United States and Great Britain. *Paediatr. Anaesth.* 1996; **6**: 187–193.
12. **Thompson N, Irwin MG, Gunawardene WMS,** *et al.* Pre-operative parental anxiety. *Anaesthesia* 1996; **51**: 1008–1012.
13. **Litman RS, Berger AA, Chibber A.** An evaluation of preoperative anxiety in a population of parents of infants and children undergoing ambulatory surgery. *Paediatr. Anaesth.* 1996; **6**: 443–447.
14. **Campbell IR, Scaife JM, Johnstone JMS.** Psychological effects of day case surgery compared with inpatient surgery. *Arch. Dis. Child.* 1988; **63**: 415–417.
15. **Bevan JC, Johnston C, Haig MJ,** *et al.* Preoperative parental anxiety predicts behavioural and emotional responses to induction of anaesthesia in children. *Can. J. Anaesth.* 1990; **37**: 177–182.
16. **Kotiniemi LH, Ryhanen PT.** Behavioural changes and children's memories after intravenous, inhalation and rectal induction of anaesthesia. *Paediatr. Anaesth.* 1996; **6**: 201–207.
17. **Kotiniemi LH, Ryhanen PT, Moilanen IK.** Behavioural changes following routine ENT operations in two-to-ten-year-old children. *Paediatr. Anaesth.* 1996; **6**: 45–49.
18. **Freeman JA, Doyle E, Ng TI,** *et al.* Topical anaesthesia of the skin: a review. *Paediatr. Anaesth.* 1993; **3**: 129–138.
19. **Lawson RA, Smart NG, Gudgeon AC,** *et al.* Evaluation of an amethocaine gel preparation for percutaneous analgesia before venous cannulation in children. *Br. J. Anaesth.* 1995; **75**: 282–285.
20. **Cray SH, Dixon JL, Heard CMB,** *et al.* Oral midazolam premedication for paediatric day case patients. *Paediatr. Anaesth.* 1996; **6**: 265–270.
21. **McCluskey A, Meakin GH.** Oral administration of midazolam as a premedicant for paediatric day-case anaesthesia. *Anaesthesia* 1994; **49**: 782–785.
22. **McGraw T.** Oral midazolam and postoperative behaviour in children. *Can. J. Anaesth.* 1993; **40**: 682–683.
23. **Friesen RH, Carpenter E, Madigan CK,** *et al.* Oral transmucosal fentanyl citrate for preanaesthetic medication of paediatric cardiac surgery patients. *Paediatr. Anaesth.* 1995; **5**: 29–31.
24. **Macaluso AD, Connelly AM, Hayes WB,** *et al.* Oral transmucosal fentanyl citrate for premedication in adults. *Anesth. Analg.* 1996; **82**: 158–161.
25. **Montenegro LM, Schreiner MS, Nicolson SC.** Perioperative problems in pediatric anesthesia. *Curr. Opin. Anesthesiol.* 1996; **9**: 221–224.
26. **Patel RI, Hannallah RS.** Anesthetic complications following pediatric ambulatory surgery: a 3 year study. *Anesthesiology* 1988; **69**: 1009–1012.
27. **Selby IR, Rigg JD, Faragher B,** *et al.* The incidence of minor sequelae following anaesthesia in children. *Paediatr. Anaesth.* 1996; **6**: 293–302.
28. **Runcie CJ, MacKenzie S, Arthur DS,** *et al.* Comparison of recovery from anaesthesia induced in children with either propofol or thiopentone. *Br. J. Anaesth.* 1993; **70**: 192–195.
29. **Morton NS, Johnston G, White M,** *et al.* Propofol in paediatric anaesthesia. *Paediatr. Anaesth.* 1992; **2**: 89–97.
30. **Murat I.** New inhalational agents in paediatric anaesthesia: desflurane and sevoflurane. *Curr. Opin. Anesthesiol.* 1996; **9**: 225–228.
31. **Black A, Sury MRJ, Hemington L,** *et al.* A comparison of the induction characteristics of sevoflurane and halothane in children. *Anaesthesia* 1996; **51**: 539–542.
32. **Sury MRJ, Black A, Hemington L,** *et al.* A comparison of the recovery characteristics of sevoflurane and halothane in children. *Anaesthesia* 1996; **51**: 543–546.
33. **Kataria B, Epstein R, Bailey A,** *et al.* A comparison of sevoflurane to halothane in paediatric surgical patients: results of a multicentre international study. *Paediatr. Anaesth.* 1996; **6**: 283–292.

34. **Lerman J.** Pharmacology of inhalational anaesthetics in infants and children. *Paediatr. Anaesth.* 1992; **2**: 191–203.
35. **Haynes SR, Morton NS.** The laryngeal mask airway: a review of its use in paediatric anaesthesia. *Paediatr. Anaesth.* 1993; **3**: 65–73.
36. **Morton NS, Benham S, Lawson RA,** *et al.* Topical diclofenac vs. oxybuprocaine for analgesia after paediatric squint correction. *Paediatr. Anaesth.* 1997 (in press).
37. **Doyle E, McFadzean W, Morton NS.** I.V. anaesthesia with propofol using a target-controlled infusion system: comparison with inhalation anaesthesia for general surgical procedures in children. *Br. J. Anaesth.* 1993; **70**: 542–545.
38. **Watcha MF, Simeon RM, White PF,** *et al.* Effect of propofol on the incidence of postoperative vomiting after strabismus surgery in pediatric outpatients. *Anesthesiology* 1991; **75**: 204–209.
39. **Morton NS.** (1994) Local anaesthesia for paediatric day-case surgery. In: *Day Case Anaesthesia and Sedation* (Ed. JG Whitwam). Blackwell Scientific Publications, Oxford. p. 332.
40. **McNicol LR.** (1994) Local anaesthesia. In: *Paediatric Day Case Surgery* (Eds NS Morton and PAM Raine). Oxford Medical Publications, Oxford. p. 24.
41. **Cook B, Doyle E.** The use of additives to local anaesthetic solutions for caudal epidural blockade. *Paediatr. Anaesth.* 1996; **6**: 353–359.
42. **Weinstein MS, Nicolson SC, Schreiner MS.** A single dose of morphine sulfate increases the incidence of vomiting after outpatient inguinal surgery in children. *Anesthesiology* 1994; **81**: 572–577.
43. **Munro HM, Riegger LQ, Reynolds PL,** *et al.* Comparison of the analgesic and emetic properties of ketorolac and morphine for paediatric outpatient strabismus surgery. *Br. J. Anaesth.* 1994; **72**: 624–628.
44. **Furst SR, Rodarte A.** Prophylactic antiemetic treatment with ondansteron in children undergoing tonsillectomy. *Anesthesiology* 1995; **81**: 799–803.
45. **Paxton LD, Taylor RH, Gallager TM,** *et al.* Postoperative emesis following otoplasty in children. *Anaesthesia* 1995; **50**: 1083–1084.
46. **Woods AM, Berry FA, Carter BJ.** Strabismus surgery and post-operative vomiting: clinical observations and review of the current literature; a medical opinion. *Paediatr. Anaesth.* 1992; **2**: 223–229.
47. **Baines D.** Postoperative nausea and vomiting in children. *Paediatr. Anaesth.* 1996; **6**: 7–14.
48. **Freeland AM.** (1996) *Evaluating the Need for a Vaseline Gauze Dressing Following Circumcision in Day Surgery.* Yorkhill NHS Trust Day Surgery Unit, Glasgow.
49. **Ridings P, Gault D, Khan L.** Reduction in postoperative vomiting after surgical correction of prominent ears. *Br. J. Anaesth.* 1994; **72**: 592–593.
50. **Anonymous.** Following up day case anaesthesia in general practice. *Drugs Ther. Bull.* 1990; **28**: 81–82.
51. **Postuma R, Ferguson CC, Stanwick RS,** *et al.* Pediatric day-care surgery: a 30 year hospital experience. *J. Pediatr. Surg.* 1987; **22**: 304–307.
52. **Scaife JM, Campbell I.** A comparison of the outcome of day-care and inpatient treatment of paediatric surgical cases. *J. Child Psychol. Psychiat.* 1988; **29**: 185–198.
53. **Atwell JD, Gow MA.** Paediatric trained district nurse in the community: expensive luxury or economic necessity? *Br. Med. J* 1985; **291**: 227–229.

CHAPTER 13

Laparoscopy

J.M. Millar

Laparoscopy has become increasingly important in day surgery, allowing minimally invasive surgery for intra-abdominal procedures to be done on a day case basis. Laparoscopic surgery, traditionally a gynaecological technique, makes feasible a seemingly unlimited range of procedures for day surgery[1–6] (*Table 13.1*).

Table 13.1. Laparoscopic procedures reported as suitable for day surgery

Gynaecological diagnosis or sterilization
Treatment of endometriosis with diathermy or laser
Removal of ovarian cyst, ectopic pregnancy, etc.
Reversal of tubal sterilization
Vaginal hysterectomy
Cholecystectomy
Hernia repair
Appendicectomy
Varicocele excision

The many advantages of laparoscopic surgery[7–10] (*Table 13.2*) have led to the increased popularity of operations like laparoscopic cholecystectomy. However, the physiological trespass and postoperative morbidity are considerable, making laparoscopy one of the most challenging day case procedures for the anaesthetist.

Table 13.2. The advantages of laparoscopic versus open surgery

Reduced postoperative pain
Improved postoperative pulmonary function
Reduced surgical morbidity
Reduced hospital stays
Earlier return to normal activities and work

Physiological changes in laparoscopy

Trendelenburg position and increased abdominal pressure from peritoneal insufflation with carbon dioxide in laparoscopy can cause cardiovascular and respiratory problems[11–14] (*Table 13.3*). The greater the intra-abdominal pressure and the steeper the head-down tilt, the greater the changes[12]. Vagal stimulation has been reported[15].

Table 13.3. Physiological changes during laparoscopy

Increased intra-abdominal pressure + steep Trendelenburg position
Reduced chest wall and lung compliance
Reduced total lung compliance (TLC) and functional residual capacity (FRC)
Altered ventilation/perfusion (V/Q) ratios
Splanchnic and aortic compression, reducing venous return
Increased systemic vascular resistance (SVR)
Cardiac output may be reduced
Vagal stimulation

The use of CO_2 as insufflating gas
Pa_{CO_2} may be increased, with acidosis
Increased postoperative pain

The Trendelenburg position *per se* does not reduce lower oesophageal sphincter pressure or reduce barrier pressure, so should not predispose to regurgitation in healthy patients[16]. Intra-abdominal pressure is not reduced by the use of neuromuscular block[17].

Although laparoscopy is said to be a less stressful procedure than open surgery, this may not be true[18]. Biochemical stress responses after laparoscopy compared with open cholecystectomy have not been shown to be reduced[10,19].

> *Although the physiological effects of laparoscopy may compromise more unfit patients[11], in the day surgery setting, they are reversible and few adverse clinical events result[15,20].*

Intraoperative risks

Some risks are related to the surgical technique, but the main issues affecting anaesthetists are the risks of aspiration of gastric contents, hypoventilation, bradycardia, and neuropathy from patient positioning (*Table 13.4*).

Table 13.4. Intraoperative risks of laparoscopic surgery

Anaesthetic
Hyper/hypotension
Dysrhythmias or bradycardia
Hypoventilation
Reflux and aspiration of gastric contents
Neuropathy from positioning

Surgical
Perforation of major blood vessel or viscus
Gas embolism
Pneumo thorax/mediastinum/pericardium
Conversion to laparotomy

Postoperative morbidity

Although the variety of laparoscopic procedures reported as suitable for day surgery is increasing, the limiting factor is the associated postoperative morbidity (*Table 13.5*).

Table 13.5. Postoperative morbidity after laparoscopy

PONV
Pain
Dizziness and fatigue
Delayed discharge
Increased overnight admission
Delayed return to normal activities postdischarge
Reduced patient satisfaction with day surgery

Laparoscopy is more likely to cause postoperative problems with delayed discharge than other day case procedures[21]. Recovery is related to the extent of the surgery[22]: the more major the laparoscopic surgery, the greater the unplanned admission or readmission rates afterwards. Admission rates of 14–17.5%, due mainly to surgical complications, but also to pain and nausea, are reported after laparoscopic cholecystectomy[1,23].

Patient satisfaction may not be as high after laparoscopic surgery as after minor day surgery. Before the introduction of propofol and the general use of NSAIDs for analgesia, 30% of patients would have preferred to spend the night in hospital after laparoscopic sterilization[24,25]. More modern anaesthetic techniques have reduced this to 8%[26].

However, even with modern anaesthesia, 18–21% would have preferred to remain in hospital for the first postoperative night after laparoscopic cholecystectomy[1,23]. Twenty-four-hour stays have been proposed as the answer to this problem[27]. However, this is 'short stay', rather than day, surgery.

> *Although more invasive procedures have been reported as suitable for day surgery, they may require longer DSU stays and have higher overnight admission rates. Patients may be less happy to be day cases for these procedures.*

Anaesthetic issues

Risk of gastric reflux and aspiration

Increased abdominal pressure and Trendelenburg position have been considered to increase the risks of passive gastric reflux[28] (*Table 13.6*). Intubation and ventilation have been recommended[29,30].

Table 13.6. Factors which may increase the risk of gastro-oesophageal reflux in laparoscopy

Atropine premedication
Steep Trendelenburg?
More than 2–3 litres inflating gas
Hiatus hernia or symptomatic reflux
Upper abdominal surgery
Obesity
Hiccup

However, Heijke *et al.* demonstrated that a small increase in gastric pressure in steep Trendelenburg position was accompanied by a corresponding increase in lower oesophageal sphincter pressure (LOSP), so that barrier pressure was unchanged[16]. It has also been suggested that increased intra-abdominal pressure flattens the abdominal oesophagus and increases LOSP[31]. Raised intra-abdominal pressure may not increase the risk of regurgitation.

The reported incidence of *aspiration* in laparoscopy is extremely low[29,32]. *Regurgitation* has been attributed to steep Trendelenburg, preoperative atropine[33] and hiccup[34]. However, in large series of unintubated patients having laparoscopy, no regurgitation or aspiration was reported[29,35].

The risks may therefore not be increased significantly. Clinical experience would support this, particularly for shorter procedures, such as laparoscopic sterilization, with minimal head down tilt and intra-abdominal pressure limited to ≤ 25 cmH$_2$O[36].

Laparoscopic cholecystectomy is an upper abdominal procedure, patients are in reverse Trendelenburg position, and the procedure takes longer. Gall bladder disease is associated with obesity, symptomatic gastric reflux and hiatus hernia. Prudence would suggest that endotracheal intubation is wise for cholecystectomy and other major laparoscopic procedures.

> *Intubation may be unnecessary for short laparoscopic procedures of <30 minutes for lower abdominal surgery, in non-obese patients with no history of gastro-oesophageal reflux. Longer operations, particularly if upper abdominal, require intubation and ventilation.*

Hypoventilation and airway obstruction

Many early reports of laparoscopic morbidity may have been related to hypoventilation or failure to maintain an adequate airway. Desmond and Gordon[30] related cardiac arrhythmias to hypoventilation, and 23% of spontaneously breathing patients in Kurer and Welch's study had airway problems[24].

The laryngeal mask airway (LMA)

In unintubated patients, the LMA maintains the airway, and may be used to support ventilation if necessary. It has been shown to be satisfactory for shorter laparoscopic procedures (<20 minutes) in non-obese patients with no symptomatic reflux[37,38]. Brimacombe and Berry have suggested conservative guidelines for the use of the LMA in laparoscopy, stressing good patient selection, correct insertion of the LMA by experienced users, adequate anaesthesia, and the avoidance of high intra-abdominal pressure, steep tilt and long procedures (>15 minutes)[39].

> *If the patient is not intubated, airway vigilance is essential and the use of the LMA is recommended. Good patient selection, correct insertion and adequate anaesthesia are essential for safety with the use of the LMA in laparoscopy.*

Bradycardia and arrhythmias

The incidence of bradycardia in laparoscopy may be as high as 30%[40]. Stretching the peritoneum with insufflating gas and applying clips in sterilization can cause sudden and severe bradycardia[40,41]. This has been related to modern, non-vagolytic anaesthetics, particularly suxamethonium, vecuronium[42], fentanyl or propofol[43], and particularly in combination[44].

Vecuronium is the drug most frequently implicated. Omitting it (Millar, unpublished observations) reduces the incidence of bradycardia in laparoscopy, but for procedures where it is used for intubation, routine prophylaxis with glycopyrrolate should be considered[42]. Atropine may be needed for sudden bradycardia.

Other arrhythmias have been reported but occur more in relation to halothane and hypercarbia[30,45].

> *Vigilance for bradycardia is essential, particularly during insufflation of the abdomen and application of clips or rings to the Fallopian tubes. Anticholinergic prophylaxis may be considered worthwhile.*

Neuropathy from patient positioning

Brachial plexus injuries can be caused by the use of shoulder supports to prevent the patient slipping off the operating table, or by the surgeon levering on the patient's extended arms on arm boards. Lithotomy poles may compress the lateral popliteal nerve.

> *Neuropathies can be avoided by using a non-slip mattress, having the patient's arms folded on the chest, and taking care with positioning of the legs, preferably using Lloyd Davis leg supports rather than lithotomy poles.*

Nausea and vomiting

The incidence of PONV after laparoscopy is so high that this procedure is commonly used to study the efficacy of antiemetics. Rates from 48 to 96% have been reported when no antiemetic efforts were made[46,47]. PONV following laparoscopy delays discharge and increases overnight admission[48,49].

The cause of this high incidence of PONV is not clear. In gynaecological laparoscopies, contributing factors are gender and the pain and spasm of the sterilization technique. The common factor in all laparoscopies is peritoneal stretching from gas insufflation. A gasless technique for laparoscopy reduced PONV from 68% to 8% and improved longer-term recovery, compared with conventional pneumo-peritoneum[50,51].

The most effective strategy for reducing PONV in laparoscopy is to avoid the use of volatile agents and to use a propofol infusion for maintenance (TIVA)[48,49,52-54]. The inclusion of nitrous oxide in a propofol infusion technique for laparoscopy has not been shown to increase PONV or to have any other effects on recovery[46,55-57].

Routine antiemetic prophylaxis has been said to be unjustified if the incidence of PONV is low[58]. The use of TIVA alone may reduce PONV sufficiently. However, for persistent PONV after the use of propofol, $5HT_3$ receptor-blocking drugs may be the most logical rescue antiemetics. Paxton *et al.* found that after propofol and isoflurane were used for laparoscopy, only ondansetron 4 mg IV significantly reduced PONV, compared with placebo, metoclopramide 10 mg IV or droperidol 1 mg IV[47]. Granisetron 20 μg kg^{-1} with dexamethasone 8 mg was more effective than granisetron alone in reducing PONV after laparoscopy[59]. To confuse the issue further, a recent study of laparoscopic cholecystectomies found that droperidol 0.625 mg IV plus metoclopramide 10 mg IV was more effective in reducing PONV than ondansetron, after propofol/desflurane anaesthesia[60]. Further studies are needed into the most effective rescue antiemetic when volatiles are omitted.

> *The best anaesthetic technique to reduce PONV after laparoscopy is the use of TIVA with propofol. Persistent PONV should probably be treated with a $5HT_3$ receptor blocker.*

Postoperative pain

Pain following laparoscopy may be difficult to control, and limits the expansion of more major day case laparoscopic surgery. Pain is initially abdominal, but shoulder pain becomes more apparent once the patient is ambulant[61]. Although laparoscopy for sterilization is associated with considerably more pain than diagnostic laparoscopy in the first 4 hours, there is no significant difference postdischarge, presumably because tubal spasm has eased[62].

There are many different causes of pain in laparoscopy. (*Table 13.7*) This means that one analgesic intervention alone is insufficient to control pain unless potent, long-acting opiates such as morphine are used. This is inappropriate, as morphine increases PONV, time to discharge and overnight admission[63–65] as well as dizziness, dysphoria and recovery times[66]. *Table 13.8* summarizes the strategies for reducing postoperative pain.

Table 13.7. Causes of pain in laparoscopy

Poor surgical technique
Volume of gas used
Type of gas used
Volume of residual gas not expelled at the end of the procedure
Extraperitoneal gas
Gas under the diaphragm
Entry port pain
Pain from intra-abdominal surgical sites
Method of tubal sterilization
Blood in the peritoneum

Table 13.8. Strategies for reducing pain in laparoscopy

Early administration of NSAID
Short-acting intraoperative opioid
Gentle surgery, avoiding extraperitoneal gas
Volume of gas used kept as low as possible
Expulsion of as much gas as possible at the end of surgery
Nitrous oxide for insufflation causes less pain than CO_2 (but supports combustion)
Local analgesia to entry port sites
Local analgesia to intraperitoneal surgical sites
Tubal clips rather than rings for sterilization
Peritoneal lavage to remove intraperitoneal blood
Postoperative pain dealt with promptly

Surgical technique

- Clinically, gentle surgical technique helps reduce pain, as does limiting the volume of gas used to distend the abdomen[50]. Gas inadvertently placed extraperitoneally can cause considerable discomfort.
- Attempts should be made to expel as much gas as possible at the end of the procedure as this reduces pain[67]. Pain has been related to the size of the residual gas bubble under the diaphragm[68] and a gas drain left in for 6 hours postoperatively was reported to reduce pain[69].
- The insufflating gas may be important. It has been suggested that carbonic acid formed from CO_2 is irritating. Nitrous oxide reduces pain when used for procedures under local anaesthesia[70,71]. CO_2 is more rapidly soluble than nitrous oxide and is safer with diathermy, or if gas embolus occurs[72].
- For laparoscopic sterilization, diathermy causes least pain; clips cause much less pain than rings[73].
- Intraperitoneal bleeding is irritant, and large amounts of residual blood or continued postoperative intraperitoneal blood loss can cause considerable pain[74]. Peritoneal lavage may help. Continuing blood loss should be excluded as a cause of severe pain that is difficult to control postoperatively.

Local analgesia

Puncture site pain. This is reduced with local analgesia, but this does not reduce analgesic requirements if pain from intra-abdominal surgical sites is not also relieved[75,76].

Shoulder pain. This may be relieved by local analgesia: the study of Narchi *et al.* showed that both lignocaine, 0.5% with adrenaline 80 ml, and bupivacaine, 0.125% with adrenaline 80 ml, reduced shoulder pain and analgesia for 48 hours postoperatively[77].

Laparoscopic sterilization. This is recognized as a painful procedure, although severe pain may be of short duration[62]. Various ways of using local analgesia have been tried (*Table 13.9*).

Table 13.9. Methods of local analgesia in laparoscopic sterilization

Instillation of local anaesthetic into Pouch of Douglas	Best
Transcervical injection of bupivacaine	↑
Infiltration of mesosalpinx	
Lignocaine gel applied to clips	

- Lignocaine gel applied to sterilization clips was ineffective in one study[78], but reduced pain and analgesic requirements in another[79]. In the second study, 84% of patients still required analgesia after lignocaine.
- Infiltration of bupivacaine into the mesosalpinx using a long spinal needle reduced pain and analgesic requirements after the use of tubal rings[80,81] but was associated with minor bleeding[80] and may be technically difficult to perform.

- Transcervical bupivacaine (0.25%, 50 ml) was an effective analgesic and simple to instil[82]. Disadvantages are the risk of spreading infection and the need for a special introducer to prevent leakage. Some peritoneal spillage of bupivacaine must occur with this technique, which may contribute to analgesia.
- Local analgesia applied to the Fallopian tubes under direct vision has been shown to be effective in procedures carried out under local anaesthesia[83]. With general anaesthesia, dripping or instilling bupivacaine, 0.25% 20 ml or 0.5% 10 ml, into the peritoneum over the Fallopian tubes relieved pain and reduced analgesia and overnight admission after diagnostic laparoscopy[84] and after laparoscopic sterilization[85]. Whether this works locally on the Fallopian tubes or, more likely, blocks the uterosacral nerves in the Pouch of Douglas, is unknown.

Laparoscopic hernia repair. Pain from this has been reduced by large quantities (100 ml) of bupivacaine 0.15% instilled into the inguinal area with the patient tipped head-up[86].

Laparoscopic cholecystectomy. The effectiveness of local analgesia is less convincing in laparoscopic cholecystectomy. Most studies have found it to be ineffective, perhaps because large volumes of diluted bupivacaine were used[87,88]. However, Pasqualucci *et al.* instilled 20 ml 0.5% bupivacaine with adrenaline both before and after surgery, and significantly reduced pain and analgesic consumption[89], so further studies using more concentrated solutions of bupivacaine are needed.

> *Bupivacaine 0.5% 10–20 ml instilled into the Pouch of Douglas during surgery is effective for painful pelvic procedures. Its effectiveness in laparoscopic cholecystectomy has not been demonstrated convincingly. The addition of adrenaline may reduce serum levels and allow greater volumes or concentrations to be used[90].*

NSAIDs

NSAIDs are deservedly popular for analgesia in laparoscopy. However, for more painful procedures they are insufficient on their own, and local analgesia and/or other analgesics are needed to control pain adequately[91–93].

There are few comparisons of different NSAIDs or different modes of administering them. Ketorolac 30–60 mg IM and/or IV at induction (larger doses than recommended in the UK)[94,95], and diclofenac 50 or 100 mg PO[96] and ibuprofen 800 mg PO given preoperatively[97], have all been shown to reduce pain after laparoscopic sterilization and cholecystectomy.

Whichever NSAID is used, sufficient time must be allowed for it to be effective when the patient wakes. Rectal diclofenac is commonly administered during surgery lasting less than 30 minutes. This is insufficient time to allow the drug to work[98].

> *NSAIDs should be given early enough to allow them to be effective when the patient wakes. Given as oral premedication they are cheap and effective. Additional analgesic measures will be needed for more painful procedures.*

Postdischarge morbidity

Although good anaesthesia and analgesia can improve recovery after laparoscopy, postoperative morbidity is still considerable. Pre-admission information on the level of discomfort that can be expected and the limitations on work and other activities is essential[99].

Discharge analgesia should be provided for a minimum of 3 days, longer for more invasive procedures[100]. Regular NSAIDs and rescue analgesia with a paracetamol/codeine preparation is usually sufficient[26].

Anaesthetic techniques

No single anaesthetic or analgesic intervention will deal with all the problems associated with laparoscopy. 'Multimodal' approaches, with antiemetic prophylaxis, NSAID, short-acting opioid, TIVA with propofol and local analgesia to the trocar sites and intraperitoneally, have reported reduced pain and nausea and increased patient satisfaction[26,101]. An anaesthetic regime which combines these is suggested in *Table 13.10*.

Table 13.10. Suggested 'multimodal' anaesthetic technique for laparoscopy

Premedication	Ranitidine 150 mg + metoclopramide 10 mg 　　PO 60–90 minutes preoperatively
NSAID	Diclofenac 50–100 mg PO *or*　　　　　　　　　　　　} 60–90 minutes preoperatively Ibuprofen 800 mg PO *or* Ketorolac 10 mg IV at induction *or* Diclofenac 100 mg PR after induction 　　(if procedure lasts >30 minutes)
Anaesthesia	Fentanyl 1.5–3 µg kg⁻¹ (or more if needed) Propofol for induction and maintenance Nitrous oxide may be used
	LMA for shorter procedures (<30 minutes) if: 　　non-obese patient (BMI <30) 　　no symptoms of gastric reflux
	Intubation and IPPV if: 　　>30 minutes 　　obese 　　symptomatic gastric reflux 　　upper abdominal procedure (cholecystectomy)
	Consider prophylaxis against bradycardia
Local analgesia	Bupivacaine 0.5% + adrenaline to entry port sites
	Bupivacaine 0.5% ± adrenaline 10–20 ml intraperitoneally 　　for laparoscopic sterilization and pelvic surgery
	? Bupivacaine 0.5% 20–30 ml to right upper quadrant for laparoscopic cholecystectomy
Rescue analgesia in recovery	Fentanyl 25–50 µg IV repeated until patient comfortable
Postoperative analgesia	Continue *regular* NSAIDs + Paracetamol 500 mg/codeine 30 mg combination if needed

IPPV, intermittent positive pressure ventilation.

Laparoscopy for tubal sterilization may be carried out successfully under local anaesthesia in well-motivated women, and has been shown to reduce recovery time, analgesia and cost[102,103]. It is not suitable when intra-abdominal manipulation or more major surgery is required, and patients may not tolerate the Trendelenburg tilt. These factors also limit the use of spinal or epidural anaesthesia.

> *Anaesthesia for laparoscopic procedures needs a multimodal approach to deal with pain, PONV and morbidity. This improves outcome, particularly after more major laparoscopic surgery.*

References

1. **Singleton RJ, Rudkin GE, Osborne GA, et al.** Laparoscopic cholecystectomy as a day surgery procedure. *Anaesth. Intens. Care* 1996; **24**: 231–236.
2. **Jain A, Mercado PD, Grafton KP, et al.** Outpatient laparoscopic appendectomy. *Surg. Endosc.* 1995; **9**: 424–425.
3. **Daniell JF, McTavish G.** Combined laparoscopy and minilaparotomy for outpatient reversal of tubal sterilization. *South. Med. J.* 1995; **88**: 914–916.
4. **Summitt RL, Stovall TG, Lipscombe GH, et al.** Randomized comparison of laparoscopy-assisted vaginal hysterectomy with standard vaginal hysterectomy in an outpatient setting. *Obstet. Gynecol.* 1992; **80**: 895–901.
5. **Obenchain TG.** Laparoscopic lumbar discectomy. *J. Laparoendosc. Surg.* 1991; **1**: 145–149.
6. **Lawrence K, McWhinnie D, Goodwin AL, et al.** Randomised controlled trial of laparoscopic versus open repair of inguinal hernia: early results. *Br. Med. J.* 1995; **311**: 981–985.
7. **MacMahon AJ, Russell IT, Ramsay G, et al.** Laparoscopic and minilaparotomy cholecystectomy: a randomized trial comparing postoperative pain and pulmonary function. *Surgery* 1994; **115**: 533–539.
8. **Grace PA, Quereshi A, Coleman J, et al.** Reduced postoperative hospitalization after laparoscopic cholecystectomy. *Br. J. Surg.* 1991; **78**: 160–162.
9. **Schulze S, Thorup J.** Pulmonary function, pain and fatigue after laparoscopic cholecystectomy. *Eur. J. Surg.* 1993; **159**: 361–364.
10. **Berggren U, Gordh T, Grama D, et al.** Laparoscopic versus open cholecystectomy: hospitalization, sick leave, analgesia and trauma responses. *Br. J. Surg.* 1994; **81**: 1362–1365.
11. **Harris SN, Ballantyne GH, Luther MA, et al.** Alterations in cardiovascular performance during laparoscopic colectomy: a combined hemodynamic and echocardiographic analysis. *Anesth. Analg.* 1996; **83**: 482–487.
12. **Fahy BG, Barnas GM, Flowers JL, et al.** The effects of increased abdominal pressure on lung and chest wall mechanics during laparoscopic surgery. *Anesth. Analg.* 1995; **81**: 744–750.
13. **Pelosi P, Foti G, Cereda M, et al.** Effects of carbon dioxide insufflation for laparoscopic cholecystectomy on the respiratory system. *Anaesthesia* 1996; **51**: 744–749.
14. **Johanssen G, Andersen M, Juhl B.** The effect of general anesthesia on the haemodynamic events during laparoscopy with CO_2 insufflation. *Acta Anaesthesiol. Scand.* 1989; **33**: 132–136.
15. **Brown DR, Fishburne JI, Robertson VO, et al.** Ventilatory and blood gas changes during laparoscopy with local anesthesia. *Am. J. Obstet. Gynecol.* 1976; **7**: 741–745.
16. **Heijke SAM, Smith G, Key A.** The effect of the Trendelenburg position on lower oesophageal sphincter tone. *Anaesthesia* 1991; **46**: 185–187.
17. **Chassard D, Berrada K, Tournadre J-P, et al.** The effects of neuromuscular block on peak airway pressure and abdominal elastance during pneumoperitoneum. *Anesth. Analg.* 1996; **82**: 525–527.
18. **Cooper GM, Scoggins AM, Ward ID, et al.** Laparoscopy – a stressful procedure. *Anaesthesia* 1982; **37**: 266–269.
19. **McMahon AJ, O'Dwyer PJ, Cruikshank AM, et al.** Comparison of metabolic responses to laparoscopic and mini-laparotomy cholecystectomy. *Br. J. Surg.* 1993; **80**: 1255–1258.
20. **Fahy BG, Barnas GM, Nagle SE, et al.** Changes in lung and chest wall properties with abdominal insufflation of carbon dioxide are immediately reversible. *Anesth. Analg.* 1996; **82**: 501–505.

21. **Chung F.** Recovery pattern and home-readiness after ambulatory surgery. *Anesth. Analg.* 1995; **80:** 896–902.
22. **Azziz R, Steinkampf MP, Murphy A.** Postoperative recuperation: relation to the extent of endoscopic surgery. *Fertil. Steril.* 1989; **51:** 1061–1064.
23. **Livingstone JI, Cahill CJ.** Day case laparoscopic cholecystectomy – a feasibility study. *Ambulatory Surg.* 1995; **3:** 179–181.
24. **Kurer FL, Welch DB.** Gynaecological laparoscopy: clinical experiences of two anaesthetic techniques. *Br. J. Anaesth.* 1984; **56:** 1207–1211.
25. **Thomas H, Hare MJ.** Day case laparoscopic sterilization – time for a rethink? *Br. J. Obstet. Gynaecol.* 1987; **94:** 445–448.
26. **Ratcliffe F, Lawson R, Millar J.** Day-case laparoscopy revisited: have post-operative morbidity and patient acceptance improved? *Health Trends* 1994; **26:** 47–49.
27. **Tuckey JP, Morris GN, Peden CJ, et al.** Feasibility of day case laparoscopic cholecystectomy in unselected patients. *Anaesthesia* 1996; **51:** 965–968.
28. **Lamberty JM.** Gynaecological laparoscopy. *Br. J. Anaesth.* 1985; **57:** 718–719.
29. **Chamberlain G, Brown JC.** (1978) *Gynaecological laparoscopy: Report of the Working Party of the Confidential Enquiry into gynaecological laparoscopy.* Royal College of Obstetricians and Gynaecologists, London.
30. **Desmond J, Gordon RA.** Ventilation in patients anaesthetized for laparoscopy. *Can. Anaesth. Soc. J.* 1970; **17:** 378–387.
31. **Jones MJ, Mitchell RW, Hindocha N.** Effect of increased intra-abdominal pressure on the lower esophageal sphincter. *Anesth. Analg.* 1989; **68:** 63–65.
32. **Wong HC, Nikana CA.** (1985) In the real world. In: *Anesthesia for Ambulatory Surgery* (Ed. BV Wetchler). JB Lippincott Co., Philadelphia, PA. pp. 357–395.
33. **Duffy BL.** Regurgitation during pelvic laparoscopy. *Br. J. Anaesth.* 1979; **51:** 1089–1090.
34. **Roberts CJ, Goodman NW.** Gastro-oesophageal reflux during elective laparoscopy. *Anaesthesia* 1990; **45:** 1009–1011.
35. **Malins AF, Cooper GM.** Laparoscopy and the laryngeal mask airway. *Br. J. Anaesth.* 1994; **73:** 121.
36. **Harris MNE, Plantevin OM, Crowther A.** Cardiac arrhythmias during anaesthesia for laparoscopy. *Br. J. Anaesth.* 1984; **56:** 1213–1217.
37. **Goodwin APL, Rowe WL, Ogg TW.** Day case laparoscopy. A comparison of two anaesthetic techniques using the laryngeal mask during spontaneous breathing. *Anaesthesia* 1992; **47:** 892–895.
38. **Swann DG, Spens H, Edwards SA, et al.** Anaesthesia for gynaecological laparoscopy – a comparison between the laryngeal mask and tracheal intubation. *Anaesthesia* 1993; **48:** 431–434.
39. **Brimacombe J, Berry A.** Airway management during gynaecological laparoscopy – is it safe to use the laryngeal mask airway? *Ambulatory Surg.* 1995; **3:** 65–70.
40. **Myles PS.** Bradyarrhythmia and laparoscopy: a prospective study of heart rate changes with laparoscopy. *Aust. N.Z. J. Obstet. Gynaecol.* 1991; **31:** 171–173.
41. **Doyle DJ, Mark PWS.** Laparoscopy and vagal arrest. *Anaesthesia* 1989; **44:** 448.
42. **Cozanitis DA, Pouttu J, Rosenberg PH.** Bradycardia associated with the use of vecuronium. A comparative study with pancuronium with and without glycopyrronium. *Anaesthesia* 1987; **42:** 192–194.
43. **Guise PA.** Asystole following propofol and fentanyl in an anxious patient. *Anaesth. Intens. Care* 1991; **19:** 116–118.
44. **Inoue K, el-Banayosy A, Stolarski L, et al.** Vecuronium induced bradycardia following induction of anaesthesia with etomidate or thiopentone, with or without fentanyl. *Br. J. Anaesth.* 1988; **60:** 10–17.
45. **Scott DB, Julian DG.** Observations on cardiac arrhythmias during laparoscopy. *Br. Med. J.* 1972; **I:** 411–413.
46. **Sengupta P, Plantevin OM.** Nitrous oxide and day case laparoscopy: effects on nausea, vomiting and return to normal activity. *Br. J. Anaesth.* 1988; **60:** 570–573.
47. **Paxton LD, McKay AC, Mirakhur RK.** Prevention of nausea and vomiting after day case gynaecological laparoscopy. A comparison of ondansetron, droperidol, metoclopramide and placebo. *Anaesthesia* 1995; **50:** 403–406.
48. **Eriksson H, Korttila K.** Recovery profile after desflurane with or without ondansetron compared with propofol in patients undergoing outpatient gynecological laparoscopy. *Anesth. Analg.* 1996; **82:** 533–538.

49. **Green G, Jonsson L.** Nausea: the most important factor determining length of stay after ambulatory anaesthesia. A comparative study of isoflurane and/or propofol techniques. *Acta Anaesthesiol. Scand.* 1993; **37**: 742–746.

50. **Lindgren L, Koivusalo A-M, Kellokumpu I.** Conventional pneumoperitoneum compared with abdominal wall lift for laparoscopic cholecystectomy. *Br. J. Anaesth.* 1995; **75**: 567–572.

51. **Koivusalo A-M, Kellokumpu I, Lindgren L.** Gasless laparoscopic cholecystectomy: a comparison of postoperative recovery with conventional technique. *Br. J. Anaesth.* 1996; **77**: 576–580.

52. **Marshall C, Jones RM, Bajorek PK, et al.** Recovery characteristics using isoflurane or propofol for maintenance of anaesthesia: a double blind controlled trial. *Anaesthesia* 1992; **47**: 461–466.

53. **Raftery S, Sherry E.** Total intravenous anaesthesia with propofol and alfentanil protects against postoperative nausea and vomiting. *Can. J. Anaesth.* 1992; **39**: 37–40.

54. **Van Hemelrijck J, Smith I, White P.** Use of desflurane for outpatient anesthesia. *Anesthesiology* 1991; **75**: 197–203.

55. **Sukhani R, Lurie J, Jabamoni R.** Propofol for ambulatory gynecologic laparoscopy: does omission of nitrous oxide alter postoperative sequelae and recovery? *Anesth. Analg.* 1994; **78**: 831–835.

56. **Jensen AG, Prevedoros H, Kullman E, et al.** Peroperative nitrous oxide does not influence recovery after laparoscopic cholecystectomy. *Acta Anaesthesiol. Scand.* 1993; **37**: 683–686.

57. **Hovorka J, Korttila K.** Nitrous oxide does not increase nausea and vomiting following gynaecological laparoscopy. *Can. J. Anaesth.* 1989; **36**: 145–148.

58. **Watcha MF, White PF.** Postoperative nausea and vomiting. Its etiology, treatment, and prevention. *Anesthesiology* 1992; **77**: 162–184.

59. **Fujii Y, Tanaka H, Toyooka H.** Granisetron–dexamethasone combination reduces postoperative nausea and vomiting. *Can. J. Anaesth.* 1995; **42**: 387–390.

60. **Steinbrook RA, Freiberger D, Gosnell JL, et al.** Prophylactic antiemetics for laparoscopic cholecystectomy: ondansetron versus droperidol plus metoclopramide. *Anesth. Analg.* 1996; **83**: 1081–1083.

61. **Dobbs FF, Kumar V, Alexander JI, et al.** Pain after laparoscopy related to posture and ring versus clip sterilization. *Br. J. Obstet. Gynaecol.* 1987; **94**: 262–266.

62. **Davis A, Millar JM.** Postoperative pain: a comparison of laparoscopic sterilisation and diagnostic laparoscopy. *Anaesthesia* 1988; **43**: 796–797.

63. **Vijay V, King TA.** Postoperative intramuscular opiates in day surgery. *J. One Day Surg.* 1995; **4**: 6–7.

64. **McEvoy A, Livingstone JI, Cahill CJ.** Comparison of diclofenac sodium and morphine sulphate for postoperative analgesia after day case inguinal hernia surgery. *Ann. R. Coll. Surg. Engl.* 1996; **78**: 363–366.

65. **Pandit SK, Kothary SP.** Intravenous narcotics for premedication in outpatient anaesthesia. *Acta Anaesthesiol. Scand.* 1989; **33**: 353–358.

66. **Lundgren S.** Comparison of rectal diazepam and subcutaneous morphine–scopolamine administration for outpatient sedation in minor oral surgery. *Acta Anaesthesiol. Scand.* 1985; **29**: 674–678.

67. **Fredman B, Jedeikin R, Olsfanger D, et al.** Residual pneumoperitoneum: a cause of postoperative pain after laparoscopic cholecystectomy. *Anesth. Analg.* 1994; **79**: 152–154.

68. **Jackson SA, Laurence AS, Hill JC.** Does post-laparoscopy pain relate to residual carbon dioxide? *Anaesthesia* 1996; **51**: 485–487.

69. **Alexander JI, Hull MGR.** Abdominal pain after laparoscopy: the value of a gas drain. *Br. J. Obstet. Gynaecol.* 1987; **94**: 267–269.

70. **Sharp JR, Pierson WP, Brady CE.** Comparison of CO_2 and N_2O-induced discomfort on pain during laparoscopy: a double blind controlled trial. *Gastroenterology* 1982; **82**: 453–456.

71. **Minoli G, Terruzi V, Spinzi GC, et al.** The influence of carbon dioxide and nitrous oxide on pain during laparoscopy: a double blind, controlled trial. *Gastrointest. Endosc.* 1982; **28**: 173–175.

72. **Yacoub OF, Cardona I, Coveler LA, et al.** Carbon dioxide embolism during laparoscopy. *Anesthesiology* 1982; **57**: 533–535.

73. **Chi IC, Cole LP.** Incidence of pain among women undergoing laparoscopic sterilization by electrocoagulation, the spring loaded clip, and the tubal ring. *Am. J. Obstet. Gynecol.* 1979; **135**: 397–401.

74. **Sivanesaratnam V, Singh A, Rachagan SP, et al.** Intraperitoneal haemorrhage from a ruptured corpus luteum. A cause of 'acute abdomen' in women. *Med. J. Aust.* 1986; **144:** 413–414.
75. **Ure BM, Troidl H, Spangenberger W, et al.** Preincisional local anesthesia with bupivacaine and pain after laparoscopic cholecystectomy. A double-blind randomized clinical trial. *Surg. Endosc.* 1993; **7:** 482–488.
76. **Maier C, Broer-Boos F, Kube D, et al.** [Wound infiltration with bupivacaine following pelviscopy does not reduce postoperative pain intensity. Results of a placebo-controlled, double blind study]. *Anaesthesist* 1994; **43:** 547–552.
77. **Narchi P, Benhamou D, Fernandez H.** Intraperitoneal local anaesthetic for shoulder pain after day case laparoscopy. *Lancet* 1991; **338:** 1569–1570.
78. **Barclay K, Calvert JP, Catling SJ, et al.** Analgesia after laparoscopic sterilisation. Effect of 2% gel applied to Filshie clips. *Anaesthesia* 1994; **49:** 68–70.
79. **Ezeh UO, Shoulder VS, Martin JL, et al.** Local anaesthetic on Filshie clips for pain relief after tubal sterilisation: a randomised double blind controlled trial. *Lancet* 1995; **346:** 82–85.
80. **Smith BE, MacPherson GH, De Jonge M, et al.** Rectus sheath and mesosalpinx block for laparoscopic sterilisation. *Anaesthesia* 1991; **46:** 875–877.
81. **Alexander CD, Wetchler BV, Thompson RE.** Bupivacaine infiltration of the mesosalpinx in ambulatory surgical laparoscopic tubal sterilization. *Can. J. Anaesth.* 1987; **34:** 362–365.
82. **Hunter A, Fogarty P.** Transcervical analgesia for laparoscopic sterilisation. *Br. J. Obstet. Gynaecol.* 1996; **103:** 378–380.
83. **Koetsawang S, Srisupandit S, Apimas SJ, et al.** A comparative study of topical anesthesia for laparoscopic sterilization with the use of the tubal ring. *Am. J. Obstet. Gynecol.* 1984; **150:** 931–933.
84. **Loughney AD, Sarma V, Ryall EA.** Intraperitoneal bupivacaine for relief of pain following day case laparoscopy. *Br. J. Obstet. Gynaecol.* 1994; **101:** 449–451.
85. **Wheatley SA, Millar JM, Jadad AR.** Reduction of pain after laparoscopic sterilisation with local bupivacaine: a randomised, parallel, double blind trial. *Br. J. Obstet. Gynaecol.* 1994; **101:** 443–446.
86. **Goulding ST, Hovell BC.** Laparoscopic inguinal hernia repair: quality of recovery following the use of intraperitoneal bupivacaine. *Ambulatory Surg.* 1995; **3:** 75–77.
87. **Schulte-Steinberg H, Weninger E, Jokisch D, et al.** Intraperitoneal versus interpleural morphine or bupivacaine for pain after laparoscopic cholecystectomy. *Anesthesiology* 1995; **82:** 634–640.
88. **Joris J, Thiry E, Paris P, et al.** Pain after laparoscopic cholecystectomy: characteristics and effect of intraperitoneal bupivacaine. *Anesth. Analg.* 1995; **81:** 379–384.
89. **Pasqualucci AD, De Angelis V, Contardo R, et al.** Preemptive analgesia: intraperitoneal local anesthetic in laparoscopic cholecystectomy. *Anesth. Analg.* 1996; **85:** 11–20.
90. **Narchi P, Benhamou D, Bouaziz H, et al.** Serum concentrations of local anaesthetics following intraperitoneal administration during laparoscopy. *Eur. J. Clin. Pharmacol.* 1992; **42:** 223–225.
91. **Hovorka J, Kallela H, Korttila K.** Effect of intravenous diclofenac on pain and recovery profile after day-case laparoscopy. *Eur. J. Anaesthesiol.* 1993; **10:** 105–108.
92. **Higgins MS, Givogre JL, Marco AP, et al.** Recovery from outpatient laparoscopic tubal ligation is not improved by preoperative administration of ketorolac or ibuprofen. *Anesth. Analg.* 1994; **79:** 274–280.
93. **Green CR, Pandit SK, Levy L, et al.** Intraoperative ketorolac has an opioid-sparing effect in women after diagnostic laparoscopy but not after laparoscopic tubal ligation. *Anesth. Analg.* 1996; **82:** 732–737.
94. **Cade L, Kakulas P.** Ketorolac or pethidine for analgesia after elective laparoscopic sterilization. *Anaesth. Intens. Care* 1995; **23:** 158–161.
95. **Liu J, Ding Y, White PF, et al.** Effects of ketorolac on postoperative analgesia and ventilatory function after laparoscopic cholecystectomy. *Anesth. Analg.* 1993; **76:** 1061–1066.
96. **Gillberg L, Harsten AS, Ståhl LB.** Preoperative diclofenac reduces post-laparoscopy pain. *Can. J. Anaesth.* 1993; **40:** 406–408.
97. **Rosenblum M, Weller RS, Conard PL, et al.** Ibuprofen provides longer lasting analgesia than fentanyl after laparoscopic surgery. *Anesth. Analg.* 1991; **73:** 255–259.
98. **John VA.** The pharmacokinetics and metabolism of diclofenac (Voltarol) in animals and man. *Rheumatol. Rehab.* 1979; **2** (Suppl.): 22–37.

99. **Donoghue J, Pelletier D, Duffield C,** *et al.* Laparoscopic surgery: the process of recovery for women. *Ambulatory Surg.* 1995; **3**: 171–177.

100. **Codd C.** Are analgesics necessary for women at home following laparoscopic gynaecological day surgery? *Nurs. Pract.* 1991; **5**: 8–12.

101. **Michaloliakou C, Chung F, Sharma S.** Preoperative multimodal analgesia facilitates recovery after laparoscopic cholecystectomy. *Anesth. Analg.* 1996; **82**: 44–51.

102. **Børdahl PE, Ræder JC, Nordentoft J,** *et al.* Laparoscopic sterilization under local or general anesthesia? A randomized study. *Obstet. Gynecol.* 1993; **81**: 137–141.

103. **MacKenzie IZ, Turner E, O'Sullivan GM,** *et al.* Two hundred out-patient laparoscopic clip sterilisations using local anaesthesia. *Br. J. Obstet. Gynaecol.* 1987; **94**: 449–453.

CHAPTER 14

Day surgery procedures

While the general principles of good anaesthesia and analgesia for day surgery are important for all types of day surgery, a knowledge and understanding of the problems of each type of surgery is necessary. This chapter identifies the specific issues related to common day surgery procedures, and suggests strategies for dealing with them.

14.1   Gynaecological procedures
14.2   General surgery procedures
14.3   Urological procedures
14.4   Plastic procedures
14.5   Orthopaedic procedures
14.6   Ophthalmic procedures
14.7   ENT procedures
14.8   Oral surgery procedures

14.1   Gynaecological procedures in day surgery
J.M. Millar

> *Female patients, so the incidence of PONV is increased. Consider pregnancy test if not menopausal or for termination of pregnancy.*

Common intrauterine procedures

- Dilatation and curettage (D&C)
- Hysteroscopy
- Evacuation of retained products of conception (ERPC)
- Termination of pregnancy (TOP)
- Endometrial ablation

Anaesthetic issues
Increased risk of acid regurgitation
- Lithotomy position[1].
- Effects of early pregnancy on gastric emptying and LOS tone[2,3].

Vagal stimulation
- Bradycardia from cervical dilation, especially if lightly anaesthetized.

Bleeding
- Uterine relaxation with volatile anaesthetics.

Emesis and pain
- Nausea and pain from prostaglandins used to facilitate TOP[4].
- PONV and pain from oxytocin or (worse) ergometrine used to contract uterus.

Fluid overload and pulmonary oedema (in endometrial ablation)
- From irrigating fluid, particularly if the fluid is pressurized or the procedure lasts longer than 45 minutes[5].

Haemorrhage and uterine perforation

Strategies
General anaesthesia
- Choose a technique with low risk of PONV, avoiding volatile agents.
- Consider routine ranitidine and metoclopramide PO on arrival (see Chapter 4).
- Propofol induction with alfentanil 7–15 µg kg⁻¹ (or consider fentanyl for cases >10 minutes).
- Propofol maintenance either by boluses or infusion.
- Nitrous oxide may help smooth anaesthetic without increasing PONV if propofol used.

Regional analgesia ± sedation
- Spinal anaesthesia or paracervical block ± propofol or midazolam sedation.
- This may be less popular with patients.

Analgesia
- Uterine pain is prostaglandin related[6], so NSAIDs are effective.
- Diclofenac, ketorolac, ibuprofen or mefenamic acid PO (or IV if relevant) work well.
- Provide NSAID for postdischarge analgesia.

Antiemetic
- Consider prophylactic antiemetic if ergometrine used.

Endometrial ablation
- Avoid glycine or 5% dextrose as irrigating fluid[5].
- Monitor fluid balance (electrolytes and serum osmolality if needed).
- Consider frusemide 20 mg IV if >1.5–2 litres in positive balance.
- Omit IV fluids to minimize fluid overload, unless bleeding.

Common laparoscopic procedures (see also Chapter 13)

- Diagnostic – infertility or pelvic pain
- Sterilization
- Treatment of endometriosis – diathermy or laser
- Intra-abdominal surgery, e.g. ovarian cysts

Anaesthetic issues
Increased risk of acid regurgitation
- Lithotomy position + head-down tilt.
- Increased intra-abdominal pressure.
- Obesity.

? Safety of LMA in laparoscopies

Vagal stimulation
- Bradycardia at abdominal distension and application of clips or rings to tubes.
- More likely if anaesthetic with no anticholinergic action is used, particularly vecuronium in association with fentanyl and/or propofol.

Intraperitoneal surgical problems
- Perforation of viscus or major blood vessel.
- Gas embolus.

Postoperative pain
- Laparoscopy usually has fairly severe pain, related to CO_2 used for inflation of abdomen and peritoneal stretching.
- Sterilization causes even more pain in the first few hours after surgery.
- By the time of discharge, sterilization pain has generally settled.
- The use of rings causes more pain than clips.
- Diathermy for sterilization is least painful but risks intraperitoneal damage.
- Large amounts of gas, failure to expel gas or extraperitoneal gas increase pain.
- Severe postoperative pain may be a sign of intra-abdominal bleeding or a perforated viscus.

PONV
- Laparoscopy, especially for sterilization, has a very high incidence of PONV.

Unplanned overnight admission
- Laparoscopies have a higher than average rate of admission because of pain and PONV.

Strategies
Combining different methods to control pain and emesis works better

General anaesthesia
- Choose a technique with low risk of PONV.
- Consider routine ranitidine and metoclopramide PO on arrival (see Chapter 4).
- Propofol induction and maintenance by infusion have been shown to reduce PONV in laparoscopy.
- Fentanyl 1.5–3 µg kg^{-1} provides intraoperative and some postoperative analgesia.
- Nitrous oxide may not increase PONV if propofol used (see Chapter 5).

Indications for use of LMA
- No symptoms of gastric reflux.
- Non-obese patient (consider distribution of fat – truncal obesity is worse).
- The procedure is of short duration – less than 30 minutes.

Neuromuscular block if needed
- Vecuronium (0.6 mg kg^{-1}) or atracurium (0.3 mg kg^{-1}) are satisfactory for short procedures (see Chapter 5).
- Consider anticholinergic prophylaxis with glycopyrrolate (or atropine) to prevent bradycardia if vecuronium used, especially with propofol and fentanyl.

Analgesia – several methods of analgesia in combination work best
- NSAIDs – diclofenac, ketorolac or ibuprofen PO or IV given early and in sufficient dose (see Chapter 9).
- Diclofenac PR given intraoperatively is not effective soon enough for a short procedure, less than 30 minutes[8].
- Perioperative opioids – see above.
- Bupivacaine 0.5% to abdominal puncture sites.
- Dissuade surgeon from using Fallope rings.
- Gentle surgery, expel as much gas as possible and avoid extraperitoneal gas.
- Intraperitoneal bupivacaine 0.5% 10–20 ml dripped into the Pouch of Douglas by surgeon for sterilization or pelvic surgery[9,10].
- If still in pain, give fentanyl 25–50 µg IV until comfortable postoperatively.
- Avoid morphine if possible.
- Provide NSAID + paracetamol/codeine combination (Tylex®, Tylenol®) for postdischarge analgesia.

Antiemetic
- Prophylactic antiemetic is not needed if propofol is used for induction and maintenance.
- If still nauseated, ondansetron may be the best rescue antiemetic[11].

Local or regional analgesia with sedation[12]
- Can be used for sterilization in well-motivated patients.
- Not suitable for procedures which require more intra-abdominal manipulation.
- Head-down position and abdominal distension may not be tolerated by patient.
- Using N$_2$O as the inflation gas reduces discomfort.

Common vulval and cervical surgery

- Bartholin's cyst or abscess
- Labial procedures, e.g. biopsy, cysts
- Cervical cone biopsy

Bartholin's cyst or abscess
- May be very painful if large.
- Local analgesia may be contraindicated if infected.
- Very large cysts or abscesses may be unsuitable for day surgery.

Labial procedures
- Local anaesthesia is essential – these can be very painful.
- Use this alone or with sedation or general anaesthesia.

Cone biopsy
- Seldom causes problems, except for bleeding.
- Local infiltration may be sufficient for laser conization[13].

References

1. **Jones MJ, Mitchell RWD, Hindocha N,** *et al.* The lower oesophageal sphincter in the first trimester of pregnancy: comparison of supine with lithotomy positions. *Br. J. Anaesth.* 1988; **61:** 475-476.
2. **Levy DM, Williams OA, Magides AD,** *et al.* Gastric emptying is delayed at 8–12 week's gestation. *Br. J. Anaesth.* 1994; **73:** 237–238.
3. **Brock-Utne JG, Dow TGB, Dimopoulos GE,** *et al.* Gastric and lower oesophageal sphincter (LOS) pressures in early pregnancy. *Br. J. Anaesth.* 1981; **53:** 381–384.
4. **Millar JM, Hall PJ.** Nausea and vomiting after prostaglandins in day case termination of pregnancy. The efficacy of low dose droperidol. *Anaesthesia* 1987; **42:** 613–618.
5. **Osborne GA, Rudkin GE, Moran P.** Fluid uptake in laser endometrial ablation. *Anaesth. Intens. Care* 1991; **19:** 217–219.
6. **Adelantado JM, Rees MCP, Lopez Bernal A,** *et al.* Increased uterine prostaglandin E receptors in menorrhagic women. *Br. J. Obstet. Gynaecol.* 1988; **95:** 162–165.
7. **Brimacombe J, Berry A.** Airway management during gynaecological laparoscopy - is it safe to use the laryngeal mask airway? *Ambulatory Surg.* 1995; **3:** 65–70.
8. **John VA.** The pharmacokinetics and metabolism of diclofenac (Voltarol) in animals and man. *Rheumatol. Rehab.* 1979; **2** (Suppl.): 22–37.
9. **Wheatley SA, Millar JM, Jadad AR.** Reduction of pain after laparoscopic sterilisation: a randomised, parallel, double blind trial. *Br. J. Obstet. Gynaecol.* 1994; **101:** 443–446.
10. **Loughney AD, Sarma V, Ryall EA.** Intraperitoneal bupivacaine for relief of pain following day case laparoscopy. *Br. J. Obstet. Gynaecol.* 1994; **101:** 449–451.
11. **Paxton LD, McKay AC, Mirakhur RK.** Prevention of nausea and vomiting after day case gynaecological laparoscopy. *Anaesthesia* 1995; **50:** 403–406.
12. **MacKenzie IZ, Turner E, O'Sullivan GM,** *et al.* Two hundred out-patient laparoscopic clip sterilisations using local anaesthesia. *Br. J. Obstet. Gynaecol.* 1987; **94:** 449–453.
13. **Helkjaer PE, Eriksen PS, Thomsen CF,** *et al.* Outpatient carbon dioxide laser excisional conization for cervical intra epithelial neoplasia under local anaesthesia. *Acta Obstet. Gynaecol. Scand.* 1993; **72:** 302–306.

14.2   General surgery procedures in day surgery
J.M. Millar

Common body surface procedures

- Lumps and bumps: sebaceous cysts, lipomata, etc.
- Breast lump biopsy/excision
- Varicose veins – ligations, avulsions and/or stripping
- Toenail avulsion or ablation
- Pilonidal sinus

Anaesthetic issues
Patients
- Women for removal of breast lumps may be extremely anxious.

Intraoperative problems
- Surgeons may prefer general or regional anaesthesia to infiltration of local anaesthetic, as this may allow better appreciation of the extent of the lesion – particularly breast lumps.
- Regional analgesia may not be feasible because of the site of the lesion.
- The prone position may be required for some varicose vein and pilonidal sinus surgery.

Postoperative problems
- Local infection may contraindicate the use of local anaesthesia, particularly in toenail and pilonidal sinus surgery.
- Wound drains may be needed after some procedures, and should generally be removed before discharge.
- Pilonidal sinus surgery may be very painful, depending on the extent of the surgery.

Strategies
Preoperative
- Sedative premedication may be required and should not be withheld from anxious patients (see Chapter 4).
- If local anaesthesia is not to be used, consider preoperative oral or early IV administration of NSAIDs to improve analgesia (see Chapter 4).

General anaesthesia
- Body surface surgery is relatively stimulating, and deeper anaesthesia may be required at the start of the procedure.
- Muscle relaxation is not required.
- The LMA is very suitable for the majority of cases in supine, lateral and 3/4 prone positions.
- For the prone position, the LMA may be used with caution in slim patients. Airway patency should be checked before surgery and it should be possible to turn the patient rapidly onto his or her side if problems occur.
- Except in high-risk patients, prophylactic antiemetics are seldom required, as these procedures are not particularly associated with increased PONV.

Local and regional anaesthesia
- Anxious patients may require sedation.
- Local infiltration is ideal for many procedures.
- Use a mixture of lignocaine 1% or 2% with adrenaline and bupivacaine for quick onset with duration of action. However, by the time the surgeon has prepared the operation site, bupivacaine is usually effective.
- The inclusion of adrenaline helps to provide a bloodless field.
- Digital or ring blocks are useful for toenail surgery. Do not use adrenaline-containing solutions.
- If infection is present in the toe, injection of local anaesthetic more proximally on either side of the metatarsal head, at a distance from the infected area, may be an option.
- Spinal or epidural anaesthesia may be used for varicose vein surgery.

Analgesia
- Persuade the surgeon to infiltrate the area with bupivacaine before the end of the procedure, even if the patient has had general anaesthesia. This is particularly useful in breast lump excision which can be painful afterwards.
- If the surgeon carries out the procedure under local anaesthesia, persuade him/her to use bupivacaine or a mixture with lignocaine as described above to allow longer duration of analgesia.
- Paracetamol/analgesic combinations are usually sufficient for postdischarge analgesia. Varicose vein surgery may require both NSAID and a paracetamol 500/codeine 30 preparation.

Hernia repairs

- Inguinal hernia – open
- Femoral hernia
- Umbilical hernia
- Epigastric hernia
- Small incisional hernia

Inguinal hernia
Anaesthetic issues
- Patients are usually male, and usually pose few anaesthetic problems.
- Ilioinguinal/iliohypogastric nerve block may result in inadvertent femoral nerve palsy. This causes difficulty in weight bearing and may delay or prevent discharge (see Chapter 10).

Surgical issues
- The advantages of open repair versus laparoscopic hernia repair are controversial.
- Laparoscopic hernia repair allows patients to return to work sooner but in general, takes longer, usually requires general anaesthesia, has more immediate recovery problems[1] and may not be cost effective[2,3]. The extraperitoneal approach may cause fewer problems than the transabdominal approach with similar surgical results[4].
- Open 'tension free' mesh repair, by contrast, is simple, recovery is uncomplicated and good long-term results have been reported[5]. Mesh repair causes less discomfort after discharge than conventional darn type repairs[6], early return to work has been reported[7], and it may allow simultaneous bilateral repairs[8].

- Many surgeons prefer to avoid muscle relaxation in open hernia repair in order to gauge the tension of the repair.
- Intraoperative antibiotics are usually required to cover the insertion of the mesh.
- Local or regional anaesthesia provide excellent analgesia while in the DSU, but once the local anaesthetic has worn off, postdischarge pain can still be considerable.

Strategies
General anaesthesia for open repair
- The LMA is ideal – many overweight middle-aged men for hernia repair have difficult airways and the LMA provides a more reliable hands-free airway than a face mask. Intubation is not necessary.
- Propofol followed by either propofol infusion or volatile agent is satisfactory.
- Small doses of alfentanil (7 µg kg^{-1}) or fentanyl (1–1.5 µg kg^{-1}) are useful to cover the insertion of the regional block or infiltration and the time until it is effective.
- The early insertion of an ilioinguinal/iliohypogastric block using bupivacaine, by the anaesthetist after induction of anaesthesia but before surgery, allows the level of anaesthesia to be reduced once the block is effective. Preoperative insertion of the block may also reduce postoperative pain[9].
- If light or sedation levels of anaesthesia are used, the adequacy of the block or infiltration should be tested and the surgeon can be asked to infiltrate more local anaesthetic if necessary.

Local and regional anaesthesia
- This is the ideal method of anaesthesia, with sedation if required – it is quick, cheap and effective, and recovery times are shortened compared with general anaesthesia[1].
- Local or regional anaesthesia is preferable to spinal or epidural anaesthesia: recovery time is shortened and postoperative pain has been shown to be reduced compared with spinal anaesthesia[10].

Infiltration
- Infiltration may be as effective as regional blockade for postoperative analgesia[11].
- Bupivacaine should be used to provide longer-lasting analgesia.

Ilioinguinal/iliohypogastric block
- This is an effective block for postoperative pain relief but extra infiltration may be needed if used without general anaesthesia.
- The genitofemoral nerve should be also be blocked by infiltrating around the pubic tubercle and along the superior margin of the pubis. Failure to do this results in pain at the medial end of the wound.
- Femoral nerve block may result from faulty ilioinguinal block technique. Injection of local anaesthetic deep to internal oblique muscle allows it to track down medially to collect around the femoral nerve[12]. This can be avoided by careful technique and by using short bevel regional block needles which allow tissue planes to be easily identified.

Postoperative analgesia
- Ilioinguinal blocks can be repeated postoperatively in the DSU although this is seldom needed if the first block has been effective.
- Patients should be warned that the local anaesthetic will wear off and that they should take analgesics as soon as they begin to feel pain.
- NSAIDs should be started before the local anaesthetic wears off. These provide good postoperative analgesia[13].

- Paracetamol 500/codeine 30 preparations may also be required postoperatively and should be taken with a dose of NSAID before going to bed the first night.
- A 5-day supply of analgesia should be prescribed to take home.

Femoral hernia repair
Anaesthetic issues
- More common in older women.
- Ilioinguinal/iliohypogastric block may not completely abolish the pain.

Strategies
- Local anaesthesia may be used with sedation if required – this is useful for less fit patients.
- If an ilioinguinal block is insufficient, it may be reinforced with extra infiltration locally.
- General anaesthesia may be used. Muscle relaxation is not necessary.

Epigastric, umbilical and incisional hernias
- If small, these are suitable to be done under local anaesthesia.
- If general anaesthesia is required, the LMA is suitable provided the patient has no symptoms of reflux and the lesion is small.
- Very large hernias may require muscle relaxation and endotracheal intubation.
- The surgeon should infiltrate with local anaesthetic, preferably before surgery.

Laparoscopic procedures (see also Chapter 13)

- Cholecystectomy
- Hernia repair

Laparoscopic cholecystectomy
Anaesthetic issues
- Association of gall bladder disease with obesity and gastro-oesophageal reflux.
- Upper abdominal surgery.
- Surgery may be prolonged.
- May need conversion to open procedure.
- PONV is common and delays discharge.
- Postoperative pain may delay discharge.
- Prolonged postoperative recovery time may be required and 24-hour stays have been recommended[14].
- This is currently a borderline procedure for day surgery.

Strategies
- Schedule early in the day to allow more time for recovery.
- Ranitidine and metoclopramide prophylaxis is recommended.
- General anaesthesia is needed.
- Endotracheal intubation is recommended.
- IV fluids are essential.
- Reduce PONV with propofol infusion and prophylactic ondansetron.
- If still nauseated, consider droperidol 10–20 μg kg^{-1} IV.
- Reduce analgesic requirements with infiltration of local anaesthetic at the entry ports.
- Intraperitoneal bupivacaine is of questionable efficacy – more studies are needed (see Chapter 13).

- Postoperative analgesia with fentanyl 25–50 µg IV until the patient is comfortable may be required.
- 5-day supply of NSAIDs and paracetamol 500/codeine 30 combinations for postdischarge analgesia.
- A follow-up telephone call the next morning is essential.

General anaesthesia for laparoscopic hernia repair
- Anaesthesia strategies as for laparoscopic cholecystectomy.
- Intraperitoneal instillation of local anaesthetic into the inguinal area with the patient head-up may be effective[15].

Common anal procedures

- Anal stretch
- Lateral sphincterotomy
- Banding or injection of haemorrhoids
- Haemorrhoidectomy

Anaesthetic issues
- Anal stretch needs deep anaesthesia to prevent laryngeal spasm.
- These operations can be <u>very</u> painful afterwards.
- Techniques and drugs which encourage urinary retention and constipation should be avoided.

Strategies
- Caudal or spinal anaesthesia, while effective, may delay discharge because of urinary retention.
- General anaesthesia is usually needed.
- Propofol anaesthesia, rapidly deepened plus a bolus of alfentanil 3–7 µg kg^{-1} just before anal stretching is effective.
- Early administration of NSAIDs and local infiltration with bupivacaine with adrenaline usually provide satisfactory pain relief.
- Avoid codeine-containing analgesics postoperatively as they are constipating. NSAIDs with non-codeine-containing paracetamol combinations may be used.
- Laxatives are also often prescribed to take at home.

References

1. **Rudkin GE, Maddern GJ.** Perioperative outcome for day case laparoscopic and open hernia repair. *Anaesthesia* 1995; **50:** 586–589.
2. **Lawrence K, McWhinnie D, Goodwin AL,** *et al.* Randomised controlled trial of laparoscopic versus open repair of inguinal hernia: early results. *Br. Med. J.* 1995; **311:** 981–985.
3. **Shrenk P, Woisetschläger R, Rieger R,** *et al.* Prospective randomized trial comparing postoperative pain and return to physical activity after transabdominal preperitoneal, total preperitoneal or Shouldice technique for inguinal hernia repair. *Br. J. Surg.* 1996; **83:** 1563–1566.
4. **Khoury N.** A comparative study of laparoscopic extraperitoneal and transabdominal preperitoneal herniorrhaphy. *J. Laparoendosc. Surg.* 1995; **5:** 349–355.
5. **Amid PK, Shulman AG, Lichtenstein IL.** An analytic comparison of laparoscopic hernia repair with open 'tension-free' hernioplasty. *Int. Surg.* 1995; **80:** 9–17.
6. **Amendolara M, Perri S, Breda E,** *et al.* [Inguinal hernioplasty: current trends]. *G. Chir.* 1995; **16:** 239–244.

7. **Kark AE, Kurzer M, Waters KJ.** Tension-free mesh hernia repair: review of 1098 cases using local anaesthesia in a day unit. *Ann. R. Coll. Surg. Engl.* 1995; **77:** 299–304.
8. **Amid PK, Shulman AG, Lichtenstein IL.** Simultaneous repair of bilateral inguinal hernias under local anesthesia. *Ann. Surg.* 1996; **223:** 249–252.
9. **Ding Y, White PF.** Post-herniorrhaphy pain in outpatients after pre-incision ilioinguinal–hypogastric nerve block during monitored anesthesia care. *Can. J. Anaesth.* 1995; **42:** 12–15.
10. **Tverskoy M, Cozacov C, Ayache M, et al.** Postoperative pain after inguinal herniorrhaphy with different types of anesthesia. *Anesth. Analg.* 1990; **70:** 29–35.
11. **Casey WF, Rice LJ, Hanallah RS, et al.** A comparison between bupivacaine instillation versus ilioinguinal/iliohypogastric nerve block for postoperative analgesia following inguinal herniorrhaphy in children. *Anesthesiology* 1990; **72:** 637–639.
12. **Rosario DJ, Skinner PP, Raftery AT.** Transient femoral nerve palsy complicating ilioinguinal nerve blockade for inguinal herniorrhaphy. *Br. J. Surg.* 1994; **81:** 897.
13. **McEvoy A, Livingstone JI, Cahill CJ.** Comparison of diclofenac sodium and morphine sulphate for postoperative analgesia after day case inguinal hernia surgery. *Ann. R. Coll. Surg. Engl.* 1996; **78:** 363–366.
14. **Tuckey JP, Morris GN, Peden CJ, et al.** Feasibility of day case laparoscopic cholecystectomy in unselected patients. *Anaesthesia* 1996; **51:** 965–968.
15. **Goulding ST, Howell BC.** Laparoscopic inguinal hernia repair: quality of recovery following the use of intraperitoneal bupivacaine. *Ambulatory Surg.* 1995; **3:** 75–77.

14.3   Urological procedures in day surgery
J.M. Millar

> Patients tend to be older and less fit, so good preoperative assessment and experienced anaesthetists are essential to reduce cancellations and complications.

Common endoscopic procedures

- Flexible cystoscopy
- Urethroscopy – dilation or excision of stenosis
- Cystoscopy – diagnostic or resection of bladder tumour
- Bladder neck incision
- Short bladder distension
- Ureteroscopy ± insertion/removal of stent
- Stone breaking (lithoclasty) or removal procedures
- Laser prostatectomy

Anaesthetic issues
Patients
- Many are elderly.
- Many require frequent repeat procedures.
- Renal function may be impaired.
- Despite this, postanaesthetic recovery is usually problem-free.

Intraoperative problems
- Light anaesthesia can produce priapism which may make the procedure difficult, hazardous, or cause it to be abandoned.
- Difficulty in predicting duration of operation with unknown extent of pathology.
- Bleeding, especially during bladder tumour resection.

Postoperative problems
- Colic may be severe after ureteric interventions, especially stone breaking or retrograde pyelograms.
- Retention of urine.
- A urinary catheter may be required.
- Clot retention may occur if no bladder irrigation is used.
- Overnight admissions are usually due to more extensive surgery than planned.

Laser prostatectomy[1]
- Pain rarely causes problems.
- The preoperative administration of NSAIDs may increase bleeding.
- Little bleeding and fluid absorption occur.
- Urinary retention is the most common problem.
- Good out of hours support and a follow-up telephone call next day are essential.

Strategies

Patient assessment
- Assign a regular, interested and experienced anaesthetist to day surgery urology.
- More patients may need individual pre-admission assessment by the anaesthetist.
- Consider creatinine and electrolyte investigation.
- Once assessed, neither elderly nor ASA 3 patients for repeat procedures cause problems.

General anaesthesia
- The LMA is ideal, particularly for procedures of indeterminate duration.
- Propofol induction and maintenance provide good conditions, although in men, PONV seldom causes problems.
- Priapism has been treated with ketamine IV, but very small doses of intracorporeal α-adrenergic agonists are the drugs of choice. Inject 1–2 ml of:
  phenylephrine (preferred) 0.5 mg diluted in 2 ml 0.9% saline[2];
  or metaraminol 0.5 mg diluted in 10 ml 0.9% saline[3];
  or adrenaline 0.01 mg (1 ml 1:100 000) diluted in 10 ml 0.9% saline[4].

Regional or local analgesia ± sedation
- Many procedures, particularly flexible cystoscopies, are ideally done under local anaesthesia.
- Women tolerate cystoscopy under local anaesthesia very well.
- Sedation or monitored anaesthetic care is often unnecessary.
- Bladder distension is uncomfortable and usually requires general anaesthesia, although intravesical bupivacaine has been used successfully with sedation[5].
- Techniques which may result in urinary retention should be avoided, e.g. spinal or caudal anaesthesia with long-acting local anaesthetic agents.

Analgesia
- Alfentanil or fentanyl intraoperatively are often sufficient, especially for diagnostic procedures.
- NSAIDs should be given in advance, either PO or IV, for painful procedures, particularly ureteric procedures, and especially lithoclasty.
- Early NSAID administration may increase intraoperative bleeding in resection of bladder tumour or prostate. If in doubt, give postoperatively if needed.
- Intravesical bupivacaine has been reported to help bladder pain[5].
- In the author's practice, instillation of bupivacaine 0.5% 20–30 ml up the ureter by the surgeon has been found to help lithoclasty pain.
- IV fentanyl may be required for ureteric colic after lithoclasty.
- Postoperatively, NSAIDs if not already given, and/or paracetamol/analgesic combinations usually suffice.

Postoperative catheters
- These may need irrigation if bleeding has been brisk.
- If a trial of removal of catheter fails, or passing urine is difficult, patients tolerate going home with catheters surprisingly well.
- This may be preferable to developing urinary retention at home.
- The patient may return to the DSU or the GP for removal of catheter 1–3 days later.

Common scrotal procedures

- Vasectomy
- Reversal of vasectomy
- Hydrocele or spermatocele operations
- Testicular biopsy

Anaesthetic issues
- Patients, especially younger men, may be very nervous.
- Pain and swelling postoperatively may be underestimated.

Strategies
General anaesthesia
- This may be needed because of patient anxiety.
- Necessary with prolonged procedures using the microscope and requiring a still patient, for example, reversal of vasectomy.

Local analgesia ± sedation
- This is the most common method for vasectomy.
- Regional anesthesia (caudal or spinal) may be used, but recovery may not be any faster.
- Genitofemoral blocks do not provide scrotal anaesthesia – the surgeon needs to infiltrate locally and into the spermatic cord.

Analgesia
- Early administration of NSAIDs with a paracetamol/analgesic combination for rescue analgesia.
- Good scrotal support is needed postoperatively.

Other common procedures

- Circumcision
- Varicocele surgery – laparoscopic or open
- Orchidectomy
- Extracorporeal shock wave lithotripsy (ESWL)

Circumcision
Patients
- Younger patients can be extremely anxious.
- Older patients tolerate local anaesthesia well.

General anaesthesia
- Propofol induction with a dorsal penile block, or local infiltration by the surgeon before surgery, allows light sedation levels of anaesthesia. This gives good intraoperative conditions with rapid, pain-free recovery.

Local anaesthesia
- Local anaesthesia with or without sedation may be used in less anxious patients.
- A dorsal block can be performed on awake patients using skin infiltration with lignocaine before attempting the block. Patients may not always tolerate it well if awake and it may be more difficult to place in an anxious patient.

- Dorsal penile blocks should be done meticulously, avoiding the dorsal vein and injection into the corpora. Do not use adrenaline-containing solutions
- Local infiltration or ring block by the surgeon is effective.
- Caudal analgesia, while effective, causes postoperative urinary retention in adults. The use of short-acting agents reduces the duration of postoperative analgesia.

Analgesia
- Dorsal block or infiltration give good postoperative analgesia for several hours.
- Local application of lignocaine gel and/or paracetamol/analgesic combination with or without NSAIDs for postdischarge analgesia.

Varicocele surgery
- This may be done laparoscopically (see Chapter 13).
- It may also be done through a groin incision. If sufficiently low, an ilioinguinal block is ideal, but for higher ligation the surgeon should be asked to infiltrate the area.

Orchidectomy
- Patients may be elderly, with prostatic carcinomatosis – careful assessment required.
- Commonly done through a groin incision.
- Ilioinguinal blocks are effective, with surgical infiltration into the scrotum.
- The most painful part is the inguinal incision, so ilioinguinal block may suffice.

Lithotripsy (ESWL)
Anaesthetic issues
- Second-generation lithotripters do not require immersion in water baths and have made lithotripsy a more suitable day case procedure.
- Flank pain at the bombardment site can be severe, and passing stone fragments can be excruciating.
- Women have more pain, perhaps because they have less muscle to cushion the shock waves.
- Pain may limit the duration of lithotripsy, necessitating repeat procedures.
- PONV is common, especially in women – rates of up to 30% have been reported[6].
- Hypertension may occur during and after the procedure.
- Autonomic hyperreflexia can be triggered in patients with spinal cord injury above T6[7].

Strategies
- ESWL is now usually performed using analgesia ± sedation.
- General anaesthesia is now uncommon.
- There must be adequately qualified supervision of the patient. Lithotripter operators are not sufficient, and patient distress and pain must not be ignored.
- Full monitoring is needed as these procedures take place in darkened rooms.
- An anaesthetist or experienced sedationist should be available to give IV analgesia ± sedation.

Patients must not be discharged until standard discharge criteria are met. They are often distressed with pain postoperatively.

Analgesia
- Diclofenac 100 mg PO or PR 30–60 minutes beforehand reduces the requirements for opioid analgesia[8,9].
- EMLA® applied locally may reduce flank pain, more so in men[10,11].

- Alfentanil/fentanyl/pethidine IV ± midazolam IV may also be needed.
- Patient-controlled analgesia (PCA) with boluses of alfentanil 25 µg with a 1 minute lockout allowed higher voltages to be used and reduced treatment times[12].
- Background infusion of alfentanil with smaller boluses has also been used[13].
- Premedication with NSAID + alfentanil PCA may be the best option.

Antiemesis
- Consider routine antiemesis, particularly in patients with risk factors for PONV.

References

1. **Keoghane SR, Millar JM, Cranston DW.** Is day case prostatectomy feasible? *Br. J. Urol.* 1995; **76:** 600–603.
2. **Muruve N, Hosking DH.** Intracorporeal phenylephrine in the treatment of priapism. *J. Urol.* 1996; **155:** 141–143.
3. **Quinney N, Lomas I.** Treatment of priapism during transurethral resection of prostate. *Br. J. Hosp. Med.* 1995; **54:** 393–394.
4. **Zappala SM, Howard PJ, Hopkins TB,** *et al.* Management of intraoperative penile erections with diluted epinephrine solution. *Urology* 1992; **40:** 76–77.
5. **Matthews RD, Nolan JF, Libby-Straw JA,** *et al.* Transurethral surgery using intravesical bupivacaine and intravenous sedation. *J. Urol.* 1992; **148:** 1475–1476.
6. **Watcha MF, White PF.** Postoperative nausea and vomiting. Its etiology, treatment, and prevention. *Anesthesiology* 1992; **77:** 162–184.
7. **Kovac AL.** Recovery room risk and outcome associated with renal extracorporeal shock wave lithotripsy. *J. Clin. Anesth.* 1993; **5:** 364–368.
8. **Dawson C, Vale JA, Corry DA,** *et al.* Choosing the correct pain relief for extracorporeal lithotripsy. *Br. J. Urol.* 1994; **74:** 302–307.
9. **Fredman B, Jedeikin R, Olsfanger D,** *et al.* The opioid-sparing effect of diclofenac sodium in outpatient extracorporeal shock wave lithotripsy (EWSL). *J. Clin. Anesth.* 1993; **5:** 141–144.
10. **Monk TG, Ding Y, White PF,** *et al.* Effect of topical eutectic mixture of local anesthetics on pain response and analgesic requirement during lithotripsy procedures. *Anesth. Analg.* 1994; **79:** 506–511.
11. **Bierkens AF, Maes RM, Hendrikx JM,** *et al.* The use of local anesthesia in second generation extracorporeal shock wave lithotripsy: eutectic mixture of local anesthetics. *J. Urol.* 1991; **146:** 287–289.
12. **Schelling G, Weber W, Mendl G,** *et al.* Patient controlled analgesia for shock wave lithotripsy: the effect of self administered alfentanil on pain intensity and drug requirement. *J. Urol.* 1996; **155:** 43–47.
13. **Kortis HI, Amory DW, Wagner BK,** *et al.* Use of patient-controlled analgesia with alfentanil for extracorporeal shock wave lithotripsy. *J. Clin. Anesth.* 1995; **7:** 205–210.

14.4   Plastic procedures in day surgery
G.E. Rudkin

> Plastic procedures are best performed under local or regional anaesthesia with minimal sedation. This results in good analgesia, smooth patient emergence, rapid recovery and discharge.

Common plastic procedures

- Skin lesion excision with flaps (small to moderate) and skin grafts
- Carpal tunnel decompression
- Tendon repairs and transfers
- Nerve repairs
- Dupuytren's contracture
- Minor hand trauma
- Liposuction
- Augmentation mammoplasty
- Mastopexy
- Rhytidoplasty (face lift)
- Otoplasty (correction prominent ears)
- Rhinoplasty
- Blepharoplasty

Anaesthetic issues
Infusion of large doses of local anaesthetic and adrenaline
- Multiple injections of local anaesthetic and adrenaline may reach maximum recommended doses.
- In the presence of inhalation agents, adrenaline can cause arrhythmias.

General anaesthesia
- With endotracheal intubation, hypertension causes congestion of the operative site, which increases intraoperative bleeding.
- Stormy emergence from continued straining, coughing and vomiting may initiate haematoma formation, and delicate suture lines may be stressed.

Analgesia
- The use of NSAIDs in plastic procedures is a controversial issue. Aspirin and non-aspirin NSAIDs prolong the bleeding time, therefore there are clinical risks of increased bleeding[1]. The risks of complications must be related to the procedure type.

Liposuction
- Blood and fluid loss
  - (i) estimation of blood and fluid loss is difficult;
  - (ii) if patients are underperfused this will pose problems for the day patient.
- Risk of fat embolus[2].

Cost-effective plastic surgery
- Prolonged procedures requiring sedation anaesthesia are often performed in 'office-based' surgeries (conducted in surgeons' private operating facility) with varying equipment, monitoring facilities and standards of nursing care[3].
- Auditing of patient satisfaction, overall costs and complication rates should be performed to determine advantages/disadvantages of managing patients in different facility types, including 'office-based' surgeries.

Strategies
General anaesthesia
- A reinforced laryngeal mask will allow turning of the head without airway compromise: useful for day case head and neck surgery.
- Use of the laryngeal mask will minimize coughing, straining and vomiting with elevation of systemic blood pressure and increased bleeding[4]. It will also avoid the hypertensive response associated with intubation[5].

Local and regional anaesthesia (see Chapter 10)
- Most plastic surgery involves superficial structures with little interference to the patients' physiological function. Hence many long procedures (4–5 hours) can be performed under a local anaesthetic with sedation.
- Close communication between the patient, anaesthetist and surgeon is essential.
- For efficiency, local anaesthetic infiltration should be injected before the surgeon scrubs.
- In most instances minimal sedation is required, with deeper sedation administered initially when local anaesthetic is infiltrated. For surgery around the head and neck safe sedation levels are mandatory, for airway control. Oxygen can be delivered by mouth (see Chapter 11) or by a funnel sitting on the patient's thorax.
- The donor site for skin grafting requires good analgesia. Choices are EMLA® cream if the site is small, local infiltration or nerve blocks. Blocks to the femoral nerve and lateral cutaneous nerve of the thigh can easily be performed singly or by a '3 in 1' lumbar plexus block[6].
- Otoplasty and rhytidoplasty are preferable under local anaesthesia with sedation to avoid haematoma formation which is common following a stormy general anaesthetic emergence.

Analgesia
- Analgesic requirements are usually minimal for most plastic procedures, due to the superficial nature of the surgery and the local/regional techniques used.
- The risk of increased bleeding in patients taking NSAIDs would suggest that patients having selected plastic procedures should not be given NSAIDs perioperatively. In these cases aspirin should also be ceased at least 10 days prior to surgery (unless medically contraindicated).
- Patients with a normal bleeding time can continue aspirin or NSAID therapy before cutaneous surgery[7]. Otley *et al.* have shown a low risk of severe complications in this patient group which is not significantly reduced by preoperative discontinuation of the drug[8].
- It is inadvisable to prescribe NSAIDs for patients having the following procedures, because if bleeding occurs it may be deleterious to the surgical outcome:
  (i)   split skin graft;
  (ii) full thickness graft;
  (iii) rhytidoplasty;

(iv) eyelid reduction;

(v) Dupuytren's contracture.

Local anaesthesia and adrenaline
- Safe doses of local anaesthetic and adrenaline should be used. However, consideration should also be given to the site of injection. In liposuction procedures, delayed uptake of local anaesthetic into the fatty tissues will occur. Peak lignocaine levels do not occur until 11–14 hours after surgery (postdischarge). Klein has shown that serum blood levels remain satisfactory even when doses as high as 35 mg kg^{-1} are used in liposuction[9].
- Patients should have ECG monitoring when adrenaline is used in the presence of inhalation agents to detect arrhythmias.

Blood and fluid replacement in liposuction
- It is difficult to estimate the total volume of blood and fluid loss, as a significant amount of fluid is lost to oedema formation following the procedure. Surgical technique will modify the blood and fluid losses. The 'tumescent' technique is where multiple injections of diluted lignocaine with adrenaline are used[10]. The purported advantages of this technique are adequate anaesthesia, less bleeding, superior aesthetic results and improved postoperative pain relief. The large amounts of local anaesthetic aspirated with this technique further adds to the difficulty of estimating the true fluid loss.
- Fluid replacement can be related to the volume of fat removed[11].

Fat removed	Replacement therapy
500–1000 ml	3000 ml crystalloid
1000–2000 ml	3000 ml colloid
2000–2500 ml	3000 ml crystalloid plus 2 Units blood

- Patients undergoing removal of 1500 ml or more of body fat have a relatively high hospitalization rate varying between 40 and 50%[3].
- Patients having an excessive amount of aspirate (>2000 ml) should not be considered as day patients.
- Estimation of blood loss approximates 80% of the total volume of aspirate (40% = blood in aspirate; 40% = volume of blood lost externally and into dead space)[12].
- To check adequacy of fluid replacement, patients must void prior to discharge.
- Fluids should be encouraged in the early postdischarge period.

Prevention of PONV
- Avoid narcotics.
- Avoid general anaesthesia.
- If general anaesthesia is necessary, prophylactic antiemetics with propofol infusion techniques should be considered.

Cost-effective surgery
- Standards of care must be assured for 'office-based surgery' with adequate monitoring, equipment and resuscitative programmes.
- Drain tubes can be removed by the GP or district nursing service, allowing more procedures to be performed on a day basis.

Discharge instructions
- Patients must receive adequate written discharge instructions addressing care of the anaesthetized limb and checks on vascular sufficiency.
- Instructions for dressing care, keeping the area dry and intact, can be vital to the success of many plastic surgery procedures.

- Adequate patient analgesia must be provided to cover donor site skin-grafting areas. Explanation that this may be more painful than the operation site is important.
- Appropriate selection of analgesics is important, avoiding NSAIDs in plastic procedures where bleeding may jeopardize the surgical outcome.

References

1. **Schafer AI.** Effects of nonsteroidal antiinflammatory drugs on platelet function and systemic hemostasis. *J. Clin. Pharmacol.* 1995; **35:** 209–219.
2. **Laub DR.** Fat embolus syndrome after liposuction: a case report and review of the literature. *Ann. Plast. Surg.* 1990; **25:** 48–52.
3. **Courtiss EH, Goldwyn RM, Joffe JM, et al.** Anesthetic practices in ambulatory aesthetic surgery. *Plast. Reconst. Surg.* 1994; **93:** 792–801.
4. **Cork RC,Depa RM, Standen JR.** Prospective comparison of the use of the laryngeal mask airway and endotracheal tube for ambulatory surgery. *Anesth. Analg.* 1994; **79:** 719–727.
5. **Fujii Y, Tanaka H, Toyooka H.** Circulatory responses to laryngeal mask airway insertion or tracheal intubation in normotensive and hypertensive patients. *Can. J. Anaesth.* 1995; **42:** 32–36.
6. **Flanagan JFK, Edkin B, Spindler K.** 3 in 1 femoral nerve block following ACL reconstruction allows predictably earlier discharge and significant cost savings. *Anesthesiology* 1994; **81:** A950.
7. **Lawrence C, Sabuntabhai A, Tiling-Grosse S.** Effect of aspirin and nonsteroidal antiinflammatory drug therapy on bleeding complications in dermatologic surgical patients. *J. Am. Acad. Dermatol.* 1994; **31:** 988–992.
8. **Otley CC, Fewkes JL, Frank W, et al.** Complications of cutaneous surgery in patients who are taking warfarin, aspirin, or nonsteroidal antiinflammatory drugs. *Arch. Dermatol.* 1996; **132:** 161–166.
9. **Klein JA.** Tumescent technique for local anesthesia; Improves safety in large volume liposuction. *Plast. Reconst. Surg.* 1993; **92:** 1085–1100.
10. **Klein JA.** Tumescent technique for regional anesthesia permits lidocaine doses of 35 mg/kg. *J. Dermatol. Surg. Oncol.* 1990; **16:** 248–263.
11. **Hetter GP.** Blood and fluid replacement for lipoplasty procedures. *Clin. Plast. Surg.* 1989; **16:** 245–248.
12. **Conlay LA.** (1995) Plastic surgery. In: *Ambulatory Anesthesiology* (Ed. KE McGoldrick). Williams and Wilkins, Baltimore, MO. pp. 452–454.

14.5   Orthopaedic procedures in day surgery
G.E. Rudkin

Regional and local techniques provide good postoperative analgesia. Consider surgeon and patient preference, procedure duration and tourniquet use. Balanced analgesia combining local anaesthetic, opioids and non-steroidal anti-inflammatory agents is needed.

Common upper limb procedures

- Shoulder, elbow and wrist arthroscopy
- Nerve/tendon repair
- Release trigger finger and de Quervain's contracture
- Closed reduction of simple fractures
- Open reduction/internal fixation of fingers
- Removal of ganglion cyst
- Carpal tunnel decompression
- Removal of orthopaedic hardware

Anaesthetic issues
Use of tourniquet
- This will alter the choice of local/regional anaesthetic technique.
- Expect patient discomfort postoperatively due to tourniquet ischaemia.

Arthroscopic shoulder surgery
- 'Barber chair' ('beach chair') position or lateral decubitus position will limit airway access and pose the added risk of air embolus. Care should also be taken in this position to prevent traction injury to the brachial plexus.

Postoperative pain
- Initially, moderate to severe pain may occur due to tourniquet ischaemia.
- Severe postoperative pain can be expected following shoulder surgery, unless supplementary local anaesthesia is provided.
- Incidence of unplanned overnight admission can be higher in arthroscopic shoulder surgery if pain is not well controlled[1].

Compartment syndrome
- This is a potential complication of any limb surgery, particularly forearm, where bleeding into a forearm compartment may cause tissue ischaemia. Excessive pain is an early sign.
- Medical staff will be alerted to this problem if the patient's pain is not controlled with routine analgesia. Regional anaesthesia may mask the pain typically seen with compartment syndrome and lead to a delayed diagnosis[2].

Strategies
General anaesthesia
- Propofol induction with alfentanil (7–15 µg kg^{-1}) or fentanyl for longer cases.
- LMA is the best choice and will provide smooth anaesthesia.

- The surgeon or anaesthetist should provide supplementary analgesia with bupivacaine, by local infiltration or nerve block at the shoulder, elbow, wrist or fingers.
- For shoulder surgery, place the head securely on a head ring with some lateral flexion, towards the operated shoulder, but preventing exaggerated flexion or extension.

Local and regional anaesthesia (see Chapter 10)
- Adequate time must be allowed for block insertion and onset time.
- Regional anaesthesia may reduce recovery room time and allow for direct transfer to second-stage recovery.
- An interscalene block is suitable for upper arm or shoulder surgery, either as a sole anaesthetic technique or combined with a general anaesthetic technique for postoperative analgesia. The anaesthetist should inform the patient and nursing staff of interscalene block side-effects such as ptosis or hoarseness. It should not be performed in those with poor respiratory reserve as unilateral diaphragmatic paresis invariably occurs[3].
- A supraclavicular brachial plexus block is a poor choice in day surgery with the associated risk of pneumothorax .
- An axillary brachial plexus block will provide good postoperative analgesia and is useful for surgery on the elbow, forearm and hand.
- Intravenous regional analgesia (Bier's block) is suitable for short superficial procedures on the hand or forearm. Anaesthesia tends to diminish after 45 minutes[4].
- Nerve blocks at the elbow, wrist or fingers are easy to perform and will provide good postoperative supplementary analgesia with the advantage of early postoperative mobilization.
- Short-acting local anaesthetic agents such as lignocaine may be considered in plexus blockade if early mobilization is required or compartment syndrome is a concern.
- Long-acting local anaesthetic agents such as bupivacaine are useful for most local/regional nerve blocks.

Tourniquet (see Chapter 10)
- Tourniquet time should be minimized: all skin marking, planning and discussion should occur before inflation of the cuff.
- Upper limit of tourniquet time is 2 hours[5]. The awake patient will tolerate a tourniquet for this period with an axillary brachial plexus block.
- 250 mmHg pressure is suitable for the adult but 300–350 mmHg may be necessary in those with muscular or obese arms or hypertensives. Alternatively 100 mmHg above systolic blood pressure is chosen[5].
- Distal forearm tourniquet is tolerated longer than upper arm tourniquet[6].
- Without plexus blockade, patient comfort time varies between approximately 30 and 45 minutes. Strategies can be adopted to increase patient comfort, such as sedation, infiltration of local anaesthetic beneath the tourniquet and exsanguination wrap[7] (wrapping entire upper extremity from fingertips to axilla with an Esmarch and then applying the tourniquet on top of the exsanguinating wrap).
- When intravenous regional anaesthesia (Bier's block) is used, a double tourniquet will improve patient comfort.

Patient postoperative instructions
- Patient instruction by physiotherapists prior to discharge will ensure optimal mobilization particularly for shoulder arthroscopy patients, reinforcing correct care and management.

- Cold packs and elevation of the limb will improve patient comfort and reduce swelling.
- Written instructions, emphasizing care of the anaesthetized limb should be given to patients who have undergone plexus anaesthesia.
- Surgeon contact is important, as pain not controllable with routine analgesia may be an initial sign of compartment syndrome.

Common lower limb procedures

- Knee, ankle arthroscopy (diagnostic and therapeutic)
- Bunionectomy
- Hammer toe correction
- Toe amputation
- Open reduction/internal fixation of ankle/foot
- Removal of selective orthopaedic hardware

Anaesthetic issues
Postoperative pain
- Patients who have had therapeutic knee arthroscopy can have severe pain postoperatively requiring opioids. Within 1–3 hours, pain is generally manageable with oral analgesics.

Use of tourniquet
- Cuff inflation pressures are generally higher than in the upper extremity, with a pressure of 150 mmHg above systolic pressure used, and maximum pressure up to 400 mmHg.

DVT risk
- Patients on the oral contraceptive pill having lower leg surgery with tourniquet, have additional risk factors for DVT.

Strategies
General anaesthesia
- LMA is most appropriate.

Local and regional techniques (see Chapter 10)
- Can be used for surgical anaesthesia or supplementary analgesia with a general anaesthetic technique.
- Knee intra-articular analgesia:
  (i) 0.5% bupivacaine (150 mg) through one of the portals; benefits are controversial[8,9];
  (ii) low dose morphine (1–2 mg); benefits are controversial[10,11];
  (iii) Mixture of 0.5% bupivacaine and low-dose morphine.
- Knee arthroscopies can be performed under local anaesthesia alone, where the knee joint is filled with 15–20 ml lignocaine 2% with adrenaline and additional local anaesthetic is infiltrated at the puncture sites[12].
- Alternatively, for knee arthroscopy a '3 in 1 block'[13] (femoral, lateral femoral cutaneous and obturator nerves) can be performed:
  (i) single injection of a large amount (>25 ml) local anaesthetic just lateral to the femoral artery; insertion facilitated by a nerve stimulator;

(ii) advantages include minimal postoperative sequelae, tourniquet not required if local anaesthetic with adrenaline is used;

(iii) shorter-acting local anaesthetics are most appropriate as longer-acting agents may delay discharge due to inability of the patient to ambulate.

- Ankle block. Most appropriate for foot procedures under a calf tourniquet. Patients tolerate a calf tourniquet extremely well for periods of up to 1 hour.
- Epidural/spinal anaesthesia:
  (i) extra time should be allocated for insertion of the block;
  (ii) risk of postdural puncture headache;
  (iii) delayed discharge can occur due to urinary retention.

Tourniquet pressures
- Use of the lowest possible cuff inflation pressure will minimize the effect of compression beneath the pneumatic tourniquet. Curved tourniquets (designed to fit conically shaped limbs) and wider tourniquets facilitate the use of lower tourniquet inflation pressures in lower-extremity surgery[14].

DVT prophylaxis
- The British National Formulary states that the oral contraceptive pill should be stopped 4 weeks before all surgery to the legs[15]. Alternative management is practised in Australia, where prophylactic anticoagulant therapy is instituted when DVT risk factors are present and the pill is not stopped (see *Table 2.4*).

Postoperative instructions
- Patient instruction by physiotherapists prior to discharge will ensure optimal mobilization particularly for knee arthroscopy patients. This will reinforce correct care and management.
- Cold-pack treatment and elevation of the limb will improve patient comfort and swelling.
- Written instructions including care of the anaesthetized lower limb should be provided to patients.
- A foot cradle can be made from a large cardboard box or pillows to keep bed covers off the limb.

References

1. **Kinnard P, Truchon R, St-Pierre A, *et al.*** Interscalene block for pain relief after shoulder surgery. A prospective randomized study. *Clin. Orthopaed. Rel. Res.* 1994; **304**: 22–24.
2. **Hyder N, Kessler S, Jennings AG, *et al.*** Compartment syndrome in tibial shaft fracture missed because of a local nerve block. *J. Bone Joint Surg. (Br.)* 1996; **78B**: 499–500.
3. **Urmey WF, McDonald M.** Hemidiaphragmatic paresis during interscalene brachial plexus block: effects on pulmonary function and chest wall mechanics. *Anesth. Analg.* 1992; **74**: 352–357.
4. **Mulroy MF** (1995) Intravenous regional anesthesia. In: *Regional Anesthesia An Illustrated Procedural Guide* (Ed. MF Mulroy). Little, Brown and Company, Boston, MA. p.184.
5. **Green DP.** (1988) General principles: the tourniquet. In: *Operative Hand Surgery* (Ed. DP Green), 2nd Edn. Churchill Livingstone, New York. Vol. II, pp. 7–26.
6. **Hutchinson DT, McClinton MA.** Upper extremity tourniquet tolerance. *J. Hand Surg.* 1993; **18A**: 206–210.
7. **Dushoff IM.** Hand surgery under wrist block and local infiltration anesthesia, using an upper arm tourniquet (letter). *Plast. Reconstruct. Surg.* 1973; **51**: 685.
8. **Smith I, Van Hemelrijck J, White PF, *et al.*** Effects of local anesthesia on recovery after outpatient arthroscopy. *Anesth. Analg.* 1991; **73**: 536–539.
9. **Henderson RC, Campion ER, DeMasi RA, *et al.*** Postarthroscopy analgesia with bupivacaine. *Am. J. Sports Med.* 1990; **18**: 614–617.

10. **Stein C, Comisel K, Haimeri E,** *et al.* Analgesic effect of intrarticular morphine after arthroscopic knee surgery. *New Engl. J. Med.* 1991; **325:** 1123–1126.
11. **Raja SN, Dickstein RE, Johnson CA.** Comparison of postoperative analgesic effects of intraarticular bupivacaine and morphine following arthroscopic knee surgery. *Anesthesiology* 1992; **77:** 1143–1147.
12. **Leou-Chyr Lin.** Arthroscopy of the knee under local anaesthesia. *J. Orthopaed. Surg.* 1995; **3:** 25–29.
13. **Flanagan JFK, Edkin B, Spindler K.** 3 in 1 femoral nerve block following ACL reconstruction allows predictably earlier discharge and significant cost savings. *Anesthesiology* 1994; **81:** A950.
14. **Pedowitz RA, Gershuni DH, Botte MJ,** *et al.* The use of lower tourniquet inflation pressures in extremity surgery facilitated by curved and wide tourniquets and an integrated cuff inflation system. *Clin. Orthop.* 1993; **287:** 237–244.
15. **British Medical Association and the Royal Pharmaceutical Society of Great Britain** (1996) *Combined Oral Contraceptives.* Surgery. British National Formulary. Vol. 32, p. 37.

14.6   Ophthalmic procedures in day surgery
G.E. Rudkin

> *The elderly eye patient is most suited to local or regional anaesthesia. This technique is reliable and safe, allowing an early return to the patient's home environment.*

Common eye procedures

- Cataract surgery
- Trabeculectomy
- Strabismus correction
- Eyelid surgery
- Ocular surface surgery
- Operations on the lacrimal apparatus
- Vitreoretinal surgery (scleral buckling and vitrectomy)
- Cryopexy and laser therapy

Anaesthetic issues
Hypertension: causes
- Anxiety.
- Antihypertensive medication not taken on the day of surgery.
- Induction of general anaesthesia.
- Phenylephrine mydriatic eye drops can cause peripheral vasoconstriction, left ventricular failure hypertension and coronary artery vasoconstriction with myocardial ischaemia.

Rise in intraocular pressure
- Occurring at laryngoscopy and intubation.
- Temporary rise following retrobulbar and peribulbar anaesthesia[1].

Oculocardiac reflex
- Bradycardia, ectopic beats or sinus arrest can occur from pressure, torsion or pulling on the extraocular muscles – most common in strabismus surgery.

Systemic complications
- Local anaesthesic toxicity from overdose or IV injection.
- Allergic and vasovagal reactions can also occur.
- Local anaesthetic injected directly into the dural cuff surrounding the optic nerve. Symptoms and signs include nausea, confusion, convulsions, unconsciousness, respiratory or cardiac arrest.
- Overdose of adrenaline.

Retrobulbar haemorrhage
- Serious complication occurring in 0.1–1.7% patients with local anaesthetic block[2].
- More likely in those receiving steroids, anticoagulants, aspirin or other NSAIDs.
- Intraocular pressure must be reduced immediately by pressure reducing devices.
- Surgery may have to be postponed.

Globe penetration (needle into the globe) or perforation (through the globe)
- Can occur with both retrobulbar or peribulbar blocks, especially with poor patient co-operation or difficult access.
- More likely in myopic eyes and those who have had retinal detachment[3]. Globes longer than 26 mm are particularly at risk.

Corneal injury
- Regional anaesthesia can suppress lacrimal gland function making the cornea more susceptible to damage.
- Damage can occur from corneal exposure, amethocaine drops (toxic to cornea), trauma (digital massage).

Optic nerve damage
- Direct optic nerve injury can occur following intraconal injection of local anaesthetic.

Extraocular muscle paresis
- High local anaesthetic concentrations result in higher incidence of myotoxicity, where recovery may not be complete in the elderly.
- Causes of postoperative ptosis are multifactorial. These include oedema of upper eyelid from local anaesthetic, effect from pressure applied to globe and upper lid, traction on superior rectus, prolonged patching.

Surgery on only remaining eye
- It is essential that sight is preserved in the remaining eye.
- Provide ideal operating conditions as successful surgery is vital.
- A low-incidence-complication block, such as topical local anaesthesia, should be considered or, in experienced hands, a peribulbar block, keeping the needle more anterior for injection of local anaesthetic.
- General anaesthesia may be considered.

Sedation
- The elderly can have unpredictable responses to sedative agents resulting in a confusional state.

PONV risk
- Greater following general anaesthesia.
- Greater with excessive manipulation of the eye, such as strabismus surgery or retinal detachment.

Strategies
Preoperative
- Establish rapport with the patient to reduce anxiety and stress.
- Instruct the patient to take prescribed antihypertensive medication on the day of surgery.
- Determine the patient's suitability for surgery under local anaesthetic:
  (i)   is there patient agreement?
  (ii) can the patient lie flat?
  (iii) can the patient lie still? (Is persistent coughing a problem?)
  (iv) can the patient obey commands?
- Local anaesthesia administration should be fully explained to the patient.
- Identify patients who may be claustrophobic so that surgical drapes can be tented well away from the face.

- Careful consideration is required before stopping anticoagulants for intraocular surgery; the risk of stopping anticoagulants may be greater than the risk of continuing.

General anaesthesia
- Propofol is advantageous as an induction agent because it minimizes pressor responses[4].
- The reinforced laryngeal mask allows airway maintenance with little risk of occlusion and ease of surgical access.
- Compared with endotracheal intubation, the LMA results in only a minimal rise in intraocular pressure during insertion and removal. There is significantly less straining, coughing and breath-holding at the end of the procedure[5].

Local/regional anaesthesia (see Chapter 10)
- Patient positioning: a head support should be used to prevent movement.
- The atmosphere in theatre should be quiet and conducive to an awake patient.
- A peribulbar technique is effective and safer than retrobulbar technique for cataract surgery[6].
- Injections should be made with the globe in primary gaze so that the optic nerve remains in the normal position.
- Short needles should be used to reduce the incidence of brain-stem anaesthesia. Needles should be no longer than 2.5 cm.
- Needle bevel facing the globe is safer.
- A short-acting agent such as lignocaine is more suitable than bupivacaine. Longer-acting bupivacaine forces the patient to keep an eye patch on longer to prevent corneal exposure.
- Topical anaesthesia with sedation has been used for cataract surgery.
- Sedation agents should be chosen judiciously; 20–40 mg propofol at the insertion of the block or 0.5–2 mg midazolam may be all that is required in the elderly with the patient awake during surgery.
- The anaesthetist must be vigilant to the patient's conscious state during surgery, preventing a sleep state. Patient comfort can be enhanced by hand holding, a warm blanket, support behind the knees and an empty bladder before surgery is commenced
- Monitoring of consciousness, respirations, oxygen saturation and cardiac rhythm is mandatory with sedation or local anaesthetic administration
- Oxygen/air mix can be administered with sedative drugs to prevent desaturation. Drapes should be tented over the patient's face to prevent claustrophobia (see Chapter 11).
- Oxygen should be administered with caution because of the ignition risk with flammable drapes and diathermy (see Chapter 11).

Intraocular pressure reducing devices
- Intraorbital and intraocular pressure can be reduced following periocular anaesthesia by the following mechanisms and devices:
  - (i) digital pressure;
  - (ii) a Honan balloon and mercury manometer. The balloon is inflated to a pressure no greater 30 mmHg total pressure (ideal 20–25 mmHg);
  - (iii) a small bag filled with mercury.
- Pressure should be applied for no longer than 5–10 minutes.
- Prime concern is the maintenance of retinal perfusion, hence the pressure and the length of its application are important.

Oculocardiac reflex
- The surgeon must promptly stop the provoking stimulus.
- Administer intravenous atropine 10–15 µg kg^{-1} and administer 100% oxygen.

Analgesia
- Analgesic requirements vary, depending on the type of surgery undertaken.
- Cataract surgery causes minimal discomfort postoperatively[7], with pain controllable by simple analgesics such as paracetamol. Very severe pain with nausea and vomiting may indicate a rise in intraocular pressure.
- Patients having strabismus surgery have more pain, and opioids are often required. A multimodal approach with NSAIDs and local anaesthetic infiltration is beneficial (see Chapter 9).

Antiemetic
- Administer prophylactic antiemetics to patients undergoing squint repair to minimize emetic sequelae.

Patient postoperative instructions
- An eye pad and shield may be applied, depending on the surgical requirements.
- Patients should not cough, strain or bend as this can increase intraocular pressure.
- Medical attention should be sought if simple analgesics do not control pain, vision deteriorates or the eye becomes red with discharge.

References

1. **Gjotterberg M, Ingemansson S.** Effect of intraocular pressure of retrobulbar injection of xylocaine with and without adrenaline. *Acta Ophthalmol.* 1977; **55**: 709–716.
2. **Cionni RJ, Osher RH.** Retrobulbar hemorrhage. *Ophthalmology* 1991; **98**: 1153–1155.
3. **Ramsay RC, Knobloch WH.** Ocular perforation following retrobulbar anesthesia for retinal detachment surgery. *Am. J. Ophthalmol.* 1978; **86**: 61–64.
4. **Lamb K, James MFM, Janick PK.** The laryngeal mask airway for intraocular surgery; effects on intraocular pressure and stress response. *Br. J. Anaesth.* 1992; **69**: 143–147.
5. **Akhtar TM, McMurray P, Kerr WJ, et al.** A comparison of the laryngeal mask airway with tracheal tube for intraocular ophthalmic surgery. *Anaesthesia* 1992; **47**: 668–671.
6. **Rubin AP.** Compications of local anaesthesia for ophthalmic surgery. *Br. J. Anaesth.* 1995; **75**: 93–96.
7. **Kaoy P. Laing A, Adams K, et al.** Ophthalmic pain following cataract surgery: a comparison between local and general anaesthesia. *Br. J. Ophthalmol.* 1991; **76**: 225–227.

14.7   ENT procedures in day surgery
M. Hitchcock

Common ear operations

- Insertion of grommets
- Myringotomy
- Tympanoplasty

Anaesthetic issues
Patients
- The majority of patients are likely to be children.

Intraoperative problems
- Operations are of short duration.
- Access to the airway is only minimally restricted.
- The use of nitrous oxide may affect the clinical findings.

Postoperative problems
- Pain and bleeding are not usually a problem.
- PONV can be problematical, especially following middle ear surgery[1]. The mechanism for this may be stimulation of the vestibular apparatus during surgery.

Strategies
- Careful assessment of children with chronic colds. Chronic non-purulent runny nose and non-productive cough are common in childhood and are no indication for cancellation of surgery (see Chapter 12).
- Analgesia: simple analgesics are usually sufficient. Consider the use of preoperative analgesia in the form of oral paracetamol, or intraoperative rectal diclofenac (only with parental consent).
- Airway management: use either a face mask or LMA, depending on the expected duration. Beware of dislodgement of the LMA on turning the head.
- The use of nitrous oxide is acceptable unless a diagnosis is being sought.
- PONV can be reduced by the use of TIVA[2]. Prophylaxis with droperidol (5–10 µg kg^{-1}) or ondansetron (4 mg in adults), is indicated, especially in patients with a history of motion sickness[3]. Although these antiemetics are less effective than drugs used to treat motion sickness, such as hyoscine, they have a more favourable side-effect profile[3].

Common nasal operations

- Reduction of fractured nose
- Septoplasty
- Nasal polypectomy
- Cautery to turbinates
- Bilateral antral washout
- Bilateral intranasal antrostomy

Anaesthetic issues
Patients
- Usually young adults.
- Beware an association between nasal polyps and NSAID-induced asthma[4].

Intraoperative problems
- Restricted access to the airway, which must be protected from both blood and mucus.
- Septoplasty and the reduction of fractured nose can cause significant bleeding.

Postoperative problems
- Septoplasty can be painful.
- Bleeding can be a problem following the reduction of fractured noses.
- Swallowed blood predisposes to nausea and vomiting.
- Nose is often packed. Warn patients beforehand.

Strategies
- Consider oral, IV or rectal NSAIDs before septoplasty.
- Surgeons will often pack the nose with cocaine-impregnated gauze before surgery to reduce bleeding and pain.
- The use of the reinforced LMA, with or without a throat pack, is safe[5] in properly selected patients.
- Controlled ventilation may be preferable for septoplasty to reduce intraoperative bleeding; spontaneous respiration is suitable for other operations.
- Alfentanil and fentanyl are the opioids of choice intraoperatively.
- Oral NSAIDs or paracetamol combinations are usually sufficient for postoperative analgesia.

Common oral procedures

- Tonsillectomy
- Adenoidectomy
- Laryngoscopy
- Laser uvulopalatoplasty

Surgical issues
Operations
- Tonsillectomy is not usually performed on a day case basis in the UK due to concerns over bleeding. However, the safety of this procedure has been demonstrated by several investigators, both in the USA and the UK[6-8].

Anaesthetic issues
Patients
- For tonsillectomy and adenoidectomy patients are usually young.
- An association exists between upper respiratory tract infections and the need for adenotonsillectomy.
- Patients for laryngoscopy can be elderly and/or smokers.
- Patients for uvulopalatoplasty may have associated sleep apnoea, and may need overnight admission for observation.

Intraoperative problems
- Restricted access to the airway, which must be protected from both blood and mucus.
- Bleeding may be affected by the use of NSAIDs, although the evidence is conflicting[9,10].
- Laryngoscopy can be very quick, but requires muscle relaxation. This procedure can also be performed under local anaesthesia with or without sedation.
- The use of lasers requires eye protection for both staff and patient.
- There is a risk of airway fires with the use of high oxygen concentrations near laser beams.

Postoperative problems
- Nausea and vomiting are common.
- Adenoidectomy and tonsillectomy are painful.
- Bleeding is a major concern following adenoidectomy and tonsillectomy[11]. Major haemorrhage can occur up to 8 hours following surgery[12].

Strategies
Preoperative
- Bleeding is more common within 6 weeks of an upper respiratory tract infection[13]. Careful preoperative assessment is mandatory (see Chapter 12).
- Patients for adenoidectomy and/or tonsillectomy require blood taken for grouping and saving.
- Although the clinical significance of altered platelet function due to NSAIDs is unclear, avoid ketorolac, especially before haemostasis is achieved[14]. Consider other oral, IV or rectal NSAIDs before adenoidectomy[10,15].
- Consider the use of prophylactic antiemetics in young adults, either oral ondansetron preoperatively, or IV droperidol at induction.

Airway management
- The use of the reinforced LMA is safe[16,17] in properly selected patients for adenoidectomy and/or tonsillectomy. It may be superior to endotracheal intubation in children, as it may reduce the incidence of laryngospasm and oxygen desaturation in the immediate recovery period.
- The reinforced LMA has also been shown to be remarkably resistant to the CO_2 laser[18], and so probably needs no additional protection, but wrap aluminium foil around the tube section if this will be near the beam.
- Laryngoscopy can also be performed through the standard LMA[19].

Anaesthesia
- TIVA offers the advantage of reduced PONV, as well as laryngeal reflex suppression during laryngoscopy.
- Rapid return of airway reflexes is essential in uvulopalatoplasty, and TIVA with propofol has been shown to be beneficial[20].
- **Avoid suxamethonium**, except in the treatment of emergencies or in patients with gastric reflux. If muscle relaxation is required, mivacurium is the drug of choice for operations of short duration.
- Alfentanil and fentanyl are the opioids of choice intraoperatively.

Analgesia
- Some surgeons infiltrate local anaesthetic around the site of surgery[21].
- Fentanyl may be required in small IV boluses in the immediate recovery period.

- Oral NSAIDs or paracetamol combinations are usually sufficient for postoperative and take-home analgesia.
- Patients who have undergone uvulopalatoplasty can be discharged with a lignocaine spray if correctly instructed in its use.

Postdischarge instructions
- Patients undergoing adenoidectomy and/or tonsillectomy must be given clear instructions about what to do if bleeding begins after discharge. It is also useful to fax the patient's general practitioner to inform him or her of any problems encountered and analgesic and antiemetic medication given. Operations such as adenotonsillectomy require good communication between all parties involved.

References

1. **Honkavaara P, Saarnivaara L, Klemola UM.** Prevention of nausea and vomiting with transdermal hyoscine in adults after middle ear surgery. *Br. J. Anaesth.* 1994; **73**: 763–766.
2. **Jellish WS, Leonetti JP, Murdoch JR, et al.** Propofol-based anaesthesia as compared with standard anaesthetic techniques for middle ear surgery. *Otolaryngol. Head Neck Surg.* 1995; **112**: 262–267.
3. **Honkavaara P.** Effect of ondansetron on nausea and vomiting after middle ear surgery during general anaesthesia. *Br. J. Anaesth.* 1996; **76**: 316–318.
4. **Power I.** Aspirin induced asthma. *Br. J. Anaesth.* 1993; **71**: 619–621.
5. **Brimacombe J, Berry A.** The laryngeal mask airway for ENT, head and neck surgery. *J. Otolaryngol.* in press.
6. **Haberman RS, Shattuck TG, Dion NM.** Is outpatient suction cautery tonsillectomy safe in a community hospital setting? *Laryngoscope* 1990; **100**: 511–515.
7. **Helmus C, Grin M, Westfall R.** Same-day-stay adenotonsillectomy. *Laryngoscope* 1990; **100**: 593–596.
8. **Kendrick D, Gibbin K.** An audit of complications of paediatric tonsillectomy, adenoidectomy and adenotonsillectomy. *Clin. Otolaryngol.* 1993; **18**: 115–117.
9. **Splinter WM, Rhine EJ, Roberts DW, et al.** Preoperative ketorolac increases bleeding after tonsillectomy in children. *Can. J. Anaesth.* 1996; **43**: 560–563.
10. **Thiagarajan J, Bates S, Hitchcock M, et al.** Blood loss following tonsillectomy in children. A blind comparison of diclofenac and papaveretum. *Anaesthesia* 1993; **48**: 132–135.
11. **Gallagher JE, Blauth J, Fornadley JA.** Perioperative ketorolac tromethamine and postoperative haemorrhage in cases of tonsillectomy and adenoidectomy. *Laryngoscope* 1995; **105**: 606–609.
12. **Yardley MPJ.** Tonsillectomy, adenoidectomy, and adenotonsillectomy: are they safe day case procedures? *J. Laryngol. Otol.* 1992; **106**: 299–300.
13. **Riding KH.** Otolaryngologic surgery. In: *Ambulatory Anaesthesia and Surgery* (Ed. PF White). WB Saunders, London. pp. 301–309.
14. **Gunter JB, Varughese AM, Harrington JF, et al.** Recovery and complications after tonsillectomy in children: a comparison of ketorolac and morphine. *Anesth. Analg.* 1995; **81**: 1136–1141.
15. **Rusy LM, Houck CS, Sullivan LJ, et al.** Double-blind evaluation of ketorolac tromethamine versus acetaminophen in paediatric tonsillectomy: analgesia and bleeding. *Anesth. Analg.* 1995; **80**: 226–229.
16. **Williams PJ, Bailey PM.** Comparison of the reinforced laryngeal mask airway and tracheal intubation for adenotonsillectomy. *Br. J. Anaesth.* 1993; **70**: 30–33.
17. **Fiani N, Scandella C, Giolitto N, et al.** Comparison of reinforced laryngeal mask airway vs endotracheal tube in tonsillectomy. *Anesthesiology* 1994; **81**: A491.
18. **Brimacombe J.** Incendiary characteristics of the laryngeal and reinforced laryngeal mask airway to CO_2 laser strike – a comparison with two polyvinyl chloride tubes. *Anaesth. Intens. Care* 1994; **22**: 694–697.
19. **Brimacombe J, Sher M, Laing D, et al.** The laryngeal mask airway: a new technique for fibreoptic guided vocal cord biopsy. *J. Clin. Anaesth.* 1996; **8**: 273–275.

20. **Hendolin H, Kansanen M, Koski E,** *et al.* Propofol–nitrous oxide versus thiopentone–nitrous oxide for uvulopalatopharyngoplasty in patients with sleep apnoea. *Acta Anaesthesiol. Scand.* 1994; **38:** 694–698.
21. **Melchor MA, Villafruela MA, Munoz B,** *et al.* Postoperative pain in tonsillectomy in general anaesthesia and local infiltration. *Acta Otorrinolaringol. Esp.* 1994; **45:** 349–355.

14.8   Oral surgery procedures in day surgery
M. Hitchcock

Commonly performed operations

- Extraction of deciduous teeth
- Orthodontic treatment
- Extraction of wisdom teeth
- Conservative treatment
- Division of tongue tie

Anaesthetic issues
Patients
- Usually young and anxious.
- May be children or young adults with special needs, e.g. Down's syndrome or cerebral palsy, who require careful preoperative assessment.
- Time available for preoperative assessment may be limited.
- Often those who can't or *won't* have their surgery done under local anaesthesia.

Intraoperative problems
- All the problems of the shared airway, with limited access to the airway and the need for airway protection, in addition to the need for good surgical access to the mouth.
- Operative time may be very short, less than 5 minutes.
- Patients undergoing surgery under local anaesthesia and sedation require appropriate monitoring and supplemental oxygen (Chapter 11).
- Surgery may take place in an unfamiliar location, removed from in-patient facilities.

Postoperative problems
- Pain can be severe.
- Swelling.
- Bleeding.

Strategies
Preoperative
- Preoperative assessment must be just as careful as for any day case. For patients with special needs this may require careful questioning of carers. Patients with cardiac lesions may need antibiotic prophylaxis.
- For very anxious patients use anxiolytic premedication. For adult patients, 10 mg temazepam is usually sufficient, but don't be afraid to give large, fit, muscular men 20 mg if you have the time to wait to ensure that this drug will be working.
- Consider the use of pre-emptive analgesia:
  (i) the use of preoperative paracetamol, either via the oral or rectal route in children;
  (ii) the use of NSAIDs, e.g. oral ibuprofen or diclofenac, rectal diclofenac, or IV ketorolac at induction[1].
- If drugs are to be given rectally, consent for this must be obtained beforehand, or the patient requested to self-medicate.

Intraoperative
- IV cannulation is almost always required, even in those patients given inhalation induction. In the latter group, sevoflurane is the drug of choice[2].

Airway management
- Avoid the use of suxamethonium, except in the treatment of emergencies or in patients with gastric reflux. Intubation can be achieved using non-depolarizing muscle relaxants, or alternatively with propofol and alfentanil alone[3].
- Airway management can take four forms:
  (i) for the very quick procedures, preoxygenation followed by an IV induction agent may be sufficient;
  (ii) nasal mask: if the procedure will take any longer than this 'quick snatch', then continued oxygenation using spontaneous respiration and a nasal mask, preferably using a total intravenous anaesthetic technique is indicated;
  (iii) reinforced LMA: for more prolonged or extensive oral surgery, the reinforced LMA, in suitable patients (Chapter 6), is almost ideal[4], as it provides excellent airway protection, is tolerated at light planes of anaesthesia without the use of muscle relaxants, does not interfere with surgical access and can safely be left in situ until the return of protective reflexes. Although the use of a throat pack may increase the incidence of postoperative sore throat, it may be useful for stabilizing the LMA[5];
  (iv) endotracheal intubation: for patients in whom use of the reinforced LMA is unsuitable, the airway must be protected using an endotracheal tube, nasal in the case of adults, oral in the case of children. Warming nasal tubes to soften them causes less trauma during insertion.

Analgesia
- Pain and swelling can be problematical in dental patients. The requirement for analgesia must be judged for each patient, but in general, if three or four deciduous teeth are being removed, analgesic requirements are usually minimal, whereas if several permanent teeth are to be removed, intravenous opioid analgesics, such as fentanyl or alfentanil are required. Consider the following:
- Intraoperative analgesia.
  (i) use intravenous fentanyl or alfentanil;
  (ii) dexamethasone is useful in that it not only reduces postoperative pain and nausea, but decreases swelling[6]. Use a single IV dose of 8 mg for a standard adult;
  (iii) **ask the surgeon to inject local anaesthetic in the area concerned if at all possible;**
  (iv) **avoid the use of morphine.**
- Postoperative analgesia:
  (i) if in severe pain on waking, use small IV boluses of fentanyl, 25 µg at 2 minute intervals until visual analogue pain scores are less than 5. Recovery staff can do this safely if the appropriate protocols are in place;
  (ii) simple analgesics are suitable for the vast majority of these patients[7], with an 'analgesic ladder' of paracetamol, co-proxamol/co-dydramol (see *Table 9.6*) and the NSAIDs.

Bleeding
- This can be evident immediately after surgery, when it usually responds to pressure on the empty tooth socket, or postdischarge. Patients should avoid hot drinks for 3–6 hours postoperatively, and must be warned about what to do if bleeding occurs once they are at home.

References

1. **Hitchcock M, Watson BJ, Davies PRF,** *et al.* Codafen continuus for dental day surgery. (Comparison of codafen versus diclofenac.) *Ambulatory Surg.* 1995; **3**: 111–114.
2. **Smith I, Nathanson MH, White PF.** The role of sevoflurane in outpatient anaesthesia. *Anesth. Analg.* 1995; **81**: 567–572.
3. **Alcock R, Peachey T, Lynch M,** *et al.* Comparison of alfentanil with suxamethonium in facilitating nasotracheal intubation in day case anaesthesia. *Br. J. Anaesth.* 1993; **70**: 34–37.
4. **Brimacombe J, Berry A.** The laryngeal mask airway for dental surgery – a review. *Aust. Dental J.* 1995; **40**: 10–14.
5. **Christie IW.** A means of stabilising laryngeal mask airways during dental practice. *Anaesthesia* 1996; **51**: 604.
6. **Baxendale BR, Vater M, Lavery KM.** Dexamethasone reduces pain and swelling following extraction of third molar teeth. *Anaesthesia* 1993: **48**: 961–964.
7. **Chye EP, Young IG, Osborne GA,** *et al.* Outcomes after same-day oral surgery: a review of 1,180 case at a major teaching hospital. *J. Oral Maxillofac. Surg.* 1993; **51**: 846–849.

CHAPTER 15

Postoperative morbidity following day surgery

M. Hitchcock

Postoperative morbidity associated with day surgery is of fundamental importance. If the expansion of day surgery continues, both in terms of the numbers of patients treated and the scope of operations undertaken, it is essential to know how patients fare after surgery, and especially after discharge. The concept underlying day surgery is that anaesthesia and surgery can be safely performed to produce the same quality of care as that achieved in any in-patient setting, and this should not be compromised by the pressure to expand day surgery or to cut costs.

Complications in day surgery are usually classified into major and minor, according to descriptions by Natof[1] (*Table 15.1*).

Table 15.1. Major and minor morbidity following day surgery

Major complication[a]	Minor complication[b]
Myocardial infarction	Pain
Pulmonary embolus	PONV
Respiratory failure	Dizziness, lethargy or drowsiness
Cerebrovascular accident	Sore throat or hoarseness
Catastrophic postoperative haemorrhage	Headache
Unrecognized damage to viscus	Infection
	Minor bleeding

[a]A major complication is one with the potential for serious harm.
[b]A minor complication is one with minimal or no potential for serious harm.

Several studies have shown that mortality is extremely rare, and major complications uncommon[2,3]. Mortality following day surgery varies between 1 in 66 500 and 1 in 11 273. The major complications after day surgery (*Table 15.1*) are distributed evenly throughout ASA groups. Using population-based epidemiological data, it has been shown that in the absence of unusual perioperative events, major morbidity occurs less often than would have been have been expected for this patient population[2]. The overall incidence of major complications following day surgery is 1 in 1455.

> *Major morbidity is uncommon after day surgery.*

Minor morbidity is very common and day surgery may be associated with a wide range of minor complications[4]. The minor morbidity reported by day case patients depends on what investigators looked for. The most common complications following day surgery are shown in *Table 15.1*. These complications are not only unpleasant for patients, but can have a profound effect on the time taken for them to recover. While 53% of all day case patients resume their normal activities on the first postoperative day, one study found that the mean number of days required was 5, with hand surgery being associated with the longest delay, at 21 days[5]. While major complications, with their potential for serious harm, are obviously important, these minor complications may cause greater concern due to their relative frequency[6].

> *Minor morbidity is not 'minor' to patients.*

Prediction of complications

The prediction of morbidity following day surgery is not straightforward. Considerable emphasis has traditionally been placed on strict patient and operative selection criteria for day surgery in the belief that this will limit postoperative problems. However, several investigators have found that many of the selection criteria which have previously limited the expansion of day surgery are of little predictive value[7] (Chapter 2).

Although general anaesthesia and some types of surgery, e.g. laparoscopic surgery, have been shown to have increased postoperative morbidity[8], in general ASA[9] status and patient fitness relate poorly to the incidence of complications after day surgery. Chung and Baylon[8] found that adverse outcomes at 24 hours after surgery were associated with general anaesthesia, non-gynaecological surgery and duration of surgery >1 hour. Meridy found that age and duration of surgery were of no predictive value[7]. Despite this, selection criteria based on age and duration of surgery are widely used.

Accurate prediction of morbidity and adverse outcome would enable selection criteria and management to be based on risk assessment for patients with specific characteristics or for specific operations.

While ASA status predicts complication rates in in-patients, there is no evidence that ASA 3 day case patients suffer a higher incidence of complications than those of ASA 1 or 2. Similarly, no evidence exists that ASA 3 day cases fare any worse than similar patients undergoing the same operation but as in-patients[6].

As most complications following day surgery are minor, it is perhaps not surprising that complications are unrelated to ASA status, which does not recognize the severity of the surgical procedure or potential hazards such as difficult intubation.

The nature and extent of surgery, and the type of anaesthesia used, exert a marked effect on the incidence of postoperative morbidity. Certain operations are often associated with postoperative morbidity[10], commonly pain or PONV. Persistent symptoms delaying home readiness have been related to both the type and duration of surgery[11]. Patients who have undergone laparoscopy or orthopaedic or general surgery have a sixfold increased risk of developing persistent symptoms. The future scope of day surgery will depend on the reduction of morbidity for these types of surgery.

Certain drugs and anaesthetic techniques are similarly associated with a greater incidence of morbidity than others (*Table 15.2*). Suxamethonium is associated with a prohibitively high incidence of muscle pains, and should be avoided in day case anaesthesia[12]. Morphine is associated with an increased incidence of PONV relative to fentanyl and alfentanil and NSAIDs[13], and endotracheal intubation causes a greater incidence of sore throat than the use of the LMA[14,15]. The relative importance of such minor morbidity in day surgery means that routine in-patient methods of anaesthetic management are not always suitable for use in day case patients if a high quality of care is to be achieved.

Table 15.2. Dos and don'ts to avoid anaesthetic-related morbidity

Do allow patients to drink up to 2 hours before surgery (black coffee is acceptable)
Do use TIVA
Do use the LMA in preference to endotracheal intubation in suitable patients
Do use the lowest effective dose of centrally acting drugs such as droperidol
Do use pre-emptive analgesia with NSAIDs or simple analgesics where possible
Do use local anaesthesia, either alone or to supplement general anaesthesia, whenever possible
Do use prophylactic antiemetics in at-risk patients
Do provide patients with accurate information regarding their surgery and a realistic description of their likely postoperative course

Don't use morphine
Don't use suxamethonium
Don't use reversal agents unless clinically indicated

> *Postoperative morbidity is generally related to the procedure undertaken and the anaesthesia used. Patient fitness is a poor predictor of complications following day surgery. ASA status is too insensitive.*

When do complications occur ?

The ability to predict when complications might occur after day surgery would enable duration of stay in the day surgery unit needed for safety to be determined. Serious postoperative complications are usually evident by the end of surgery, or within the first 3 postoperative hours[16].

However, time taken for potential complications to become evident can be much longer. Patel and Hanallah have shown that while postoperative haemorrhage after day case tonsillectomy was uncommon, with an incidence of 0.7%, it occurred up to 8 hours after surgery[17]. To ensure that day case tonsillectomy is as safe as possible, a recovery stay of at least 8 hours is recommended; this may have cost implications[18].

> *A third of all postoperative complications occur over 48 hours after surgery[2]. Studies of postoperative morbidity limited to the first 24 hours after surgery may underestimate morbidity.*

How long does morbidity following day surgery last?

Phillip[19] has shown that 86% of day case patients complain of at least one minor sequela after discharge, and this persists for 1 day in 59% of patients, for 2 days in 28%, and for 3 days or longer in 14%.

> *Minor morbidity following day surgery may not be transient and can have implications for the time taken to return to work and the burden of care placed on community health services.*

Unplanned admission

Most studies of morbidity following day surgery have concentrated on its role in unplanned hospital admission[20]. Although this ignores morbidity occurring following discharge, unplanned admission is important as it represents a fundamental failure in the provision of day surgery. Not only does it have significant financial implications, but it conceals the number of patients who go home with postoperative morbidity which is not quite bad enough to merit admission, but is still considerable.

The incidence of unplanned admission varies between 0.1 and 5%[7,21]. Surgical factors are responsible for much of this; one study found that more extensive surgery than anticipated, rather than surgical misadventure, accounted for 63.2% of unanticipated admissions[21]. Pre-existing medical diseases and perioperative complications accounted for 19.9%, social reasons a further 4.7%, and anaesthesia-related reasons 12.7%.

Increased community health service workload

The extent of the burden placed on general practitioners and community services depends on the quality of day surgical care provided. High quality day surgery performed in a dedicated unit means that although 48% of patients will require some form of community health care following discharge, this may be simply additional information given over a telephone regarding the removal of sutures[22]. The increased workload placed upon general practitioners in this way may be as little as 4 minutes per patient over the first 5 days following surgery[22].

Minor morbidity – factors and management

The most common problems after day surgery which can be influenced by the anaesthetist are pain, PONV and recovery problems such as drowsiness, dizziness and lethargy. Other side-effects may be less likely to affect overall outcome but may not be easy to prevent.

Pain
It has been claimed that two-thirds of all unplanned admissions following day surgery are due to uncontrolled pain[7], and more recent audits have shown that moderate to severe pain occurs in 30% of day case patients[23]. The prevention, assessment and management of pain following day surgery are dealt with in Chapter 9.

> Pain is a common form of morbidity following day surgery.

Postoperative nausea and vomiting (PONV)
PONV is a frequent problem following day surgery and anaesthesia[24]. Many factors, both surgical and anaesthetic, in addition to patient characteristics, are implicated in its aetiology[25]. Prevention of PONV requires careful assessment of the anticipated risk of PONV and the adaptation of the anaesthetic technique to avoid those anaesthetic factors known to increase its incidence. These issues are dealt with in Chapter 8. The importance patients attach to the prevention of PONV should not be underestimated[26].

Other minor morbidity
Headache. Headache ranks among the most frequent minor postoperative sequelae. The use of volatile anaesthesia, tracheal intubation, and relative dehydration may be implicated[27]. Patients accustomed to high caffeine intake may develop withdrawal headaches due to preoperative fasting[28], and the prophylactic use of caffeine tablets has been shown to effective in reducing their incidence[29].

Drowsiness and dizziness. Drowsiness following day surgery is not uncommon, with an incidence of between 11 and 23%[30,31]. Prolonged drowsiness is related to the duration of surgery, to the anaesthetic drugs used, or to the side-effects of supplementary drugs, for example, opioids or antiemetics[32,33]. Propofol has been repeatedly shown to produce rapid clear-headed recovery relative to other intravenous induction agents and volatile agents[34–36], and as such is the drug of choice for both induction and maintenance of anaesthesia. All supplementary drugs acting centrally used should be short acting and, where their use is unavoidable, they should be used in the lowest effective dose[37]. The newer volatile agents, desflurane and sevoflurane, have been shown to cause less residual drowsiness than other volatiles, but have the same incidence of PONV[38,39].

Sore throat. The incidence of sore throat is related to the use of endotracheal tubes, and the use of the LMA in suitable patients may reduce this[13,14] (Chapter 6). The use of unhumidified anaesthetic gases may also be important, and this effect can be reduced by the use of filters.

Patient dissatisfaction. Postoperative pain and PONV, the types of morbidity which cause the greatest patient dissatisfaction, are also the commonest. In addition, PONV has been shown to be the form of morbidity patients are most concerned to avoid[26]. Overall, however, patients are highly satisfied with day surgical treatment[41], and as the types of morbidity that occur are not exclusive to day surgery and seldom improve due to specific in-patient treatment, it can be argued that, provided the severity and duration of these problems are acceptable, patients prefer to go home following their operation. Further research is required to determine what level of morbidity patients regard as compatible with discharge.

> *Most morbidity that occurs following day surgery is minor in that it has little or no potential for serious harm. However, minor morbidity is of major importance to patients. Although the type of surgery performed exerts a marked effect on the incidence of morbidity, so too does anaesthesia. While morbidity-free day surgery is an ideal, the appropriate choice of anaesthetic drugs and techniques may reduce the incidence of morbidity to acceptable levels.*

References

1. **Natof HE.** (1985) Complications. In: *Anaesthesia for Ambulatory Surgery* (Ed. BV Wetchler). JB Lippincott Co., Philadelphia, PA. p. 321.
2. **Warner MA, Shields SE, Chute CG.** Major morbidity and mortality within one month of ambulatory surgery and anaesthesia. *J. Am. Med. Assoc.* 1993; **270:** 1437–1441.
3. **Natof HE.** FASA survey results revised, as reported by Wetchler BV, Outpatient Anaesthesia. No double standard. *Anesth. Patient Safety Found. Newsletter* 1987; **2:** 8.
4. **Duncan PG, Cohen MM, Tweed WA, et al.** The Canadian four-centre study of anaesthetic outcomes: III. Are anaesthetic complications predictable in day surgical practice ? *Can. J. Anaesth.* 1992; **39:** 440–448.
5. **Vaghadia H, Smythe S.** Long term follow-up after ambulatory surgery: b) return to function. *Abstracts of Society of Ambulatory Anaesthesia Meeting*, Chicago, 1994.
6. **Hitchcock M, Ogg TW.** (1996) Follow-up and postdischarge complications. In: *Ambulatory Anaesthesia and Surgery* (Ed. PF White). WB Saunders, London. pp. 526–533.
7. **Meridy HW.** Criteria for selection of ambulatory surgical patients and guidelines for anaesthetic management: a retrospective study of 1553 cases. *Anesth. Analg.* 1982; **61:** 921–926.
8. **Chung F, Baylon GJ.** Persistent symptoms delaying discharge after day surgery. *Can. J. Anaesth.* 1994; **40:** A21.

9. **American Society of Anesthesiologists** New classification of physical status. *Anesthesiology* 1963; **24**: 111.
10. **Madsen MR, Jensen KEJ.** Postoperative pain and nausea after laparoscopic cholecystectomy. *Surg. Laparosc. Endosc.* 1992; **2**: 303–305.
11. **Chung F.** Recovery pattern and home-readiness after ambulatory surgery. *Anesth. Analg.* 1995; **80**: 896–902.
12 **Alcock R, Peachey T, Lynch M,** *et al.* Comparison of alfentanil with suxamethonium in facilitating nasotracheal intubation in day case anaesthesia. *Br. J. Anaesth.* 1993; **70**: 34–37.
13. **Weinstein MS, Nicholson SC, Schreiner MS.** A single dose of morphine sulphate increases the incidence of vomiting after outpatient inguinal surgery in children. *Anesthesiology* 1994; **81**: 572–577.
14. **Alexander CA, Leach AB.** Incidence of sore throats with the laryngeal mask. *Anaesthesia* 1989; **44**: 791.
15. **Lee SK, Hong KH, Choe H,** *et al.* Comparison of the effects of the laryngeal mask airway and endotracheal intubation on vocal function. *Br. J. Anaesth.* 1993; **71**: 648–650.
16. **Koka BV, Jeon IS, Andre JM,** *et al.* Postintubation croup in children. *Anesth. Analg.* 1977; **56**: 501.
17. **Patel RI, Hanallah RS.** Anaesthetic complications following paediatric ambulatory surgery: a 3 year study. *Anesthesiology* 1988; **69**: 1009–1012.
18. **Sung YF, Reiss N, Tillette T.** The differential cost of anaesthesia and recovery with propofol–nitrous oxide anaesthesia versus thiopental sodium–isoflurane–nitrous oxide anaesthesia. *J. Clin. Anesth.* 1991; **3**: 391–394.
19. **Philip BK.** Patients' assessment of ambulatory anaesthesia and surgery. *J. Clin. Anesth.* 1992; **4**: 355–358.
20. **Gold BS, Kitz DS, Lecky JH,** *et al.* Unanticipated admission to the hospital following ambulatory surgery. *J. Am. Med. Assoc.* 1989; **262**: 3008–3010.
21. **Levy ML.** Complications: prevention and quality assurance. *Anesth. Clin. North Am.* 1987; **5**: 137–166.
22. **Fletcher J, Dawes M, McWilliam J,** *et al.* Day surgery and community health services workload: a descriptive study. *Br. J. Gen. Prac.* 1996; **46**: 477–478.
23. **Hitchcock M, Ogg TW.** Quality assurance in day case anaesthesia. *Ambulatory Surg.* 1994; **2**: 193–204.
24. **Watcha MF, White PF.** Postoperative nausea and vomiting: its aetiology, treatment and prevention. *Anesthesiology* 1992; **77**: 162–184.
25. **Lerman J.** Surgical and patient factors involved in postoperative nausea and vomiting. *Br. J. Anaesth.* 1992; **69** (Suppl. 1): 24S–32S.
26. **Orkin F.** What do patients really want? Preferences for immediate postoperative recovery. *Anesth. Analg.* 1992; **74**: S225.
27. **Nikolajsen L, Larsen KM, Kierkegaard O.** Effect of previous frequency of headaches, duration of fasting and caffeine abstinence on perioperative headache. *Br. J. Anaesth.* 1994; **72**: 295–297.
28. **Weber JG, Ereth MH, Danielson DR.** Perioperative ingestion of caffeine and postoperative headache. *Mayo Clin. Proc.* 1993; **68**: 842–845.
29. **Hampl KF, Schneider MC, Ruttimann U,** *et al.* Perioperative administration of caffeine tablets for prevention of postoperative headaches. *Can. J. Anaesth.* 1995; **42**: 789–792.
30. **Chung FF, Un V, Theodorou-Michaloliakou C.** Adverse outcomes after outpatient anaesthesia: III The effects of anaesthetic agents. *Can. J. Anaesth.* 1993; **40**: A22.
31. **Swann DG, Spens H, Edwards SA,** *et al.* Anaesthesia for gynaecological laparoscopy – a comparison between the laryngeal mask airway and tracheal intubation. *Anaesthesia* 1993; **48**: 431–434.
32. **Davis PJ, McGowan FX, Landsman I,** *et al.* Effect of antiemetic therapy on recovery and hospital discharge time. *Anesthesiology* 1995; **83**: 956–960.
33. **Melnick B, Sawyer R, Karambelkar D,** *et al.* Delayed side-effects of droperidol after ambulatory general anaesthesia. *Anesth. Analg.* 1989; **69**: 748–751.
34. **Heath PJ, Ogg TW, Gilks WR.** Recovery after day-case anaesthesia. A 24-hour comparison of recovery after thiopentone or propofol anaesthesia. *Anaesthesia* 1990; **45**: 911–915.
35. **Millar JM, Jewkes CF.** Recovery and morbidity after day case anaesthesia. A comparison of propofol with thiopentone–enflurane anaesthesia with and without alfentanil. *Anaesthesia* 1988; **43**: 738–743.

36. **Pollard BJ, Bryan A, Bennett D,** *et al.* Recovery after oral surgery with halothane, enflurane, isoflurane or propofol anaesthesia. *Br. J. Anaesth.* 1994; **72**: 559–566.

37. **Melnick BM.** Extrapyramidal reactions to low-dose droperidol. *Anesthesiology* 1988; **69**: 424–426.

38. **Ghouri AF, Bodner M, White PF.** Recovery profile following desflurane–nitrous oxide versus isoflurane–nitrous oxide in outpatients. *Anesthesiology* 1991; **74**: 419–424.

39. **Huang S, Wong CH, Yang JC,** *et al.* Comparison of emergence and recovery times between sevoflurane and propofol as maintenance in adult outpatient surgery. *Anesthesiology* 1994; **81**: A6.

40. **Black N, Sanderson C.** Day surgery: development of a questionnaire for eliciting patients' experiences. *Qual. Health Care* 1993; **2**: 157–161.

41. **Ratcliffe F, Lawson R, Millar J.** Day-case laparoscopy revisited: have postoperative morbidity and patient acceptance improved ? *Health Trends* 1994; **26**: 47–49.

CHAPTER 16

Patient recovery and discharge

G.E. Rudkin

Dedicated DSUs have indisputable advantages over their hospital-integrated counterparts. Although the increased initial capital outlay has been recognized, the dedicated unit offers higher quality of service at lower running costs. The development of a team spirit is more likely amongst nurses in a dedicated facility, allowing more efficient use of nurses, easier recruitment and better organization[1]. A recently published multicentre study conducted in Australia and New Zealand highlighted differences in the standards achieved between freestanding (self-contained) and non-dedicated facilities (i.e. hospital integrated with either a dedicated day surgery recovery area or in-patient mixed recovery room). Hospital-integrated units with a mixed recovery room had the least favourable outcome results[2].

> *There are distinct advantages in having a dedicated recovery area for day patients: a better quality of care and increased efficiency in patient throughput with its inherent cost advantages.*

Phases of patient recovery

Patient recovery from anaesthesia must be evaluated in terms of both speed and quality. It can be separated into three main phases: early, intermediate and late[3] (*Figure 16.1*).

Assessment of early recovery involves the measurement of physiological parameters such as blood pressure and respiration rate and a basic appraisal of alertness (*Table 16.1*).

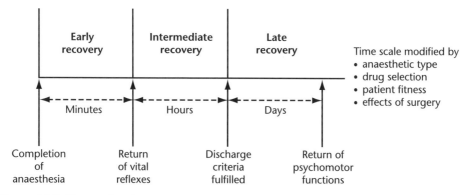

Figure 16.1. Phases of patient recovery.

Table 16.1. Tests of early recovery

Eyes open
Date of birth
Orientation (place, date, name of head of country)
Able to obey commands
Aldrete postanaesthesia score (activity, respiration, circulation, consciousness, colour)[4]
Steward score (consciousness, colour)[5]
Modified Steward score[6,7]
Excitement score[8]

Intermediate recovery lasts until the patient has reached 'home readiness', that is, he or she is clinically stable and able to rest at home under the care of a responsible adult[9]. It is only at the end of the late recovery phase, when all psychomotor functions have returned to normal, that the patient is deemed 'street fit'[10].

With the introduction of shorter-acting anaesthetic agents such as propofol, patients can pass rapidly through the different phases of recovery, and the late recovery period is reduced from days to hours. However, more outcome studies are required to further quantify the full impact of these newer drugs on complete day patient recovery.

> The time spent in each phase of recovery may be influenced by both the drugs and techniques used by the anaesthetist. Rapid initial wake-up may not correlate with a return to normal function.

Staged recovery room facilities

Definitions of recovery facilities or postanaesthesia care units (PACU) vary in different countries. For convenience, terminology used will refer to first- and second-stage recovery facilities.

First-stage recovery
This is commonly referred to as the 'recovery room'. It is the acute care recovery ward and demands the same high standards of nursing care and monitoring as for in-patient recovery.

Aim. Patient to reach a level of recovery where close nursing staff supervision is no longer necessary.

Patient end points.
- Stable vital signs.
- Recovered protective reflexes.
- Able to obey commands.

Second-stage recovery
This is commonly referred to as the 'ward' or 'step-down unit'.

Aim. Patient to reach a level of recovery where they can safely be discharged from the day surgery facility with a suitable adult carer. There should be minimal nausea and vomiting and pain able to be managed in the home environment.

Patient end point. Discharge criteria met.

There are differences in the structured care provided by nursing staff in the two stages of recovery (*Table 16.2*). Ideally, for ease of patient transfer and anaesthetist and surgeon access, the patient recovery area should be in close proximity to the operating room. Nursing staff benefit from physically adjoining first- and second-stage recovery facilities because staff can move easily from one area to the other, depending on patient needs.

Table 16.2. Comparison of staged patient recovery care

First stage	Second stage
High nurse:patient ratio	Low nurse:patient ratio
15 minute patient observations	Observation on arrival, half-hourly and discharge
Intravenous (IV) therapy administered	Oral food and fluid offered (supplemented with IV fluids as necessary)
Drugs administered IV	Drugs encouraged orally (supplemented with IV drugs as necessary, e.g. antiemetics)
No carers allowed entry	Carers may accompany patients and receive discharge instructions
Acute care scoring system, e.g. Aldrete	Day surgery discharge scoring system, e.g. PADSS

PADSS, postanaesthesia discharge scoring system.

Monitoring and safety
Appropriate monitoring of the patient in the recovery period is important from a safety aspect, particularly as longer and more complex procedures are being performed in day surgery. The same safety standards apply as for in-patient recovery where patients are managed by suitably qualified staff. Recovery room staff should be familiar with day patient requirements and priorities, and progress patients through the early stages of recovery until discharge with minimal complications. They must recognize the importance of personalized patient care and the institution of early protocols for nausea and vomiting and pain management following surgery[11,12]. There has been a recent trend to reduce patients' recovery room times to a minimum so that costs are minimized.

> *Refined surgical techniques, newer short-acting anaesthetic drugs, improved regional and sedation techniques and reliable discharge criteria may shorten recovery times. However, primary considerations must be patient safety and comfort.*

Guidelines for patient assessment through recovery room phases
In the past it has been popular for day surgery staff to keep patients in the recovery room for specified periods of time and then assess fitness for discharge. This is time-based recovery of patients. However, it is an inappropriate method of recovery room care for

two reasons. Firstly because of the vast individual variation in patient well-being following surgery or procedural work; and secondly, due to the advent of minimally invasive surgery, the introduction of short-acting anaesthetic agents and infusion techniques, most patients can safely progress faster through recovery room stages than the predetermined times set down.

The alternative and recommended method of patient assessment in the recovery room is criteria-based recovery. This method allows patients to progress through each stage of recovery and discharge at their own speed, according to specified criteria.

The transfer from first-stage recovery room to second-stage recovery is made when patients meet specific criteria (*Figure 16.2*):

- stable vital signs;
- recovered protective reflexes;
- obey commands.

In some facilities a well-recognized postanaesthesia recovery scoring system is used, such as the Aldrete scoring system[13,14] where staff assign scores to patient activity, respiration, circulation, consciousness and skin colour[4].

These scoring systems cannot be used for day surgery patient discharge, as they do not address patient ambulation, pain or emesis. Evaluation of patient discharge may be based on discharge criteria which should be met, using an objective scoring system of functions such as ambulation and pain control to ensure safe recovery and discharge following anaesthesia.

Should we use any other methods of assessment in recovery?

Psychomotor tests and driving simulators can be used to assess a patient's overall recovery. However, these tests are complex, require skilled operators, take considerable

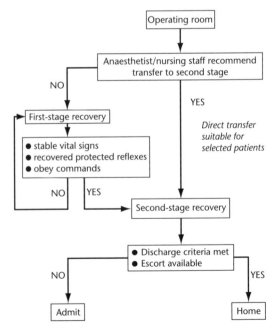

Figure 16.2. Flow chart for staged patient transfer in the recovery room.

time to implement and are generally not useful to apply to routine clinical practice[15,16]. Nevertheless, these tests remain useful as research tools for the objective assessment of new drugs and techniques used on day surgery patients prior to their discharge home.

Direct patient transfer from operating theatre to second-stage recovery room

More recently there has been a trend for selected patients to transfer directly to second-stage recovery from the operating theatre (*Figure 16.2*). Patients who are suitable for direct transfer to second-stage recovery are shown in *Table 16.3*.

Table 16.3. Patient suitability for direct transfer to second-stage recovery

Patients who have received local anaesthesia only
Patients who have received local anaesthesia and minimal sedation with short-acting drugs
Patients who have received regional anaesthesia such as upper or lower limb extremity blocks either alone or in combination with minimal sedation using short-acting drugs (not spinal or epidural anaesthesia)

Before deciding on direct transfer, the anaesthetist or surgeon should have ascertained that the patient:

- is awake;
- is alert;
- is responsive;
- has stable vital signs;
- is able to move with minimal assistance;
- has manageable pain;
- has no nausea and vomiting.

The anaesthetist, in conjunction with day surgery nursing staff, should make the decision as to who is suitable for direct second-stage transfer.

Common recovery room problems

Recovery room problems vary depending on the phase of the patient's recovery. Common first-stage recovery room problems include uncontrolled pain, nausea, vomiting and changes in blood pressure, both low and high. Patients in second-stage recovery pose additional problems such as syncope, which Wetchler describes as symptoms of dizziness, drowsiness, weakness and hypotension, either singly or in combination[17]. Syncope can be dealt with quickly by Trendelenburg tilt, oxygen administration, fluids and a vasopressor such as ephedrine. Implementing a management plan as soon as possible avoids delaying discharge or subsequent admission.

Factors affecting patient recovery period

The duration of the patient's stay in the first- and second-stage recovery rooms following surgery varies with the specific surgical case mix and anaesthetic techniques used in the particular facility. In a study by Chung, using a day surgery discharge criteria scoring system, 82% of patients were safely discharged 1–2 hours following their surgery, and 95.6% of patients discharged within 3 hours[9]. Patients undergoing dilatation and curettage and cataract extractions under local anaesthesia were discharged faster than patients undergoing laparoscopy, orthopaedic or general surgical procedures. Patients undergoing these latter procedures also had a sixfold increased risk of developing postoperative symptoms up to 24 hours following surgery.

In an Australian outcome study of 6000 day cases, the mean recovery times were longer after general anaesthesia compared with patients undergoing local or regional anaesthesia. Recovery times were significantly longer after gynaecological laparoscopy than after other common day surgery procedures. Patient recovery times did not correlate with patient age and only weakly correlated with procedure duration[13].

Nausea and vomiting, as well as pain, should be minimized following surgery. Cardosa *et al.* showed that, in a study of 465 day patients undergoing knee arthroscopies, postoperative pain, nausea and vomiting significantly prolonged postoperative recovery times, with most delay associated with nausea and vomiting[18]. It is important to be aware that there are financial costs incurred by patients experiencing prolonged postoperative nausea and vomiting[19].

With the introduction of more complex and painful procedures it is expected that recovery room times may be significantly longer for certain surgery, such as laparoscopic cholecystectomy. Published reports have also shown that patients undergoing this procedure have a higher admission rate[12].

Procedure cost effectiveness must be addressed. If a day surgery unit is running at full capacity it may be more cost-effective to perform a larger number of shorter surgical procedures than longer surgical procedures such as laparoscopic cholecystectomy. Alternatively the cost effectiveness of longer procedures may be justified by avoiding overnight stays with higher nursing costs.

Marais *et al.* have shown that nursing salaries constitute half of all day surgery costs[20]. Reduction in recovery room times can therefore provide a more cost-effective service. Data collected on specific times that patients spend in various stages of day surgery should be benchmarked for specific procedures as a guide for other day care facilities, providing criteria are met for patient safety and comfort. It would be anticipated that with the introduction of Chung's modified discharge criteria[14], and continuing improvements in surgery and anaesthetic drugs and techniques, patient recovery times could be further reduced.

> *Recovery times are primarily affected by the surgical procedure and the anaesthetic technique. More complex procedures with longer surgical and recovery room times can now be performed safely in day surgery. However, the cost effectiveness of performing these procedures needs to be assessed.*

Administrative challenges relating to the recovery room

It is important that lines of responsibility and authority are clearly set out, particularly regarding the decision for admission, medical management of unstable patients and responsibility for discharge. However, the ultimate responsibility and authority lies with the medical director. An anaesthetist is most suited as a medical director, having expertise in preoperative assessment, anaesthesia, recovery room care and the ability to make patient discharge decisions.

The day surgery team, consisting of the medical director, anaesthetists, surgeons and nursing staff, should be responsible for setting the operational policy, including practical protocols such as how and where the patient is transferred if admission is required. These policies must undergo regular review and modification because of the changing criteria and newer procedures in an expanding day surgery population group.

The day surgery team is also responsible for audit, staff development and instituting programmes to update staff recovery emergency skills and performance evaluation.

Patient discharge

There are distinct advantages in the use of defined criteria or a scoring system for patient discharge; they are important for patient comfort, safety and for medico-legal reasons. A written discharge policy, preferably involving 'signing out' the patient, is good practice and a requirement of most accreditation bodies. Korttila has compiled a set of day surgery discharge criteria and several variations on these have been developed (*Table 16.4*)[3].

Table 16.4. Guidelines for safe discharge

Vital signs stable for at least 1 hour
The patient must be
    oriented to person, place, time
    able to tolerate orally administered fluids[a]
    able to void[b]
    able to dress
    able to walk without assistance
The patient must not have
    more than minimal nausea or vomiting
    excessive pain
    bleeding
The patient must be discharged by both the person who gave anaesthesia and the person who performed the surgery, or their designees
Written instructions for the postoperative period at home, including a contact place or person, need to be reinforced
Patients must have a responsible 'vested' adult to escort them home and to stay with them at home

Reproduced from **Korttila K.** (1995) Recovery from outpatient anaesthesia. *Anaesthesia* 1995; **50** (Suppl.): 22–28 (Table 4) with permission from Academic Press.
[a]Drinking is recommended before discharge but is not mandatory.
[b]Voiding is recommended as a criterion for discharge but is not mandatory. It should be required after spinal or epidural blocks and pelvic-related surgery.

Important aspects of a discharge scoring system are that it:

- is valid and reliable;
- is simple;
- is practical;
- is easy to remember;
- is quantitative/objective;
- provides a uniform assessment of all patients;
- enables a routine of repeated re-evaluation for home readiness;
- is of added medico-legal benefit;
- has a proven safety record with evaluated criteria.

One recent discharge scoring system which fits the above criteria is that introduced by Chung: the modified PADSS[14] (*Table 16.5*). Once the patient is in second-stage recovery, home readiness can be evaluated by PADSS. If this is satisfied twice at 30 minute intervals, the patient can be considered for discharge.

Table 16.5. Modified postanaesthesia discharge scoring system (PADSS)

1. *Vital signs*
   2 = within 20% of preoperative value
   1 = 20–40% of preoperative value
   0 = 40% of preoperative value
	4. *Pain*
	   2 = minimal
	   1 = moderate
	   0 = severe

2. *Ambulation*
   2 = steady gait/no dizziness
   1 = with assistance
   0 = none/dizziness
	5. *Surgical bleeding*
	   2 = minimal
	   1 = moderate
	   0 = severe

3. *Nausea/vomiting*
   2 = minimal
   1 = moderate
   0 = severe	

The total score is 10. Patients scoring ≥9 are considered fit for discharge.

However, it is to be emphasized that any discharge criteria must be used with common sense and clinical judgement; the patient should feel well enough to go home. The very anxious patient may have raised blood pressure on admission which normalizes postoperatively, this must be taken into consideration for vital signs scoring. Clinical judgement is used with moderate surgical bleeding, where surgical review prior to patient discharge may be appropriate.

Voiding is not included in this discharge criteria. Patients must be informed that if they have any difficulty voiding to contact their GP or hospital. However, the ability to void is *mandatory* in patients who have undergone spinal or epidural anaesthesia and advisable in those who have had herniorrhaphy[3] or some urological procedures.

The advantage of the modified PADSS discharge scoring system is that it is useful for those patients who have undergone regional, general or sedation anaesthesia. They are thereby able to move through recovery to safe discharge at their own pace.

Symptoms may develop or recur after meeting the discharge criteria but prior to actual discharge[9]. Delayed discharge has been shown to be due to unavailable escort, recurrence of symptoms and persistent adverse symptoms. Day surgery staff should anticipate these problems and minimize their occurrence by good preoperative assessment, appropriate anaesthesia and early institution of recovery room protocols.

> *The prompt and safe discharge of patients can help reduce costs and improve unit efficiency.*

What instructions should be given to the patient at discharge?

All patients who have received anaesthetic drugs should receive general safety instructions to be observed for at least 24 hours. Patients should not:

- drive a car or motor bike, or ride a bicycle;
- drink any wine, beer or spirits;
- make important decisions (such as signing important papers);
- travel alone by public transport;
- cook or use hazardous machinery (this includes household appliances such as kettles);

- engage in sport, heavy work or heavy lifting;
- take sedative drugs that are not authorized by a medical practitioner.

In addition, patients should receive specific instructions relating to their surgery. All instructions should be given to the patient and guardian in written and verbal form. It is advisable for staff in day surgery units to devise their own, specific discharge instructions for surgical procedures, as these vary between surgeons, units and countries. Information sheets should be provided to patients both in advance of surgery and at discharge to help them prepare for their postoperative course, particularly with respect to analgesic requirements and anticipated return to work. The discharge information sheets should be succinct and easily understood.

Guidelines for writing patient information are given in Chapter 3.

> *When writing discharge instruction sheets keep the reader in mind at all times. Design and layout is as important as the content. If the information appears complicated or unimportant it is unlikely to be read.*

When can patients drive?

Patients must be clearly instructed not to drive a motor vehicle for at least 24 hours. If not warned, patients may drive themselves to the hospital and be tempted to drive home again following surgery.

Despite the introduction of newer, short-acting drugs where the recovery of driving skills may return to normal earlier, it is prudent to maintain these driving guidelines for patient safety and for medico-legal reasons. However, these shorter-acting drugs should further improve outcome by providing fast exit and early return to normal daily activities[21]. Patients with psychomotor impairment may be prone to accidents during transportation or at home[22,23].

Recovery from anaesthetic drugs may be delayed by alcohol intake, sedatives or strong analgesics, and for this reason patients should only take medications as prescribed by their medical officers.

Take-home analgesia

Patients must be fully instructed both verbally and in writing about the appropriate analgesia following their surgery. It is important that patients feel comfortable with their take-home analgesia[24]. Where two or more different analgesics are offered (e.g. NSAID, opioid and simple analgesic) the patient must clearly understand which tablet to take and when, relating it to the severity of pain. A useful way of supplying combined medication for maximal efficacy is to provide combination packs to patients (i.e. combination NSAID and opioid). Separate instruction leaflets may also be helpful (*Table 16.6*).

Patients must also have a clear understanding of the side-effects of analgesics. The possibility of constipation (often related to opioids) and simple management strategies for problems should be explained. Staff should also instruct patients to report any other, more severe side-effects to a medical officer immediately.

> *Postoperative pain following day surgery is a common problem. Prescribing appropriate analgesia, together with clear instructions, is crucial.*

Table 16.6. Example of patient instruction sheet for combination analgesia

---

PAIN KILLERS TO TAKE HOME AFTER DAY SURGERY

You have been given 2 types of pain killer to take home

Diclofenac should be taken <u>regularly</u>: 1 tablet every 8 hours
Start as soon as you feel any pain or before you go to bed. This means that you stay more comfortable and don't wake up with pain in the night

If you still have pain, you may take in addition to diclofenac:
Paracetamol 500 mg/codeine phosphate 30 mg tablet (Tylex or Panadeine Forte) 1–2 capsules every 4 hours. Do not take more than 8 tablets in 24 hours

We recommend that you take both pain killers before going to bed on the first night after your operation to make sure that you have a pain-free night

DO NOT EXCEED THE RECOMMENDED DOSES

If you are still in pain despite taking the tablets you have been given, please contact your own doctor or telephone the Day Surgery Unit

NB Tylex or Panadeine Forte contains paracetamol so do not take additional paracetamol

---

Who is a 'responsible' guardian?

This term can be interpreted and applied in various ways. Each unit must have its own policies and criteria, together with direction for staff[25]. A 'responsible' carer is a competent (*i.e. not mentally handicapped*) person over 16 years of age who is physically able.

Issues to address are as follows.

- Who judges the acceptability of the responsible adult?
- What control do day surgery staff have over patient plans after discharge?
- Should a patient be allowed to leave if staff know that the guardian will not stay with the patient at home?
- Where do liability and responsibility lie when suspected unacceptable home circumstances exist?

Who should discharge the patient?

It is not necessary for a medical officer to be present when a patient is discharged, although it is recognized that the discharge should be authorized by the surgeon and anaesthetist (or their designated alternatives) after discharge criteria have been met[26]. Nursing staff should implement these criteria and discharge patients according to a strict plan.

Management of complications following discharge from a day surgery unit

Patients can suffer complications following discharge from day surgery, such as haemorrhage, uncontrollable pain, vomiting and syncope. It is therefore recommended that patients should travel for no longer than 1 hour.

Contact telephone numbers of the surgeon and/or the facility, and the after-hours number of the emergency service should be given to the patient at discharge. Patients must also have ready access to a telephone.

A communication sheet should also be given to the patient stating the operation performed, anaesthesia type, discharge drugs and instructions, and any complications that occurred. This is an important communication link if the patient needs to contact his local GP. If there is a computer network available to the patient's GP, this information should be transferred from the DSU at patient discharge.

Postoperative telephone calls
There are significant advantages in contacting day surgery patients following their surgery. For the patient this provides an opportunity for continuity of care, and for the staff it is a means of patient feedback of the care provided. Staff should ask appropriate day surgery questions and open-ended questions pertaining to the surgery performed, allowing the patient to provide valuable comments (*Table 16.7*).

Postdischarge care alternatives
Increasing numbers of patients request nursing and medical support following their day surgery. The West Australian Consumers' Council (1994) conducted a short survey, placed in the daily newspaper in Perth (Australia), and reported that:

- 44% of the 932 respondents would not be able to arrange help at home and someone to care for them after day surgery;
- 77% expected a nurse to visit them at home after surgery and 52% expected a doctor to visit them.

Table 16.7. Guidelines for postoperative telephone calls

Question	Elaboration
How would you rate your pain today?	Pain score at rest Pain score at mobilization
Is your pain medication effective?	Yes/no/not required
What are your pain medication requirements?	
Do you have any troublesome effects following your pain medication?	Ask for specific side-effects (e.g. constipation from codeine-related drugs)
Do you have any nausea or vomiting?	Yes/No (medication required?)
Do you have any bleeding?	Yes/No **If yes:** Number of pads soaked? Number of dressings changed?
Do you have any concerns about your wound?	
Do you feel drowsy?	e.g. Are you steady on your feet?
Do you have a temperature/fever/chills?	
Have you had any significant problems necessitating a visit to a hospital or GP?[a]	

[a]Specific questions should be asked relevant to the surgical procedure or anaesthesia, e.g. headache after spinal anaesthesia.

Some patients undergoing day surgery require postdischarge care for the following reasons[27]:

- lack of social support systems;
- unsuitable home environment, e.g. stairs to climb;
- complex postoperative care, e.g. wound or catheter care, extended pain relief;
- personal coping deficits, e.g. anxiety, depression, memory problems.

These patients should be identified in advance and only admitted to day surgery if postoperative care has been arranged.

Extended recovery care facilities. These facilities provide nursing care for extended periods of time after surgery. The 23-hour recovery care centres are a popular option in North America for insurance reimbursement reasons. The care provided includes nursing, issue of medication and meals, access to emergency response personnel and professional care following surgery[25,28]. Families are encouraged to be with the patients. The evaluation of patients in a day surgery setting for a period of time before a final decision is made regarding discharge creates the 'observation concept'. The 23-hour observation units for day surgery patients have the following advantages in situations where:

- home and social circumstances negate acceptance for day surgery;
- patients require monitoring for medical instability;
- patients require more controlled analgesia for more painful procedures such as anterior cruciate repairs and vaginal hysterectomies.

It is important to monitor the cost efficiency of these units and also patient satisfaction, both during their 23-hour stay and the immediate postdischarge period, to determine whether this method of patient care is superior to in-patient management.

Hospital at Home nursing care. This alternative provides hospital-based nurses who visit patients in their own homes following day surgery[29]. Plans for Hospital at Home nurses should be made prior to the day of surgery to increase the likelihood of having a nurse assigned.

Hospital at Home nurses can provide:

- continuity of care (availability 7 days a week);
- short-term nursing care availability (<7 days);
- specialist nursing staff under the direction of the hospital consultant or GP.

Areas of care include:

- care of wound, catheter, dressing and drain;
- administration of medication and advice;
- patient education.

Costs for the provision of this service must be taken into consideration. Costs include nursing time per visit, equipment used, car hire, petrol and mobile phone services. Comparative average costs (data from The Queen Elizabeth Hospital, Woodville, South Australia) are as follows.

- Hospital at Home nursing visit, AU$25.
- Overnight stay in low nursing staff/patient ward, AU$80.
- Acute care bed, AU$200.

In the future, new modes of administering analgesics, such as ambulatory patient-controlled analgesia, may be instances where Hospital at Home nurses can assist in extending services to patients.

Medical hotels. This is an option for patients who may have travelled a long distance for surgery or who have no one to assist them at home. There are cost advantages to this system as opposed to in-patient management[30]. Usual admission criteria are that patients care for themselves and use the available emergency care only when necessary. Meals and medications may be provided or may be the responsibility of the patient.

Traditional hospitalization. When alternative settings are not available or are not adequate, hospitalization is an option, albeit a costly one. There are cost implications in keeping a bed available, and bed availability is often a problem. An alternative cost-effective option is to manage a ward with a low nurse to patient ratio, for those patients who can partly cater for themselves where constant monitoring is not required. This can significantly reduce the overhead costs.

> *Safe and practical discharge criteria and patient follow-up are crucial for high-quality day care.*

References

1. **Audit Commission** (1990) *A Short Cut to Better Services. Day Surgery in England and Wales.* HMSO, London.
2. **Rudkin GE, Bacon AK, Burrow B,** *et al.* Review of efficiencies and patient satisfaction in Australian and New Zealand day surgery units: a pilot study. *Anaesth. Intens. Care* 1996; **24:** 74–78.
3. **Korttila K.** Recovery from outpatient anaesthesia. *Anaesthesia* 1995; **50** (Suppl.): 22–28.
4. **Aldrete JA, Kroulik D.** A postanesthetic recovery score. *Anesth. Analg.* 1970; **49:** 924–934.
5. **Steward DJ.** A simplified scoring system for the post-operative recovery room. *Can. Anaesth. Soc. J.* 1975; **22:** 111–113.
6. **Spear RM, Yastor M, Borkowitz ID,** *et al.* Preinduction of anesthesia in children with rectally administered midazolam. *Anesthesiology* 1991; **74:** 670–674.
7. **Lebovic S, Reich DL, Steinberg G, Vela FP, Silvay G.** Comparison of propofol versus ketamine for anesthesia in paediatric patients undergoing cardiac catheterization. *Anesth. Analg.* 1992; **74:** 490–494.
8. **Rita I, Seleny FL, Mazurek A,** *et al.* Intramuscular midazolam for paediatric preanesthetic sedation: a double blind controlled study with morphine. *Anesthesiology* 1985; **63:** 520–531.
9. **Chung F.** Recovery pattern and home-readiness after ambulatory surgery. *Anesth. Analg.* 1995; **80:** 896–902.
10. **Chung F.** Are discharge criteria changing? *J. Clin. Anesth.* 1993; **5** (Suppl 1): 64S–68S.
11. **Bran DF, Spellman JR, Summitt RL.** Outpatient vaginal hysterectomy as a new trend in gynaecology. *AORN J.* 1995; **62:** 810–814.
12. **Singleton RJ, Rudkin GE, Osborne GA,** *et al.* Laparoscopic cholecystectomy as a day surgery procedure. *Anaesth. Intens. Care.* 1996; **24:** 231–236.
13. **Osborne GA, Rudkin GE.** Outcome after day-care surgery in a major teaching hospital. *Anaesth. Intens. Care* 1933; **21:** 822–827.
14. **Chung F.** Discharge criteria – a new trend. *Can. J. Anaesth.* 1995; **42:** 1056–1058.
15. **Korttila K.** (1990). Recovery period and discharge. In: *Outpatient Anesthesia* (Ed. P White). Churchill Livingstone, New York. pp. 369–396.
16. **Wetchler BV** (Ed.) (1991) *Anesthesia for Ambulatory Surgery,* 2nd Edn. JB Lippincott Co., Philadelphia, PA. p. 415.
17. **Wetchler BV** (Ed.) (1991) *Anesthesia for Ambulatory Surgery,* 2nd Edn. JB Lippincott Co., Philadelphia, PA. p. 403.

18. **Cardosa M, Rudkin GE, Osborne GA.** Outcome from day-case knee arthroscopy in a major teaching hospital. *Arthroscopy* 1994; **10**: 624–629.
19. **Carroll NV, Miederhoff PA, Cox FM, *et al.*** Costs incurred by outpatient surgical centers in managing postoperative nausea and vomiting. *J. Clin. Anesth.* 1994; **6**: 364–369.
20. **Marais LM, Maher MW, Wetchler BV, *et al.*** Reduced demands on recovery room resources with propofol (Diprivan) compared to thiopental–isoflurane. *Anesthesiol. Rev.* 1989; **16**: 29–40.
21. **Korttila KT.** Post-anaesthetic psychomotor and cognitive function. *Eur. J. Anaesthesiol.* 1995; **12** (Suppl. 10): 43–46.
22. **Carroll NV, Miederhoff P, Cox FM, *et al.*** Postoperative nausea and vomiting after discharge from outpatient surgery centers. *Anesth. Analg.* 1995; **80**: 903–909.
23. **Korttila K.** (1988) How to assess recovery from outpatient anesthesia. In: *ASA Refresher Course in Anesthesiology* 16 (Ed. PG Barash). American Society of Anesthesiologists, IL. pp. 133–144.
24. **Rudkin GE.** Patient choice in sedation anaesthesia and recovery room analgesia. *Ambulatory Surg.* 1994; **2**: 75–80.
25. **Burden N.** Discharging patients: innovative postoperative care. *Ambulatory Surg.* 1993; **1**: 70–76.
26. **Australian and New Zealand College of Anaesthetists** (1995) *Guidelines for the Perioperative Care of Patients Selected for Day Care Surgery.* Bulletin, Review P15, pp. 62–63.
27. **Redmond MC.** Phase III recovery: referral options in postoperative discharge planning. *J. Post. Anesth. Nursing* 1994; **9**: 353–356.
28. **Clement P, Sangermano C.** Twenty-three hour recovery: observation versus hospitalization. *Semin. Periop. Nursing* 1992; **1**: 261–267.
29. **Montaito M, Dunt D.** Delivery of traditional hospital services to patients at home. *Med. J. Aust.* 1993; **159**: 263–265.
30. **Jarrett PEM, Wallace M, Jarrett MED, *et al.*** Experience of a hospital hotel. *Ambulatory Surg.* 1996; **4**: 1–3.

CHAPTER 17

Balancing cost and quality in day surgery

G.E. Rudkin

Orkin has identified the issues of cost and quality in defining 'value-based care' as the best patient outcome at a reasonable cost[1]. This is mathematically expressed as:

$$Value = Quality/Cost.$$

Quality is determined by the overall satisfaction of the patient's expectations. The patient's satisfaction is determined by factors as diverse as individual wealth, political stability and the medico-legal systems. It is also influenced by clinical performance. Quality clinical indicators measure the quality of clinical performance and cost indicators are the cost of providing these services.

There is a close linkage between quality and cost[2], although direct relationships do not necessarily apply between quality care delivered and cost, as poor quality care can, in fact, be more costly. For example, inadequate patient assessment may mean that complications such as hypertension are not managed properly preoperatively, resulting in patient complications or cancellation on the day, both incurring added costs.

The implementation of value-based care as defined by Orkin requires a practical framework. Groups with vested interests in day surgery, such as administrators, surgeons, anaesthetists, nurses and patients, need to be active participants. This team approach will help solve what is medicine's major dilemma in providing value-based care: a balance between cost and quality.

When is the treatment cost not worth the quality of the outcome?

The challenges in value-based care are increasingly evident in day surgery where more patients who are 'less fit' are undergoing more complex surgical procedures. In order to provide value-based care, we are seeing the quality of care improved with streamlined assessment systems and more appropriate selection of anaesthetic drugs and techniques to provide a problem-free recovery period. The cost indicator is increasingly evident with the continued health budget constraints. However, we must be able to justify both the level of quality provided and the costs incurred.

> *Value-based care, by definition, has neither the quality nor the cost as the single overriding factor in determining the processes of anaesthetic delivery in day surgery.*

Day surgery facilities, whether private or public, large or small, need to monitor the processes that determine their value-based care. The process may be described as: audit, continuous quality improvement programmes, quality assurance and cost–benefit analysis.

> *In the published literature there is a preponderance of models and a shortage of standards or benchmarks for these models.*

A practical model for improving your value-based care

Donabedian's triad of structure, process and outcome is a practical model[3] (*Table 17.1*). This model suggests that problems are 'system-based', rather than attributable to poor performance by individuals. Regular system review and modification of activities will assist teams to achieve improvements in the value of the care provided: 'to do better what is currently being done'.

Table 17.1. Triad of structure, process and outcome

Structure:	the organization and the physical and human resources of the day surgery centre *(e.g. the day surgery anaesthetist is absent from an assessment clinic which is then run by an inadequately trained person)*
Process:	how the organization functions to provide the health care *(e.g. the assessment report failed to indicate that the patient was continuing aspirin medication)*
Outcome:	the effect of structure and process on the patients *(e.g. surgery is cancelled on the day of surgery)*

The systematic improvement in the value of day surgery services needs to be both organized and adequately resourced (e.g. facilities, staff and equipment). Effective improvement starts with the facility's overall strategic planning process and requires a value-based care plan to be integrated within the facility's operational plan. A multidisciplinary team, including surgeons, anaesthetists, nurses and administrators, should be involved in the process. It is critical that the group meet regularly and report on a regular basis to senior management who have line responsibility and are capable of implementing changes. The programme should include mechanisms for setting priorities, providing feedback and reviewing and evaluating effectiveness on a regular basis. There is a need for:

- planned collection of information used in processes;
- documentation of activities;
- communication of results to providers and consumers of the service;
- feedback to all users and those with staff and line responsibility.

This feedback is imperative so that the team may see 'how we can do better what we are doing now'.

Quality clinical indicators

A quality clinical indicator is defined as a 'measure of the clinical management and outcome of care'. Many quality clinical indicators have been identified which might effectively and economically assess the quality of service in day surgery centres[4,5]. The following four commonly used clinical indicators are useful for accreditation purposes and for their adaptability to various healthcare systems with differing levels of standards and sophistication.

- Cancellation on the day of surgery.
- Return to theatre.
- Delayed discharge.
- Unplanned overnight admission.

In addition to these quality clinical indicators, the team may also include some of the following:

- surgical delay;
- preoperative waiting times;
- patient discharge delay;
- patient satisfaction;
- postoperative infection rate;
- readmission within 28 days.

Cost indicators

Obtaining cost indicators can be complex as the team must decide the extent to which it will include costs beyond the facility's immediate responsibility: for example, transferred costs of readmission, or treatment by another facility, or the cost to the patient of a delayed return to work.

Some commonly used cost indicators are as follows:

- overall cost of facility;
- cost by surgical procedure;
- cost by staff group;
- consumable cost by staff group;
- post discharge costs.

However, the best framework for managing costs is to group them according to the staff that control them (*Table 17.2*). A staff group without discretion to control costs cannot be responsible for them.

Table 17.2. Example of discretionary costs

Staff group	Costs at the discretion of the staff group
Administrator	Dedicated or non-dedicated unit staffing levels
Surgeon	Laparoscopic or open inguinal hernia repair
Anaesthetist	General anaesthesia or regional anaesthesia drug costs
Nurse Stage 1 recovery	Pain management by intravenous or oral route
Nurse Stage 2 recovery	Speed of discharge

When managing cost indicators, it is critical to identify who has the discretion to control the cost. Then focus specifically on that group.

For each quality clinical indicator and cost indicator, baseline standards or benchmarks should be established, performance evaluated and corrective actions initiated. Repetition of the quality activity cycle will show whether issues have been solved, a situation improved or further action is necessary (*Figure 17.1*).

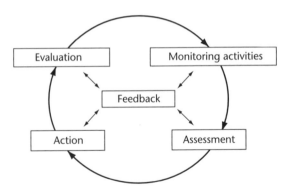

Figure 17.1. Full cycle of an effective value-based care process.

Measurement of patient satisfaction

Staff from day surgery facilities commonly review patient satisfaction. Generally, reports confirm high patient satisfaction of the day surgery service[6]. However, these figures should be interpreted with caution, as generally there is a lack of expertise in the design and execution of patient survey work in day surgery.

It is important to monitor patients as they have a crucial role in setting the criteria for evaluating service quality[6]. In addition, poor-quality care which reduces satisfaction may, in turn, adversely affect health outcomes[7]. Patient satisfaction surveys appear to value patient opinion but are often used to justify services, given that satisfaction levels are usually high (85% satisfaction, or thereabouts, is standard). The challenge for staff designing patient satisfaction questionnaires is to seek comments from dissatisfied patients and to explore reasons for them.

A patient satisfaction instrument is of value only if it provides information that is useful in improving quality. To do this, it has to get to candid assessments of what patients think. It needs to get past the gratitude response. The survey must be:

- reliable: whether a measure of the same case will produce the same results on successive survey;
- valid: whether a measure assesses what it purports to;
- feasible: whether it is practical to use.

It is important to define the aims of the patient satisfaction survey. Ask questions on topics that you are able to influence or change. Lack of attention to design and to the capacity to obtain useful data means that much money, time and effort can be wasted without achieving the aims. *Table 17.3* gives guidelines for improved design in patient questionnaires.

Published cost and quality reports

One of the issues facing day surgery, with respect to improving the value of care, is the absence of relative benchmarks or standards for specific quality clinical indicators and cost indicators. These may differ between private and public day surgery facilities. Further benchmarking needs to be performed and published for the benefit of day surgery teams. However, the parameters that may affect the translation of published benchmarks from one unit to another must be considered (*Table 17.4*).

Table 17.3. Guidelines for 'improved design' in day surgery patient questionnaires

Define the target sample size, ensuring representatives and spread of conditions
Do not exclude the 'disadvantaged' patient, e.g. non-English speaking
Consider involving a neutral party to distribute the questionnaire. Health staff may bias the sample by omitting patients they judge to be unsuitable
Respondents are less prepared to be critical if they know that the health staff will see their questionnaires
Anonymity is important
Consider designing a short, general questionnaire supplemented by subsidiary questionnaires where dissatisfaction is shown to occur
Include open-ended questions, as they produce more negative ratings and comments than closed questions[8]
Consider qualitative research (in-depth interviews with patients) as a key input to the development of a pilot survey. Patient interviews reveal higher rates of problems than questionnaires
50% or less is not an acceptable response rate. Much higher rates should be achieved
Follow-up cards or calls are recommended to improve response rates
Response rate for mail surveys are significantly higher than phone surveys; however, there are more missing data from mail surveys
Carers of relatives or friends may rate care more negatively than patients[8] – patients and carers have differing needs. Separate questions to both groups may be appropriate
Decide what you will do with the results. Disseminate the information to patients and staff. Publish the results

Table 17.4. Factors that may modify benchmarks for specific clinical indicators

Country, state/province, cultural variations
The corporate objective of the facility: private, or public where teaching is involved
Facility type: freestanding and non-dedicated facilities
Varying levels of clinical skills and resources
Case mix
Frequency of the occurrence of the clinical procedure being measured
Patient expectation: user pay or free service

Facility type

There has been a recent trend for many surgical procedures, particularly plastic cosmetic procedures, to be performed in the 'surgeon's office' under local anaesthetic and sedation. Procedures performed in this way include varicose vein surgery[9], laparoscopic surgery[10], breast augmentation and mastopexy[11]. Investigators have shown that a genioplasty can be performed at half the price in a 'surgeons' office' as compared with a day surgical suite[12].

A multicentre study in Australia and New Zealand compared free-standing (purpose-built self-contained day surgery facility) and hospital-integrated day surgery facilities, where day patients were recovered in a shared recovery room with in-patients or in dedicated day surgery recovery areas. This study demonstrated significantly improved efficiency and patient satisfaction when in-patients and day patients were not mixed[13].

Assessment

There has been a recent trend to introduce pre-admission assessment clinics which have been shown to reduce cancellations and hospital admissions on the day of surgery and to be cost effective[14]. Significant cost savings have also been identified by ordering day patient preoperative tests on clinical indication rather than routine preoperative testing[15].

Anaesthetic drug selection and technique

The cost of an anaesthetic drug may be more complex than its purchase price. Anaesthetic economies may incur much greater costs in other budgetry areas. PONV is a good example of this. Carroll *et al.* showed that the incidence of PONV substantially increased the costs incurred by out-patient surgical centres[16].

The cost effectiveness of the anaesthetic agent should also be considered. Watcha and Smith reported that droperidol and ondansetron were more effective than metoclopramide, but that prophylactic droperidol was more cost effective than ondansetron[17]. Drugs must not be reviewed in isolation, as the anaesthetic technique itself may impact on the degree of nausea and vomiting. Recently, Gan *et al.* have shown that in patients undergoing breast surgery, propofol infusion was more effective than ondansetron in minimizing the incidence of PONV and the use of rescue antiemetics in the early postoperative period[18]. Propofol infusions have also been shown to be cost-neutral when compared with inhalation techniques for shorter day surgery procedures[19].

> *TIVA with propofol may be the most cost-effective choice for day surgery procedures where there is a high risk of PONV. Droperidol or ondansetron are suitable choices for rescue medication.*

Studies have shown that the cost of regional anaesthesia (spinal and epidural) and nerve blocks tends to be less than general anaesthesia, even when pre-assembled kits, special block needles and sedation were included[20]. Other quality indicators should be considered, such as reduction in postoperative complications, reduced recovery time and improved postoperative analgesia with regional techniques. Where regional techniques were employed, Flanagan *et al.* reported that by utilizing a femoral nerve block for anterior cruciate ligament reconstruction, patient hospital stay can be minimized with significant cost savings[21].

However, despite the overall reduced costs for regional techniques, patient choice is important. Ferry and Rankin evaluated safety, cost effectiveness and patient acceptability for a wide variety of gynaecological procedures, including endometrial resections, using local analgesia. Cost benefits, patient acceptance and a reduction in operating list waiting time were demonstrated[22]. Reports of safe, quick and adequately performed laparoscopic tubal ligation under local anaesthesia have been shown to be cost effective[23], but investigators must have parallel studies into quality care to be certain that the value of care is not being eroded.

Results from a cost analysis study of total intravenous anaesthesia compared with more traditional volatile anaesthesia in day surgery showed comparable costs for the two techniques, particularly where day case operations were of less than 30 minutes' duration[19]. Although the costs of anaesthetic drugs are important, this must be put into the overall cost equation as they are only a small percentage of the total costs of the surgical procedure[24]. Other efficiency factors must be analysed in day surgery, such as turnaround time and recovery room stay[25].

Today, it must be demonstrated that a new drug is worth the extra cost in relation to its clinical benefits. The increasing importance of pharmaco-economics is highlighted by the fact that, in Australia, economic evaluation has become part of the drug approval process[26,27].

Patient recovery

The choice of surgical technique for a particular procedure has been shown to influence patients' postoperative period. A study of perioperative outcome after day case laparoscopic versus open inguinal hernia repair showed significantly shorter recovery room times, fewer perioperative complications and less analgesia required in the open inguinal hernia repair group compared with the laparoscopic group[28].

Marais *et al.* have shown that nursing salaries constitute half of all day surgery costs[29]. Reduction in the time that patients spend in the recovery room can therefore provide a more cost-effective service. It would be anticipated that with the introduction of Chung's modified discharge criteria[30] and continuing improvements in surgery, anaesthetic drugs and techniques, patient recovery times could be reduced even further.

The need to improve value-based care has been highlighted in a recently published study. Data collected on 465 day patients undergoing knee arthroscopy demonstrated that pain and PONV management were of prime concern in the recovery room and significantly delayed patient recovery[31].

Unanticipated hospital admissions and re-admissions

Several published studies have measured unanticipated hospital admission rates on the day of surgery[32–34]. Rates vary from 0.1% to 2.4%, depending on case mix. However, few centres have reviewed patient re-admissions. A follow-up study in the first 14 days after surgery showed that the incidence of major postoperative complications necessitating patient re-admission was similar to the unanticipated admission rate, and most of these were due to surgery-related causes[35]. Twersky *et al.*[34] reported a re-admission rate of 3.13% and these were also due mainly to surgery-related causes. Re-admission rates vary according to surgical procedure. Investigators demonstrated a 0.86% re-admission rate within 28 days following knee arthroscopic surgery[31], a 0.7% re-admission rate following extraction of third molars[36] and others have reported a disproportionately higher percentage of re-admissions following ophthalmological surgery[37].

Follow-up information

There is a paucity of published information on patient follow-up, providing challenges for teams in day surgery facilities. In one study researchers reviewed 6000 consecutive day surgery patients, showing that at early follow-up 4.0% of patients had presented to a local medical practitioner and 3.1% to a hospital accident and emergency service, usually for minor problems[32]. This study reinforces the necessity for all day surgery patients to receive adequate documentation about their responsibilities after discharge. It also emphasizes the need to educate GPs in day surgery management. There is often poor communication between hospitals and GPs, and this is an area where major improvements can be made. Feedback to GPs should include the procedure and special investigations performed, the drugs prescribed and any treatment and further care required.

Does a focus on value-based care improve the value of care?

Those who have participated in gathering cost and quality information report that when quality and cost indicators are measured, the value of care improves . Day surgery staff should be encouraged to focus on providing value-based care by balancing quality and cost through structured team processes.

> *Value-based care analysis is the key for day surgery teams so that ' they can do better what is currently being done'.*

References

1. **Orkin FK.** Moving toward value-based anesthesia care. *J. Clin. Anesth.* 1993; **5**: 91–98.
2. **Orkin FK.** (1997) Value-based care. In: *Ambulatory Anesthesia and Surgery* (Ed. PF White). WB Saunders, London. p. 673.
3. **Donabedian A.** (1985) *Explorations in Quality Assessment and Monitoring.* Health and Administration Press, Ann Arbor, MI. Vols 1–3.
4. **Roberts L.** Clinical indicators for quality assurance in ambulatory surgery. *Ambulatory Surg.* 1994; **2:** 5–6.
5. **Roberts L.** Accreditation of ambulatory surgery centres utilizing universally acceptable clinical indicators – is it achievable? *Ambulatory Surg.* 1994; **2**: 223–226.
6. **Zeitaml VA, Parasuraman A, Barry LL.** (1990) *Delivering Quality Service: Balancing Customer Perceptions and Expectations.* The Free Press, New York.
7. **Westbrook J.** Patient satisfaction: methodological issues and research findings. *Aust. Health Rev.* 1993; **16**: 75–88.
8. **Aharony L, Strasser S.** Patient satisfaction: what we know about and what we still need to explore. *Med. Care Rev.* 1993; **50**: 49–79.
9. **Ricci S, Georgiev M.** Office varicose vein surgery under local anesthesia. *J. Dermatol. Surg. Oncol.* 1992; **18**: 55–58.
10. **Schultz LS.** Cost analysis of office surgery clinic with comparison to hospital outpatient facilities for laparoscopic procedures. *Int. Surg.* 1994; **79**: 273–277.
11. **Conlay LA.** (1995) Plastic surgery. In: *Ambulatory Anesthesiology. A Problem-oriented Approach* (Ed. KE McGoldrick). Williams and Wilkins, Baltimore, MD. pp. 455–456.
12. **Van Sickels JE, Tiner BD.** Cost of a genioplasty under deep intravenous sedation in a private office verses general anesthesia in an outpatient surgical centre. *J. Oral Maxillofac. Surg.* 1992; **50**: 687–690.
13. **Rudkin GE, Bacon AK, Burrow B,** *et al.* Review of efficiencies and patient satisfaction in Australian and New Zealand day surgery units: a pilot study. *Anaesth. Intens. Care* 1996; **24**: 74–78.
14. **Pollard JB, Zboray AL, Mazze RI.** Economic benefits attributed to opening a preoperative evaluation clinic for outpatients. *Anesth. Analg.* 1996; **83**: 407–410.
15. **Rudkin GE, Osborne GA, Doyle CE.** Assessment and selection of patients for day surgery in a public hospital. *Med. J. Aust.* 1993; **158**: 308–312.
16. **Carroll NV, Miederhoff PA, Cox FM.** Costs incurred by outpatient surgical centres in managing postoperative nausea and vomiting. *J. Clin. Anesth.* 1994; **6**: 364–369.
17. **Watcha MF, Smith I.** Cost-effectiveness analysis of antiemetic therapy for ambulatory surgery. *J. Clin. Anesth.* 1994; **6**: 370–377.
18. **Gan TJ, Ginsberg B, Grant AP,** *et al.* Double-blind, randomized comparison of ondansetron and intraoperative propofol to prevent postoperative nausea and vomiting. *Anesthesiology* 1996; **85**: 1036–1042.
19. **Hitchcock M, Rudkin G.** The real cost of total intravenous anaesthesia: cost versus price. *Ambulatory Surg.* 1995; **3**: 43–48.
20. **Greenberg CP, Brown AR.** (1997) Cost Containment – Utilization of Techniques, Personnel, Equipment and Supplies. In: *Ambulatory Anesthesia and Surgery* (Ed. PF White). WB Saunders, London. p. 640.

21. **Flanagan JFK, Edkin B, Spindler K.** 3 in 1 femoral nerve block following ACL reconstruction allows predictably earlier discharge and significant cost savings. *Anaesthesiology* 1994; **81:** A950.
22. **Ferry J, Rankin L.** Low cost, patient acceptable, local analgesia approach to gynaecological outpatient surgery. A review of 817 consecutive procedures. *Aust. N.Z. J. Obstet. Gynaecol.* 1994; **34:** 453–456.
23. **Poindexter AN, Abdul-Malak M, Fast JE.** Laparoscopic tubal sterilization under local anesthesia. *J. Obstet. Gynaecol.* 1990; **75:** 5–8.
24. **Macario A, Vitez TS, Dunn B,** *et al.* Where are the costs in perioperative care? Analysis of hospital costs and charges for inpatient surgical care. *Anesthesiology* 1995; **83:** 1138–1144.
25. **Tuman KJ.** (1994) Cost containment/efficiency in perioperative care. In: *ASA Refresher Course in Anesthesiology* 23 (Ed. PG Barash). American Society of Anesthesiologists, IL. pp. 231–246.
26. **Henry D.** Economic analysis as an aid to subsidization: the development of Australian guidelines for pharmaceuticals. *Pharmaco. Econ.* 1992; **1:** 54–67.
27. **Mitchell A.** Update and evaluation of Australian guidelines: government perspective. *Med. Care* **34** (Suppl.): ds216–ds225.
28. **Rudkin GE, Maddern GJ.** Peri-operative outcome for day-case laparoscopic and open inguinal hernia repair. *Anaesthesia* 1995; **50:** 586–589.
29. **Marais LM, Maher MW, Wetchler BV,** *et al.* Reduced demands on recovery room resources with propofol (Diprivan) compared to thiopental–isoflurane. *Anesthesiol. Rev.* 1989; **16:** 29–40.
30. **Chung F.** Discharge criteria – a new trend. *Can. J. Anaesthesiol.* 1995; **42:** 1056–1058.
31. **Cardosa M, Rudkin GE, Osborne GA.** Outcome from day-case knee arthroscopy in a major teaching hospital. *Arthroscopy* 1994; **10:** 624–629.
32. **Osborne GA, Rudkin GE.** Outcome after day-care surgery in a major teaching hospital. *Anaesth. Intens. Care* 1983; **21:** 822–827.
33. **Fancourt-Smith PF, Hornstein J, Jenkins LC.** Hospital admissions from the Surgical Day Care Centre of Vancouver General Hospital 1997–1987. *Can. J. Anaesth.* 1990; **37:** 699–704.
34. **Twersky RS, Abiona M, Thorne AC,** *et al.* Admissions following ambulatory surgery: outcome in seven urban hospitals. *Ambulatory Surg.* 1995; **3:** 141–146.
35. **Rudkin GE, Osborne GA, Paix AD** (1993) *Challenges in Day Surgery.* Abstracts of The Australian and New Zealand College of Anaesthetists, Adelaide.
36. **Chye EPY, Young IG, Osborne GA, Rudkin GE.** Outcomes after same-day oral surgery: a review of 1,180 cases at a major teaching hospital. *J. Oral Maxillofac. Surg.* 1993; **51:** 846–849.
37. **Paix A, Rudkin GE, Osborne GA.** Ambulatory surgery complications and patient fitness. *Ambulatory Surg.* 1994; **2:** 166–170.

CHAPTER 18

The future of day surgery and anaesthesia

T.W. Ogg

Throughout the world spending on health care has assumed great political significance. Twenty years ago, few people could have forecast the explosion of free-standing ambulatory facilities in the USA nor the expansion of European day surgery, that has been fuelled by the introduction of purchaser-provider health systems. The possibilities seem unlimited for the future for day surgery. All countries with established day care programmes should actively encourage others to follow their example. Many countries are only now realizing the importance of providing surgery on a day case basis. This chapter will outline some of the predicted advances in the field over the next 20 years with emphasis on the possible surgical, anaesthetic and administrative changes. By the year 2000 it has been predicted that 50% of all non-emergency surgery in Britain should be performed on a day basis[1]. Are all health-care professionals aware of this projection and will they be able to meet these targets?

Long waiting lists for elective surgery have now brought public opinion into the health debate[2]. Indeed, day surgery is patient-led and studies have shown a high degree of consumer satisfaction amongst day surgery patients[3,4]. Furthermore, it may be argued that the delivery of health care has been influenced by the success of day surgery, resulting in a shift of patient treatment from the hospital to the community. Despite this major achievement, there is an immense variation in the amount of day surgery practised within districts, regions and countries. The future goal should be to reverse this situation with planned programmes of day surgery being established, but this will only occur if attention is given to quality assurance, education for all staff, and ongoing research. Even in the 1990s there is scant economic evidence to prove that increases in day surgery will reduce the need for in-patient beds[5].

Surgical advances: minimally invasive surgery (MIS)

The gynaecologists were the pioneers of laparoscopic surgery, and ovarian surgery, laparoscopic myomectomy and pelvic lymphadenectomy are now carried out as MIS[6]. In general surgery, laparoscopic appendicectomy is a routine procedure, and MIS is ideal for the simple patch repair of perforated duodenal ulcers[7]. Although day case laparoscopic cholecystectomy has its advocates, its future is uncertain[8]. The urologists too have replaced open surgery with percutaneous endoscopic lithotomy and few complications have been reported[9]. In the future, many transurethral resections of prostate will be performed on a day basis.

It took some time before other surgeons appreciated the gynaecological initiative in the development of laparoscopic surgery, but now that MIS has been adopted world-wide and has already revolutionized conventional surgical practice, the future is bright. The technology to develop new visual systems and endoscopic instruments will be employed to make smaller and smaller electronic cameras. Surgeons will then be able to work via a magnified, high-definition camera monitor, thus allowing all operating theatre staff to participate in the operation with subsequent educational benefit. In addition, simple surgical suturing could be replaced by either mechanical stapling or radio-frequency heat energy. Lasers too should be in common use for the dissolution of urinary calculi, and the destruction of tumours will be performed by photodynamic treatment[10].

Radiologists are likely to be performing increased amounts of their current interventional work-load, and their involvement in bile duct stenting for malignancy and coronary artery disobliteration will prove popular. However, whether the next 20 years will see the application of robotics to interventional therapy remains to be seen. Micro-engineering is now based on crystal technology and shortly microscopic electric motors of less than 1 mm in size will be marketed[11]. These instruments will be capable of introduction into every body cavity thereby performing surgery impossible by macroscopic means today.

Training implications will be enormous, and already the Royal Colleges of Surgeons in the UK have developed simulator laboratories[12]. These should continue to flourish and the future of all MIS education for surgeons, anaesthetists and nurses will have to be tailored accordingly. However, there will still be a need for conventional surgery to be taught and programmes of audit, education and research will have to compare the results of both surgical methods.

Day case anaesthesia advances

Many anaesthetists have accepted the leading role in the organization of day surgery units. Advances in clinical pharmacology, monitoring and equipment design have all been harnessed by these specialists wishing to provide safe, prompt and cost-effective care for the majority of their patients. Advances in day case anaesthesia will continue with the development of new anaesthetic induction drugs, inhalation agents, and equipment. In addition widespread use of sedation and regional anaesthesia will probably evolve. In future there will be a pressing need to introduce far better drugs to alleviate PONV and pain.

Whether TIVA will eventually replace the volatile inhalation anaesthetic agents for the maintenance of day case anaesthesia remains to be seen. The combination of propofol with the opioid alfentanil or fentanyl provides excellent anaesthetic results[13]. Recently, the real cost of TIVA has been studied and the results suggest that it is comparable to the more traditional volatile anaesthetics, especially when administered to day case operations lasting less than 30 minutes[14]. In future, the development of target infusion anaesthesia will smooth the maintenance of day case anaesthesia[15].

The synthetic opioid alfentanil has become deservedly popular for day surgery with its duration of action being one-third that of fentanyl. The recent introduction of remifentanil has shown that this drug has a rapid onset time but a short duration of action. In future, any anaesthetist tempted to use remifentanil for day surgery should remember to provide adequate postoperative analgesia. Further opioid advances may become available with the introduction of trefentanil and mirfentanil; the former has characteristics intermediate between alfentanil and remifentanil[16]. Recently esmolol has been used as an adjunct for laparoscopic sterilization instead of fentanyl and, in addition to providing a rapid recovery and minimal nausea and vomiting, it provided a satisfactory alternative to fentanyl[17].

Techniques involving TIVA will require syringe pumps for the induction and maintenance of anaesthesia, thereby maintaining a steady state. Before recommending the universal adoption of TIVA, it would be prudent to embark on relevant training programmes. Finally, it is acknowledged that many countries will be unable to supply and service these infusion pumps, thus limiting the future adoption of these techniques, although the cost of these may be less than the cost of acquiring modern vaporizers and the monitoring and scavenging equipment required to use them.

Will there be a need for new volatile anaesthetic agents?
In the future, volatile anaesthetics with even lower blood gas solubility coefficients will be marketed for day case anaesthesia. Desflurane has been commercially available in the USA and Europe since 1993. This inhalation anaesthetic has the properties to make it a useful day case anaesthetic, e.g. low blood and tissue solubility account for its rapid uptake and elimination. However, desflurane produces a high incidence of PONV but, in keeping with its overall molecular stability, it may still find a place in day surgery because it is stable in closed circuit techniques with soda lime[18].

Sevoflurane has been used in Japan since 1982 but it is not the ideal day case anaesthetic. It is a fluorinated ether with low blood/gas and oil/gas coefficients. Gaseous induction with sevoflurane is both pleasant and rapid so perhaps it will find a place in paediatric anaesthesia[19]. However, it is degraded to form an olefin called Compound A and this may limit its use with the closed circuit. To date, no human morbidity has been reported from this degradation product but rats have developed tubular necrosis after prolonged exposure to sevoflurane. Neither sevoflurane nor desflurane, with a high incidence of emesis, has been found to produce a marked improvement over previous inhalational anaesthetics.

Anaesthetic pollution
Measurable anaesthetic pollution may occur in anaesthetic induction rooms, operating theatres and recovery areas[20]. In Britain the regulatory body for the Control of Substances Hazardous to Health (COSHH) has issued upper limits of exposure for some volatile gases.

In busy day surgery units the problem of anaesthetic pollution may be increased by the high patient throughput and by the need to induce paediatric anaesthesia via a face mask. Only a few anaesthetists have turned to TIVA and it would, indeed, be premature to forecast the demise of inhalational anaesthetics within the day unit setting. There is a paucity of sound scientific studies to answer many of the unsolved problems relating to the adverse effects on humans of anaesthetic pollution.

Muscle relaxants
There is an definite need for a short-acting non-depolarizing muscle relaxant free from the not inconsiderable risks and side-effects of suxamethonium.

Mivacuronium chloride, a non-depolarizing muscle relaxant which undergoes hydrolysis by plasma cholinesterase, has a duration of activity of 15–20 minutes, and may not require reversal of its effects. It may, therefore, be regarded as a suitable day case muscle relaxant[21]. The other non-depolarizer worthy of mention is rocuronium bromide. At the initial recommended dose of 0.6 mg kg^{-1}, good intubating conditions were obtained in 80% of patients at 60 seconds with a mean duration of activity of 22 minutes[22]. These characteristics may make rocuronium suitable for rapid sequence intubation for intermediate day surgery.

It remains to be seen whether cisatracurium will establish itself in day care. It is a purified preparation of one of the isomers of atracurium and is eliminated by Hoffmann degradation. Since cisatracurium has a rapid and predictable recovery with minimal histamine release, it may prove useful for day surgery[23].

Will the future see more local and regional anaesthesia with sedation techniques?

Factors delaying patient discharge from day units include slow anaesthetic recovery, PONV and uncontrolled pain. Thus in many countries the use of cost-effective regional anaesthesia makes good sense as these techniques may reduce these postoperative complications. PONV is the source of much day case dissatisfaction[24] and an overall reduction of postoperative emesis is recorded after regional anaesthesia, especially if opiates are avoided[25].

Most anaesthetists will employ upper and lower extremity nerve blocks with the long-acting local anaesthetic bupivacaine, 0.25–0.75%, thereby producing reliable postoperative analgesia for 4–24 hours[26]. In addition, the infiltration of hernia repair wounds has much to recommend it, especially as it has been reported that opiate requirements also fall following this procedure[27]. However, what anaesthetists will be seeking in future for extensive day operations will be a new local anaesthetic with an activity duration of between 24 and 48 hours and no tissue toxicity. Alternatively, newer methods of continuous wound irrigation with infusion systems may also be beneficial, provided their safety is proven[28]. It is by no means futuristic to suggest that experienced day unit nursing staff could train and supervise their community counterparts in the administration of these methods, thus resulting in an excellent postoperative pain relief service.

In several European countries spinal and epidural blockade are widely practised although discharge times may be delayed as a result of motor blockade. Nevertheless there is evidence to suggest that discharge times of 2 hours following chloroprocaine and 3 hours after lignocaine are attainable[29]. Future day unit design will assume importance and a separate area for local blocks should be incorporated so that valuable operating theatre time is not lost. Inevitably, experience will improve the anaesthetic block success rate and patient acceptance will also increase if the benefits of these procedures are explained by enthusiastic surgeons and anaesthetists.

Opposition to spinal anaesthesia in the past on account of post-lumbar puncture headache is no longer valid. This may be reduced to less than 1% by the use of 25–26-gauge spinal needles and by restricting the spinal technique to older, less mobile day cases[30]. The use of the new, rounded bevel spinal needles has even been reported to have reduced the incidence of spinal headache in younger cases[31].

With the use of improved short-acting sedation drugs, much of general anaesthesia administered today will be replaced by monitored sedation in combination with local and regional anaesthetic techniques. For the future we are likely to see the introduction of new modes of administration of sedative agents into clinical practice, such as patient controlled sedation techniques. Up until now these have been primarily research initiatives.

Complications

PONV and unrelieved pain are common reasons for in-patient hospital admission after day surgery[32]. These complications will have economic implications and, in future, anaesthetists should channel their energies into preventing such morbidity. Appropriate anaesthetic techniques such as TIVA with propofol and alfentanil, the insertion of the LMA, avoidance of muscle relaxant reversal and excellent postoperative local anaesthetic blocks should all be practised[33]. Ongoing audit will also allow the comparison of the incidence of PONV following the use of different anaesthetic techniques and, if day case anaesthesia is to be taken seriously, scientific, double-blind, randomized trials will have to be conducted. PONV is a multifactorial problem and all day unit personnel should play a part in the reduction of this complication. It is acknowledged that the expensive ondansetron, a highly selective $5HT_3$ antagonist, is an effective antiemetic[34] but PONV may be significantly reduced by good patient selection and appropriate anaesthesia and analgesia. Anaesthetists will have to ask themselves why some day units can report a PONV incidence of 5% while they themselves tolerate rates of 45–50%[35].

Postoperative analgesia also requires serious consideration in view of an increase in the extent of day operations. Pre-emptive analgesia has not been as successful as when first introduced and further controlled studies will be required to decide whether to continue analgesic treatment prior to the development of pain[36]. The value of local anaesthetic blocks has already been mentioned, and community nurses could be trained to administer top-up local solutions, either in the home or patient hotel environment.

Controversy still surrounds the use of the NSAIDs. However, there is a need for powerful non-opioid analgesia in future day surgery and they may either be prescribed alone or used to reduce the opiate requirements for inguinal hernia repair or varicose vein stripping. The complications following the use of NSAIDs are well documented and in future the administration of these drugs intravenously may prove more convenient and less unpleasant than either intramuscular or rectal administration[37]. All day units should establish their own protocols for pain management. Furthermore, units should standardize and audit their analgesic treatments for mild, moderate and severe pain. In future, anaesthetists ought to reconsider the use of alternative analgesic methods, for instance heat, hypothermia, acupuncture, hypnosis and transcutaneous electrical stimulation. Lastly, more studies should evaluate transdermal fentanyl patches, buccal, intranasal, subcutaneous and oral slow-release preparations[38].

Future day surgery projects

Facilities
The debate as to whether to encourage the growth of British free-standing DSUs is still open. Over the past 20 years the expansion of these units in the USA has been impressive and 2000 units have so far been registered. This has been followed by the development of 23-hour recovery units for ambulatory surgical patients and these should make a considerable impact on both hospitals and free-standing day units. *Table 18.1* outlines the recommendations published by the British Association of Day Surgery (BADS) with regard to the running of these free-standing units. In addition, it appears likely that day units will have to extend their working hours to evenings and weekends, thus benefiting patients unwilling to miss their work for minor surgery. The downside of this suggestion will probably be the resultant increase in running costs for these sessions.

Patient hotels
At present there is a need to redefine what day surgery really is, and the definition outlined in Chapter 1 still stands. However, there have been recent reports of major surgical procedures such as partial thyroidectomy, breast reduction and parotidectomy being performed on an ambulatory basis, with the support of 23-hour recovery facilities. From a European point of view this is short-stay surgery, and not the original concept of day surgery.

The answer to this may be patient hotels[39]. It has been estimated that 14% of all in-patients, depending on the speciality, could be suitable candidates for patient hotel accommodation[40]. Any hotel scheme could form an integral part of a progressive hospital's business plan. Benefits will be maximized where both the bed management

Table 18.1. The recommendations for free-standing units (British Association of Day Surgery)

1. A medical member of staff should remain on the premises until all day cases are discharged
2. The nursing staff and operating department assistants should be experienced in day surgery. They should be trained in operating theatre techniques, anaesthesia and recovery
3. A preoperative assessment facility should be provided
4. An arrangement with an in-patient hospital should be established in the event of emergency admissions
5. Transport arrangements for emergency transfers to an in-patient hospital should be established
6. A quality assurance programme should be in place

system and the arrangements for discharging patients are reviewed prior to any development.

Day surgery will continue to expand, so planners should consider the number of in-patient beds planned for any new hospital complex. There is enough evidence to suggest that 60% of all elective surgery could safely be treated on a day basis. Therefore future hospitals should decrease in size and day unit complexes ought to replace them. Facilities should accommodate space for MIS, interventional radiology, paediatric and adult day surgery, chronic pain treatment and endoscopy. Ideally such a unit should be sited on the ground floor of a hospital complex, near to good parking facilities. In addition, for this venture to succeed, substantial teaching space should be allocated, as the future of any successful day unit will depend on an active programme of quality assurance, education and research.

Economics

Any future attempt to study the relative costs of day versus in-patient surgery should include all the relevant costs. Day units should be planned on sound financial grounds and clinical directors should be allocated their individual budgets so that they may have some control over their finances and benefit from improved efficiency schemes. Already there have been studies with reported average day unit cost savings of between 19% and 68%[41] when compared with in-patient surgery for similar procedures. However, one of the future dangers for day surgery is that its expansion could be driven by cost savings rather than by quality. Purchasers of health care should therefore be advised to study the quality outcome following day surgery as well as the cost. Countries who lag behind in the day surgical field should work to remove these obstacles. Usually these will include such barriers as health-care insurance and apathy from hospital doctors and managers. Finally, many would agree that the expansion of day surgery has been one of the most significant advances in health provision over the past decade, and many countries will surely benefit from the introduction of day surgery in the future.

A teamwork approach is required, with training programmes on technological advancement and the holistic approach to day surgery. Movement of hospital-based nurses into the community will continue, where they will supervise postoperative analgesic and monitoring programmes. The future success will be through the collaboration of medical, nursing and administrative staff.

References

1. **National Health Service Executive Day Surgery Task Force.** (1993) *Day Surgery*. HMSO, London.
2. **Sierra E, Pi F, Domingo J,** *et al.* Ambulatory surgery to cope with long patient waiting lists. *Ambulatory Surg.* 1995; **3**:19–22.
3. **Linden I, Bergbom Engberg I.** Patient's opinions and experiences of ambulatory surgery – a self care perspective. *Ambulatory Surg.* 1995; **3**: 131–139.
4. **Theus RJ, Go PMNH, Van Wijmen F.** Quality assessment in a day surgery unit. *Ambulatory Surg.* 1995; **3**: 195–198.
5. **Edwards N.** Day for night. *Health Serv. J.* 1996; **2 May**, 24–26.
6. **Sutton C.** Laparoscopic surgery in gynaecology. *Hospital Update*, 1993; **March:**143–152.
7. **Monson JRT.** Advanced techniques in abdominal surgery. *Br. Med. J.* 1993; **307**: 1346–1350.
8. **Livingstone JI, Cahill CJ.** Day case laparoscopic cholecystectomy – a feasibility study. *Ambulatory Surg.* 1995; **3**: 179–182.
9. **Wickham JEA.** Treatment of urinary tract stones. *Br. Med. J.* 1993; **307**: 1414–1417.
10. **Dougherty TJ.** Photosensitisation of malignant tumours. *Semin. Surg. Oncol.* 1986; **2**: 24–37.
11. **Studt T.** Micro machines. *Res. Devel. Mag.* 1990; **Dec**: 36–38.
12. **Cushieri A.** Minimal access surgery; the birth of a new era. *J. R. Coll. Surg. Edinb.* 1990; **35**: 345–347.
13. **Carroll PH, Ogg TW.** Recovery after day surgery with intravenous anaesthetic agents. *Ambulatory Surg.* 1996; **4**: 19–23.
14. **Hitchcock M, Rudkin G.** The real cost of total intravenous anaesthesia: cost versus price. *Ambulatory Surg.* 1995; **3**: 43–48.
15. **Bovill JG.** New delivery systems for anaesthesia. *Curr. Opin. Anaesthiol.* 1995; **8**: 287–291.
16. **Bovill JG.** New drugs. *Curr. Opin. Anaesthiol.* 1996; **9**: 318–322.
17. **Bagshaw RJ, Conahan TJ, Delling C,** *et al.* Esmolol as an anaesthetic adjunct in ambulatory surgery. *Ambulatory Surg.* 1995; **3**: 13–17.
18. **Smith I, White PF.** New anaesthetics, analgesics and muscle relaxants for ambulatory surgery. *Curr. Opin. Anaesthiol.* 1995; **8**: 298–303 .
19. **Smith I, Nathanson M, White PF.** Sevoflurane – a long awaited volatile anaesthetic. *Br. J. Anaesthesia* 1996; **76**: 435–445.
20. **Health and Safety Commission** (1996) *Anaesthetic Agents: Controlling Exposure under COSHH.* Health Services Advisory Committee, Bristol.
21. **Caldwell JE.** New muscle relaxants. *Curr. Opin. Anaesthesiol.* 1995; **8**: 356–361.
22. **Chetty MS, Pollard BL, Wilson A,** *et al.* Rocuronium bromide in dental day case anaesthesia – a comparison with atracurium and vecuronium. *Anaesth. Intens. Care* 1996; **24**: 37–41.
23. **Savarese JJ, Deriaz H, Mellinghoff H,** *et al.* The pharmacodynamics of cisatracurium in healthy adults. *Curr. Opin. Anaesthesiol.* 1996; **9** (Suppl. 1): S16–S22.
24. **Watcha MF.** Nausea and vomiting: choice of drugs and treatment. *Curr. Opin. Anaesthesiol.* 1996; **9**: 300–305.
25. **Barker JP, Vafidis GC, Hall GM.** Post-operative morbidity following cataract surgery: a comparison of local and general anaesthesia. *Anaesthesia* 1996; **51**: 435–437.
26. **Green G, Jonsson L.** Nausea: the most important factor determining length of stay after ambulatory surgery. *Acta Anaesthesiol. Scand.* 1993; **37**: 742–746.
27. **Munro HM, Riegger LQ, Reynolds PI,** *et al.* Comparison of the analgesic and emetic properties of ketorolac and morphine for paediatric outpatient strabismus surgery. *Br. J. Anaesth.* 1994; **72**: 624–628.
28. **Harrison CA, Morris S, Harvey JS.** Effect of ilioinguinal and iliohypogastric nerve block and wound infiltration with 0.5% bupivacaine on post-operative pain after hernia repair. *Br. J. Anaesth.* 1994; **72**: 691–693.
29. **Neal JM, Deck JJ, Lewis MA,** *et al.* A double-blind comparison of epidural 2-chloroprocaine versus lidocaine for outpatient knee arthroscopy. *Anesthesiology* 1993; **79**: A12.
30. **Mulroy MF, Wills RA.** Spinal anesthesia for outpatients: appropriate agents and techniques. *J. Clin. Anesthesiol.* 1995; **7**: 622.
31. **Buettner J, Wresch KP, Klose R.** Postdural puncture headache: comparison of 25 gauge Whitacre and Quincke needles. *Reg. Anesthesiol.* 1993; **18**: 166.

32. **Twersky RS, Abiona M,Thorne AC,** *et al.* Admissions following ambulatory surgery: outcome in seven urban hospitals. *Ambulatory Surg.* 1995; **3:** 141–146.
33. **Ogg TW, Watson BJ.** (1995) Aspects of day surgery and anaesthesia: a multidisciplinary approach. In: *Anaesthesia Rounds* (Ed. TW Ogg). The Medicine Group (Education) Ltd, Abingdon, Oxon. pp. 11–19.
34. **Wetchler BV, Sung YF, Duncalf D,** *et al.* Ondansetron decreases emetic symptoms following laparoscopy. *Anesthesiology* 1990; **73:** A36.
35. **Watson BJ, Hitchcock M, Swailes R,** *et al.* Nausea and vomiting after day surgery under general anaesthetic. A multicentre survey of symptoms after discharge. *Ambulatory Surg.* 1997; in press.
36. **Dahl JB.** The status of pre-emptive analgesia. *Curr. Opin. Anaesthesiol.* 1995; **8:** 323–330.
37. **Hitchcock M, Ogg TW.** (1994) Acute post-operative pain management in day-case surgery patients. In: *Pain Management* (Ed. F Camu). Adis International, Chester. pp. 1–12.
38. **Bovill JG.** New delivery systems for anaesthesia. *Curr. Opin. Anaesthesiol.* 1995; **8:** 287–291.
39. **Jarrett PEM, Wallace M, Jarrett MED,** *et al.* Experience of a hospital hotel. *Ambulatory Surg.* 1996; **4:** 1–3.
40. **NHS Management Executive, Value for Money Unit** (1992) *Patient Hotels: A Quality Alternative to Ward Care.* HMSO, London.
41. **Jarrett PEM.** Day surgery – the future. *Ann. Chirug. Gynaecol.* 1995; **84:** 379–383.

Index